A Clinician's Guide to CBT for Children to Young Adults

A Clinician's Guide to CBT for Children to Young Adults

A Companion to *Think Good, Feel Good* and *Thinking Good, Feeling Better*

Second Edition

Paul Stallard

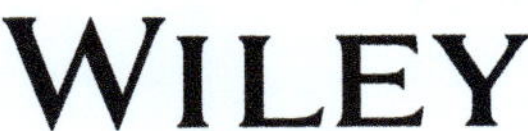

Contents

6 D: Discovery — 111

7 E: Emotions — 133

8 F: Formulations   149

About this book

This book provides practical ideas about how to use cognitive behavioural techniques (CBT) with children, adolescents, and young adults. The book is organised around a competency framework and highlights the underlying philosophy, process, and core skills of undertaking CBT with this client group. The ideas can be used as part of an individual intervention for those with psychological problems or as a group-based prevention programme to promote helpful 'life skills' to build resilience.

The CORE philosophy of CBT, namely a Child-centred, Outcome-focused, Reflective, and Empowering approach, is described. Attention is paid to the PRECISE process of working with children, adolescents, and young adults. This is based on Partnership working, pitched at the Right developmental level, promoting Empathy, Creativity, Investigation, and Self-efficacy, and which is Engaging and enjoyable.

Finally, the specific core skills, the ABCs of CBT, are described. These are defined as Assessment and goals, Behavioural, Cognitions, Discovery, Emotions, Formulations, General skills, and Home assignments. Each skill is described with practical examples provided of how these can be applied in work with children, adolescents, and young adults.

When discussing specific skills and techniques, reference is made to relevant worksheets which are available in *Think Good, Feel Good* (TGFG) for children and young adolescents and *Thinking Good, Feeling Better* (TGFB) for older adolescents and young adults.

Acknowledgements

There are many people who have contributed to the ideas contained in this book. Instead of providing an endless list of names, I would quite simply like to thank everyone I have had the privilege to work with. In particular, all the children, young people, and amazing colleagues I have been fortunate to work with during my career. They have inspired and challenged me in equal measure.

I would like to thank my family, Rosie, Luke, and Amy, for their unwavering encouragement, support, and enthusiasm for this project.

Finally, I would like to thank those who read this book. I hope that these materials will help you to develop your practice and to make a real difference to the lives of the young people you work with.

Online resources

All the text and workbook resources in this book are **available free, in colour, to purchasers** of the print version. To find out how to access and download these flexible aids to working with your clients visit the website

www.wiley.com/go/cliniciansguide2e

The online facility provides an opportunity to download and print relevant sections of the workbook that can then be used in clinical sessions with young people. The materials can be used to structure or supplement clinical sessions or can be completed by the young person at home.

The online materials can be used flexibly and can be accessed and used as often as required.

Introduction and overview

Cognitive behaviour therapy (CBT) is a generic term used to describe a variety of interventions that focus on the relationship between cognitions, emotions, and behaviours. These interventions are based on the shared premise that emotional distress is generated by the way we think about particular events that occur. Some ways of thinking are dysfunctional and unhelpful and can lead to the emergence of psychological problems. These unhelpful patterns are maintained by attention and memory biases, emotional responses, and maladaptive ways of behaving such as avoidance.

Traditional CBT interventions focus on identifying, directly challenging, and reappraising dysfunctional cognitions and through so doing reduce emotional distress and unhelpful behaviours. Recent models, often termed third wave, focus on changing the nature of the relationship with these thoughts rather than changing their specific content. Thoughts are understood as mental activity rather than defining reality, with mindfulness, acceptance, compassion, and distress tolerance helping to minimise the emotional distress they generate.

CBT as an intervention

CBT has been well evaluated and has established itself as the most extensively researched of all the child psychotherapies (Graham 2005). Systematic reviews consistently demonstrate that CBT is effective for the treatment of a range of emotional problems in children, adolescents, and young people, including post-traumatic stress disorder (PTSD; Gutermann et al. 2016; Morina et al. 2016; Smith et al. 2019); anxiety (Bennett et al. 2016; James

A Clinician's Guide to CBT for Children to Young Adults: A Companion to Think Good, Feel Good and Thinking Good, Feeling Better, Second Edition. Paul Stallard.
© 2021 John Wiley & Sons Ltd. Published 2021 by John Wiley & Sons Ltd.
Companion website: www.wiley.com/go/cliniciansguide2e

et al. 2015); depression (Oud et al. 2019; Zhou et al. 2015), and obsessive-compulsive disorder (OCD; Öst at al. 2016). Research is beginning to document the benefits of third wave CBT interventions such as mindfulness (Dunning et al. 2019; Klingbeil et al. 2017), dialectical behaviour therapy (McCauley et al. 2018), and acceptance and commitment therapy (Hancock et al. 2018).

Brief models of CBT, such as single-session exposure therapy for the treatment of specific phobias, have been found to be highly effective (Öst & Ollendick 2017). Similarly, brief parent-guided CBT has been found to be effective in the treatment of anxiety disorders (Cartwright-Hatton et al. 2011; Creswell et al. 2017). Finally, model-specific interventions, such as cognitive therapy for social anxiety (Leigh & Clark 2018) or single-session exposure therapy for specific phobias (Davis et al. 2019), have found encouraging results.

This substantial and consistent evidence has resulted in CBT being recommended by expert groups such as the UK National Institute for Health and Clinical Excellence and the American Academy of Child and Adolescent Psychiatry for the treatment of young people with emotional disorders including depression, OCD, PTSD, and anxiety. This growing evidence base has also promoted the development of national training programmes in CBT. In the UK, the successful Improving Access to Psychological Therapies (IAPT) programme has been extended to children and young people (Shafran et al. 2014).

CBT as a preventative intervention

In addition to being an effective treatment, CBT has proven to be effective in the prevention of mental health problems such as anxiety and depression (Calear & Christensen 2010; Neil & Christensen 2009). Preventive programmes offer the potential to reduce the severity of symptomology of those already displaying problems whilst enhancing the resilience of those who are not currently symptomatic. The results of prevention programmes are encouraging and suggest that school-based anxiety and depression prevention based on CBT is effective (Dray et al. 2017; Hetrick et al. 2015; Stockings et al. 2016; Werner-Seidler et al. 2017).

Typically, preventative programmes are provided in schools either to whole classes of young people (e.g. universal approach) or to young people identified as at risk of developing or experiencing problems (e.g. targeted approaches). School-based programmes have good reach, and integrating them into the school curriculum can help to reduce the stigma attached to mental health so that worries and problems can be more openly acknowledged and discussed (Barrett & Pahl 2006). Reviews suggest that classroom-based approaches designed to improve mental health and well-being are effective both as universal and as targeted programmes (Šouláková et al. 2019; Stockings et al. 2016).

There are many CBT anxiety and depression prevention programmes, with the most well evaluated being FRIENDS for Life (Barrett 2010), Penn Resilience Programme (Jaycox et al. 1994), Coping with Stress Course (Clarke et al. 1990), Resourceful Adolescent Program (Shochet et al. 1997), and the Aussie Optimism Programme (Roberts 2006). Whilst the results are generally positive, not all evaluations of these programmes have shown positive effects. The intervention leader requires careful consideration. Whilst teachers and school staff are well placed to deliver these programmes, studies have shown that they may not necessarily be as effective as trained mental health leaders (Stallard, Skrybina, et al. 2014; Werner-Seidler et al. 2017). It is therefore important to consider the knowledge, support, and supervision of those delivering these programmes.

CBT with younger children

Whilst CBT can routinely be used with children from the age of seven years, comparatively few studies have evaluated the effectiveness of CBT with children under the age of 12 (Ewing et al. 2015). Most studies tend to involve young adolescents aged 12–17. Randomised controlled trials evaluating CBT for the treatment of depression rarely include children under the age of 12 (Forti-Buratti et al. 2016). For example, Yang et al. (2017) undertook a review and meta-analysis of CBT for the treatment of depression in children (defined as under the age of 13) and identified only nine studies, with six of these being conducted before the turn of the century.

In terms of anxiety, a few specific programmes for young children have been developed. These include Being Brave (Hirshfeld-Becker et al. 2010), Taming Sneaky Fears (Monga et al. 2015), and the school-based universal prevention programme Fun Friends (Pahl & Barrett 2010). Results from these studies are limited but nonetheless encouraging.

A few researchers have developed and explored the effectiveness of CBT with young children with PTSD (Dalgleish et al. 2015; Salloum et al. 2016). For example, Scheeringa et al. (2011) reported the feasibility of a trauma-focused CBT intervention with children aged three to six who had experienced a life-threatening event and found a large reduction in PTSD symptoms at six months. Research with OCD is similarly limited, although once again the results are promising. In one of the few studies, Freeman et al. (2014) found that 72% of children aged five to eight with OCD were assessed as 'much improved' after completing a 14-session family-based CBT programme.

It cannot be assumed that because CBT is effective with young adolescents that it will also be effective with young children. Developmental factors need to be considered and the role of parents/carers requires careful attention. Nonetheless, although research is limited, the results are encouraging and are consistent with those obtained with older samples.

CBT with children and young people with learning difficulties

There is evidence that CBT can be effective with young people with learning difficulties, particularly those with high-functioning autistic spectrum disorder (ASD; Perihan et al. 2019). For example, studies have demonstrated that CBT programmes for young people with ASD do have a beneficial effect on reducing symptoms of anxiety (Storch et al. 2013; Van Steensel & Bogels 2015; Wood et al. 2009) and OCD (Vause et al. 2018).

Researchers have highlighted how CBT needs to be modified to accommodate the young person's specific learning difficulties (Attwood & Scarpa 2013; Donoghue et al. 2011). This involves attending to factors such as communications/language abilities, interpersonal/social abilities, cognitive and behavioural inflexibility, and sensory sensitivities (Scarpa et al. 2017). In terms of communication, adaptations might include the use of simple, precise, and concrete language and the greater use of more non-verbal visual techniques such as pictures, worksheets, or visual prompts (e.g. writing the aim/focus of each session on a board). The young person's special interests can be integrated into the intervention through the development of metaphors or use of rewards. Interpersonal skills with young people with ASD maybe more limited, so greater attention needs to be paid to the assessment and development of core skills such as 'mind reading' to aid understanding of how people might think and feel. Once again, the process can be made concrete through the use of role plays. Cognitive flexibility can be promoted using self-talk where different options are verbalised and modelled or through multiple choice questions which encourage awareness and consideration of alternative strategies. For behavioural inflexibility, interactions during clinical sessions may need to be modified to be more consistent with the expectations of the young person. For example, Donoghue et al. (2011) note that the usual social exchanges at the start of therapy sessions may create anxiety and suggest that the therapist adopts a more task-focused approach. Similarly, anxiety associated with change can be minimised by using the same room to meet, having a clear session routine/structure, and establishing a clear length for the meeting. In terms of sensory issues, it may be necessary to reduce the length of the session, change the lighting, remove visual material from the room, or use relaxation skills to help reduce sensory overload. Finally, generalisation from clinical sessions to the young person's everyday environment can be facilitated through the involvement of parents, mobile phones to send prompts and reminders, and digital cameras to capture difficult situations (Donoghue et al. 2011).

Research with young people with other disorders is more limited. For visually impaired young people, tactile prompts can be used to remind the young person of the steps involved in managing anxiety (Visagie et al. 2017). For those with moderate learning difficulties, skills such as problem solving can be broken down into simple steps (Stop, Plan, Do) and limited decision-making options (e.g. you can do either X or Y).

Technologically delivered CBT

There is increased interest in the use of technology to support and deliver CBT to children and adolescents. Technology offers the potential to reach geographically isolated populations; flexible access; increased convenience; fewer visits to specialist clinics; greater privacy and anonymity; enhanced treatment fidelity; rapid scalability; and low-cost delivery (Clarke et al. 2015; MacDonell & Prinz 2017). It is also very acceptable and particularly appealing to adolescents, who are typically early adopters and regular users of new technologies (Johnson et al. 2015; Wozney et al. 2018).

Internet or technologically delivered CBT programmes have attracted much interest and have demonstrated encouraging results (Grist el al. 2019; Pennant et al. 2015; Vigerland et al. 2016). Digital technologies deliver interventions via computers, or through web-based platforms via mobile tablets or smartphones (Hollis et al. 2017). The structured nature of CBT lends itself well to digital delivery, resulting in several computerised CBT interventions being developed. For example, the face-to-face CBT anxiety programme *Cool Teens* can be effective when delivered via a CD-ROM with minimal therapist support (Wuthrich et al. 2012). Similarly, online CBT anxiety programmes such as *BRAVE* were found to be very acceptable to young people and as effective as face-to-face CBT (Spence et al. 2011). In terms of depression, encouraging results have been reported for *Stressbusters*, a computerised CBT program (Smith et al. 2015; Wright et al. 2017) and a computer game (*SPARX*) when used both as an intervention and as a prevention programme (Merry, Hetrick, et al. 2012; Merry, Stasiak, et al. 2012; Perry et al. 2017).

Reviews indicate that technologically delivered CBT is effective (Grist et al. 2019) and is now recommended in the United Kingdom as a first line treatment for mild to moderate depression (NICE 2019). Other technologies such as apps, virtual reality, and games have seldom been developed or evaluated.

Involving parents

Parents have a central role in supporting their child, and by involving them in the intervention important parental behaviours and contextual factors can be addressed. Their involvement can therefore facilitate generalisation, practice, and reinforcement of new skills in the young person's everyday life. However, there is no consistent evidence to suggest that involving parents in CBT programmes results in better outcomes (Breinholst et al. 2012). For example, reviews have shown that CBT for anxiety is effective with and without parental involvement (Higa-McMillan et al. 2016; Reynolds et al. 2012). Neither the age of the young person nor whether both parents are involved appears to be related to enhanced outcomes (Carnes et al. 2019; Manassis et al. 2014). Similarly, school-based CBT anxiety prevention programmes have been found to be effective without any parental involvement (Stallard, Skryabina, et al. 2014). However, assessing the benefits of parental involvement is complex and the potential beneficial impact on parents or other family members has seldom been assessed (Breinholst et al. 2012). In addition, whilst the additional short-term benefits may not be evident, parental involvement in CBT may support the longer-term maintenance of treatment gains (Manassis et al. 2014).

There has been less research focusing on parental involvement in depression programmes. In a review, Oud et al. 2019 found that parental (caregiver) involvement may enhance outcomes compared to child-only CBT. The way in which parents are involved in programmes has received limited attention and may explain some of the differences between studies. Stallard (2005) described four models of parental involvement: facilitator, co-clinician, clinician, and co-client. The most limited involvement is that of the facilitator where parents attend one or two review meetings with their child. The focus of the intervention is on the child's problems, with parents receiving information about the intervention and the skills their child will be developing. As co-clinicians, parents are more actively involved in treatment. They attend each session with their child, either for the whole session or joining for the last 15 minutes. The intervention remains focused on the child's problems, but parents have greater awareness of the skills their child is acquiring and so can prompt and encourage generalisation. This role is further enhanced when parents are involved as clinicians. In this role parents are provided with the information and support required to teach their child CBT skills. Finally, parents may be involved as a co-client. This model recognises that parents may be behaving in a way that contributes to their child's problems. The intervention therefore helps the child to develop and practise skills to deal with their anxiety whilst parents learn new ways of encouraging and rewarding their child for facing their worries.

In summary, parental involvement needs to be considered on a case-by-case basis and a decision made about whether parental involvement may be beneficial and, if so, how parents/carers need to be involved (Carnes et al. 2019).

The competencies to deliver child-focused CBT

There are many materials and structured workbooks available which provide helpful ideas about how CBT can be undertaken with children and young people. These include specific manuals such as the Coping Cat programme for young people with anxiety (Kendall 1990); How I Ran OCD Off My Land (March & Mulle 1998), and the Adolescent Coping with Depression Course (Clark et al. 1990). In addition, there are materials to help young people with social skills problems (Spence 1995) and chronic fatigue syndrome (Chalder & Hussain 2002) and anxiety and depression prevention programmes such as Friends for Life (Barrett 2010). There are also books that provide practical ideas about how CBT can be adapted for use with children and young people (Friedberg & McClure 2015; Fuggle et al. 2012; Stallard 2019a) and how CBT can be used as a modular approach which flexes according to how the young person responds (Chorpita 2007). Finally, there are self-help books for parents to help them overcome their child's fears or worries (Cartwright-Hatton et al. 2010; Creswell & Willetts 2018) or to help their depressed teenager (Reynolds & Parkinson 2015)

Such good quality child-friendly materials make available many helpful ideas about how to introduce and use specific CBT strategies with children and young people. However, comparatively less attention has been paid to how these techniques are used, that is, the process of undertaking CBT with children, adolescents, and young adults. Attending to the process of CBT is essential and ensures that the theoretical model and the core principles that underpin CBT are preserved. This will ensure that CBT is used in a coherent and theoretically robust way thereby avoiding a simplistic approach in which individual strategies are used in a disconnected and uninformed way.

Think Good, Feel Good (Stallard 2002a, 2019a) and *Thinking Good, Feeling Better* (Stallard 2019b) provide a number of practical ideas about how some of the specific techniques of CBT could be conveyed to and adapted for use by children, adolescents, and young adults. This book looks behind these strategies to focus upon the process that underpins their use. This book is not intended to be prescriptive and does not advocate a particular style. Instead it aims to promote awareness of some of the key issues that need to be considered and integrated into CBT in a way that is engaging and helpful for the young person and their carer whilst maximising the effectiveness of the intervention.

Assessing competence

A clear strength of CBT is the underpinning philosophy and theoretical model. The philosophy underpins the collaborative process of self-discovery whilst the theoretical model informs and guides the use of specific techniques. It is therefore important to develop a good understanding of the basic model and to ensure that the process and rationale for use of specific techniques is understood and competently executed.

The most widely used tool for measuring CBT competence with adults is the Cognitive Therapy Scale–Revised (CTS-R) (Blackburn et al. 2001). This is a revised version of the original Cognitive Therapy Scale developed by Young and Beck (1988). The CTS-R consists of 12 items which assess important generic CBT skills. These include four general skills (feedback; collaboration; pacing and efficient use of time; and interpersonal effectiveness) and seven specific CBT skills (eliciting appropriate emotional expression; eliciting key cognitions; eliciting behaviours; guided discovery; conceptual integration; application of change methods; and homework setting). The remaining item, agenda setting, overlaps both sets of items and is included in the general and specific sub-scales.

The suitability of the CTS-R to assess competencies when using CBT with children and adolescents has been questioned (Fuggle et al. 2012). In particular, the authors argue that the CTS-R is not appropriate because:

- Important systemic influences on the onset and maintenance of the young person's problems need to be acknowledged and the role of the carers/ family in CBT considered.

- The young person's cognitive, emotional, linguistic, and reasoning ability are developing, and CBT needs to be appropriately adapted to be consistent with their abilities.

- Creative non-verbal methods may be required to convey the concepts of CBT to young people in clear and understandable ways.

- The process of undertaking CBT with young people and their carers needs greater specification.

Specific CBT competence scales for use with children and young people have been developed and evaluated. Of those available, the majority assess competence in delivering a specific manualised programme or treatments for specific disorders. For example, Mcleod et al. (2019) developed a scale to assess competence delivering the Coping Cat anxiety programme, Bjaastad et al. (2016) the FRIENDS anxiety programme, and Gutermann et al. (2015) for assessing competence in treating PTSD. Although there are some differences in the competencies that have been identified, there are several shared dimensions. For instance, in a Delphi study, Sburlati et al. (2011) identified various generic therapeutic competencies (e.g. practising professionally, knowledge of children and adolescents, building a positive relationship, conducting a thorough assessment), CBT-specific competencies (e.g. understanding CBT theory, developing a CBT formulation, working collaboratively), and specific CBT techniques (e.g. managing negative thoughts, changing maladaptive behaviours, managing maladaptive mood). McLeod et al. 2018 identified four categories of competence for delivering anxiety interventions. These are interventions that are common to CBT programmes (e.g. maintaining focus on CBT model, homework review, etc.), interventions specific to anxiety programmes (e.g. relaxation, fear ladder, exposure), how the intervention is delivered (coaching, modelling, rehearsal), and overall ratings of skilfulness and responsiveness. Whilst there are some specific differences, there tends to be a consensus that undertaking CBT with children and young people requires competencies both in the method of delivery (e.g. the therapeutic process) and in the application of specific CBT techniques.

Cognitive Behaviour Therapy Scale for Children and Young People

The absence of a psychometrically robust scale developed specifically to assess general CBT competence with children and young people led to the development of the Cognitive Behaviour Therapy Scale for Children and Young People (CBTS-CYP) (Stallard, Myles, et al. 2014). The aim was to develop a scale to assess the overall quality of CBT, not to assess in detail the way that specific techniques like exposure are conducted.

In terms of development, it was firstly decided to build upon the CTS-R. The CTS-R is widely used and considered to provide a comprehensive overview of the generic skills required to competently practise CBT with adults (Fairburn & Cooper 2011; Kazantzis 2003; Keen & Freeston 2008). Secondly, the CTS-R assesses the specific use of CBT methods as well as general skills that facilitate their effective delivery. It was therefore decided that the CBTS-CYP would contain items that assessed competence both in the application of specific methods and in the process of using CBT with children and young people. Thirdly, upon reviewing the CTS-R, it was decided that all items should be included in the CBTS-CYP, modified as appropriate to reflect the use of CBT with children and young people. Similarly, the framework for defining competence proposed by Dreyfus (1986) and adapted into a seven-point Likert scale on the CTS-R was adopted for use in the CBTS-CYP. Fourthly, the CTS-R is widely used by CBT training courses to assess competence. In order to maintain consistency with the CTS-R, it was decided to adopt the same thresholds for assessing competency, that is, score 2 or more on each item and a total score of 50% or more. Finally, it was decided that the scale would be developed to assess both verbal and non-verbal behaviours and so could be used like the CTS-R to assess both audio and video recordings of clinical sessions. It was anticipated that specific items would not necessarily be mutually exclusive. For example, a formulation requires the development of a shared conceptualisation in which important cognitions, emotions, and behaviours are bound together within the CBT model. The elicitation and identification of key cognitions and processes would therefore be expected to be associated with the formulation. Similarly, CBT typically involves developing an understanding of the links between cognitions, emotions, and behaviours and as such there will inevitably be overlap between these different aspects of the cognitive behavioural model.

In addition to competencies in the application of core methods, the use of CBT with young people also requires competencies in the way that CBT is provided. CBT is predicated on a process of collaborative empiricism, a process which requires greater attention when working with children, adolescents, and young adults. These competences relating to the therapeutic process have been defined by the acronym PRECISE (Stallard 2005).

- ▶ **P:** The therapeutic process involves the young person and their family working in a **partnership** with the clinician. The partnership is based upon collaborative empiricism and highlights the active roles of the young person and their parents/carers in securing change.

- ▶ **R:** The intervention is pitched at the **right developmental level** to ensure that it is consistent with the young person's cognitive, linguistic, memory, and perspective-taking abilities.

- ▶ **E:** A warm, caring, respectful, and **empathic relationship** is established.

- ▶ **C:** The concepts of CBT are **creatively** and flexibly conveyed in a way that matches the young person's interests and understanding.

- ▶ **I:** **Investigation** and self-discovery are encouraged through the adoption of a curious and reflective approach.

- ▶ **S:** **Self-efficacy** is promoted as the young person is helped to discover and build upon their strengths, skills, and ideas.

- ▶ **E:** Sessions are **enjoyable and engaging** in order to maintain the young person's motivation and commitment to change.

The CBTS-CYP assesses the above seven PRECISE process items and the following eight method items, referred to as the ABCs of CBT.

- **A:** *Assessment*, and the ability to establish clear goals and to appropriately use diaries, questionnaires, and rating scales for assessment.

- **B:** Use of *behavioural techniques* such as graded exposure, behavioural activation, and activity scheduling to facilitate therapeutic change.

- **C:** Use of *cognitive techniques* to identify cognitions, to promote cognitive awareness, to challenge, to reframe, or to develop mindfulness, acceptance, and compassion.

- **D:** Facilitating *discovery* using techniques such as the Socratic dialogue, behavioural experiments, and prediction testing.

- **E:** Use of *emotional techniques* to identify and manage strong, unpleasant emotions.

- **F:** Ability to construct a case *formulation* which highlights the relationships between events, cognitions, emotions, physiological responses, and behaviour.

- **G:** *General skills* to effectively manage sessions such as agenda setting, session planning, and managing challenging behaviour

- **H:** Appropriate use of *home assignments* with clear goals and purpose.

The first version of the CBTS-CYP consisted of 14 items, with home assignments initially being subsumed within the discovery competence. Following review, these were separated, with the current iteration, like the CTS-R, having home assignments as a separate and discrete set of competencies. Table 1.1 summarises how the CTS-R items map on to the 15 items of the CBTS-CYP.

In an initial evaluation of the CBTS-CYP, video clips of clinicians undertaking CBT were assessed by independent raters (Stallard, Myles, et al. 2014). Face validity and internal reliability were high, and convergent validity with the CTS-R was good. It compared well with the CTS-R in discriminative ability and demonstrated an increase in skills through a course of CBT training.

The CBTS-CYP can be used for clinical reflection and self-assessment. It should be completed in an open and honest way so that strengths, weaknesses, and development needs can be identified. These competencies can then be self-monitored and reflected upon after clinical sessions as a way of developing practice.

A copy of the CBTS-CYP is included in Chapter 12. The subsequent chapters will explore each competence in detail and provide specific examples.

Table 1.1 Comparison of items on the CBTS-CYP and CTS-R.

CBTS-CYP process item	Equivalent CTS-R item
Partnership working (P) Establishes a collaborative partnership with the child/young person (and, as appropriate, their carers) in which they are actively engaged in working together towards a set of joint goals and targets	Collaboration
Right developmental level (R) Engages with the child/young person and family at a level and in a manner that is consistent with their developmental level and understanding	None
Empathy (E) Empathises with the child/young person and their carers/family through the development of a genuine, warm, and respectful relationship	Interpersonal effectiveness
Creative (C) Adapts the ideas and concepts of CBT to facilitate the understanding of and engagement in therapy of the child/young person and their parents/carers	None
Investigation (I) Adopts an open and curious stance that facilitates guided discovery and reflection	Feedback
Self-efficacy (S) Adopts an empowering and enabling approach in which self-efficacy and positive attempts at change are promoted	None
Enjoyable and engaging (E) Makes therapy sessions appropriately interesting and engaging	None
CBTS-CYP methods item	
Assessment and goals (A) Establishes clear goals for the intervention and appropriately uses diaries, questionnaires, and rating scales for assessment	None
Behavioural techniques (B) Demonstrates appropriate use of a variety of behavioural techniques to facilitate therapeutic change	Eliciting behaviours Application of change methods
Cognitive techniques (C) Demonstrates appropriate use of a variety of cognitive techniques to facilitate therapeutic change	Eliciting key cognitions Application of change methods

Table 1.1 (Continued)

CBTS-CYP process item	Equivalent CTS-R item
Discovery (D) Appropriately uses a variety of methods to facilitate self-discovery and understanding	Guided discovery
Emotional (E) Appropriately uses a variety of emotional techniques to facilitate therapeutic change	Eliciting appropriate emotional expression Application of change methods
Formulation (F) Facilitates the development of a coherent understanding which highlights the relationships between events, cognitions, emotions, physiological responses, and behaviours	Conceptual integration
General skills (G) Sessions are well prepared and conducted in a calm and organised way	Agenda setting and adherence Pacing and efficient use of time
Home assignments (H) Uses home assignments to gather data and transfer skills between clinical sessions and everyday life	Homework setting

CORE philosophy

In addition to the process and core methods of undertaking CBT with children, adolescents, and young people, it is helpful to remain aware of the underlying philosophy.

This is the **CORE** philosophy which is

- ▶ **C: *Child-centred***

- ▶ **O: *Outcome-focused***

- ▶ **R: *Reflective***

- ▶ **E: *Empowering***

Figure 1.1 provides a visual summary of the core philosophy, therapeutic process, and methods that embrace CBT with children, adolescents, and young people.

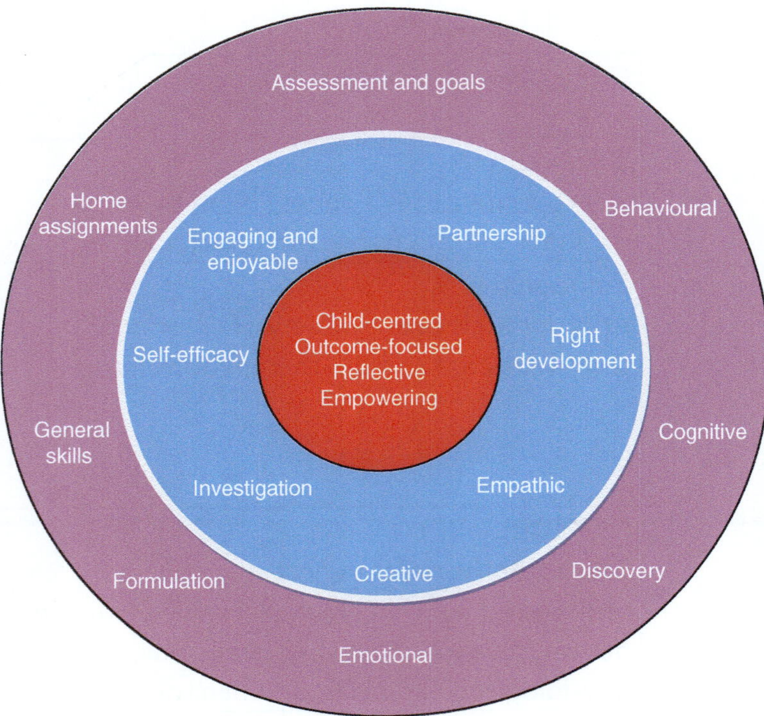

Figure 1.1 Core philosophy, therapeutic process, and methods of undertaking CBT with children, adolescents, and young adults.

Child-centred

The CORE philosophy clearly places the young person at the very centre of the intervention. Children and young people are a vulnerable group and for this reason it is important to ensure that they are safe, that potential risks are minimised, and that they are appropriately protected from potential harm. There is a need to remain mindful of potential physical, emotional, or sexual harm or exploitation from adults or peers either in person or via the Internet and to take appropriate action to safeguard the young person.

The child-centred philosophy also ensures that the intervention remains focused on the young person and their problems. Maintaining this focus is important, particularly if parents/carers have their own problems or needs which may dominate clinical sessions and overshadow those of the young person. Parent problems may need to be directly addressed, particularly if they are significantly impacting on the young person's problems or progress. This needs to be discussed with the parent/carer, whose problems and needs should be acknowledged, and, where appropriate, signposted or referred for direct help in their own right.

Parents/carers or other adults may have their own views about what needs to change, and this may not necessarily be shared by the young person. These views are important, and they need to be heard and acknowledged. However, adult goals may be held and 'parked' and returned to at a later stage. The initial focus, wherever possible, should remain on directly engaging the young person and on identifying and working towards their goals. However, the young person's goals need to be positive and helpful and should not compromise their health or safety in any way. For example, a young person with an eating disorder may choose a goal to maintain (rather than increase) a medically concerning body weight. This would be an inappropriate goal which would compromise the young person's physical health. This needs to be openly discussed, the reasons why this cannot be supported clarified, and alternative goals identified.

In terms of process, a key objective of the child-centred approach is the active involvement of the young person in therapy sessions. To maximise engagement, it is important that the young person is provided with plenty of opportunities to contribute during sessions, thereby signalling that their contributions are welcomed, heard, and valued. Clinical sessions therefore need to be conducted in ways that are sensitive to the young person's level of development and which are consistent with their cognitive, social, and emotional maturity. This will be discussed in more detail when considering the competencies required for partnership working and for pitching the intervention at the right developmental level.

In summary, the child-centred focus ensures that the young person is safe, that their problems are the primary focus, and that the intervention is carefully attuned to their developmental level to maximise understanding, engagement, and participation.

Outcome-focused

The CORE philosophy promotes a hopeful, future-orientated approach with a clear emphasis on outcomes, goals, and objective measurement. From the first session, the young person is encouraged to think about the future, their goals, and how things would be different if they no longer had their problems.

Typically, young people do not refer themselves for help and may not necessarily share the concerns and goals of those who referred them. This is often exemplified with school non-attendance, where the objective of the parent and school in securing the young person's school attendance may not be the main priority of, or indeed a goal shared by, the young person.

Young people may also be unable to think about how things could be different or identify any goals. This is a common problem with young people who become very familiar with their current situation and are unable to think about how this could change. Similarly, previous experience with adults may lead young people to assume a passive role in which they expect others to identify their problems and to tell them how they need to change, without necessarily having any ownership of either the problem or the change process.

Helpful techniques for eliciting goals are discussed in Chapter 3 (Assessment and goals). For example, the miracle question offers a future-orientated way of helping the young person to consider what their life may be like if all their problems miraculously disappeared overnight. This visualisation of a problem-free future offers the potential to identify what might need to change to achieve this. In many cases, desired outcomes may appear daunting or feel too large or unachievable, and this can be demotivating. In order to maintain motivation, outcomes can be broken down into a series of smaller, more manageable, goals. The successful achievement of each goal takes the young person closer towards their overall objective. Goals should be specific, measurable, achievable, relevant, and timely (SMART), thereby clearly and positively identifying what the young person hopes to achieve. The identification of clear goals ensures that the intervention remains focused and that the young person and clinician are explicitly working towards agreed objectives.

In order to maintain momentum, progress should be regularly assessed using rating scales and routine outcome measures. These provide a way of quantifying change and of capturing small, but important, changes that highlight progress. Similarly, the absence of change should prompt a curious discussion with the young person where this is acknowledged, possible reasons or barriers explored, and a plan agreed.

In summary, this future-orientated approach focusing on outcomes is positive and empowering and from the outset builds a sense of hopefulness and a focus on change. The use of goals and routine outcome measures helps to clarify and quantify achievements, and ensures that the intervention remains focused and the young person motivated.

Reflective

CBT is a reflective process in which the young person is encouraged through an open and curious approach to discover insights into their problems and difficulties and to find potential solutions and strategies that are helpful.

The CBT framework provides a simple model for bringing together different aspects of the young person's experience that may feel random or unconnected. By encouraging the young person to attend to their thoughts, feelings, and behaviours, they are helped to understand the basic premise of the CBT model, that is, that they are connected and interlinked. Typically, this culminates in the development of a problem formulation where the young person discovers that the way they think is associated with how they feel and what they do. This understanding is empowering and can help to develop self-efficacy as the young person and their parents are encouraged to use this understanding to consider how the current unhelpful cycle could change.

The process of reflection and discovery is encouraged using the Socratic dialogue. This process is discussed in more detail in Chapter 6 (Discovery) and involves an open and curious approach where questions guide the young person to attend to new or overlooked information. The dialogue encourages reflection and consideration of what might happen if they responded differently to their thoughts and feelings. For example, a Socratic dialogue with a depressed girl might help her to attend to times when she has been successful thereby challenging her belief that she is a failure. Similarly, a Socratic dialogue with an anxious boy might help him attend to times or places where he has successfully managed his anxiety, leading to reflection about potential coping skills.

This reflective process is embedded in clinical sessions by regularly encouraging the young person to reflect and to summarise what they have discovered and how they might be able to use and apply this. Diaries, home assignments, and behavioural experiments all provide opportunities for reflection.

▶ What have you found out?

▶ What does this mean?

▶ How does this help?

The CORE philosophy promotes a process of reflection and self-discovery which encourages the young person to develop new insights and understandings.

Empowering

The final pillar of the CORE philosophy is that of empowerment, a process which helps the young person to become stronger and more confident, to discover what works for them, and to explore and develop solutions to their problems. Empowerment therefore increases understanding and helps the young person to recognise their skills and strengths and their ability to positively influence their well-being. In effect, the young person is empowered to become their own therapist and to draw on their strengths and ideas to overcome their difficulties.

Empowerment is a strengths-based, positive approach that involves the enhancement of three inter-related processes. The first, self-awareness, helps the young person to understand themselves, their values, their strengths, the way they think, and how they feel and behave. Through the development of self-awareness, young people are better equipped to identify and positively respond to potential problems at an early stage. Self-awareness is promoted through an educative process where the young person acquires new knowledge, insights, and meanings. The development of the formulation, for example, is an educative process where thoughts, feelings, and behaviours are brought together in a coherent way that helps the young person to make sense of their experiences. The young person is the 'expert' of their own experiences, with the clinician providing the framework within which these experiences can be organised. Understanding the relationship between the key elements of the CBT model helps the young person to discover how their current problems have developed and how they are being maintained. Once understood, the formulation can be used by the young person as a structure for thinking about what needs to change to break out of this unhelpful cycle. The young person is empowered to consider whether they might need to change their relationship with their thoughts, how they can manage or tolerate unpleasant feelings, or how they could behave in different ways.

The second process, self-efficacy, relates to how effectively young people use their skills, strengths, and personal resources to positively secure their goals and resolve their difficulties. The CORE philosophy aims to strengthen self-efficacy and the belief that the young person has strengths and skills that can be positively used to improve their well-being. Enhancing self-efficacy can be motivating and empower greater engagement. A key aspect of self-efficacy is the accurate recognition of one's own strengths, skills, and abilities. The Socratic process can help young people attend to situations where they have coped/ been successful and identify what they did on those occasions that was helpful. Self-efficacy can be developed by inviting the young person to consider how these skills could be used in other situations or to help with other problems. Similarly, self-monitoring provides useful feedback about helpful skills and strategies that may already be within the young person's repertoire. Highlighting these can strengthen the young person's beliefs that they can overcome their problems and do something to improve their well-being.

Finally, self-control is the ability to regulate behaviour, emotions, and thoughts. Through CBT, the young person develops effective self-management skills which help them to feel more confident, in control, and able to deal with future challenges. This concept of self-control is promoted throughout CBT through the development of skills. Active skills can include the development of emotional management techniques or thought challenging that promote greater control by actively attempting to challenge and change distressing emotions or thoughts. Behavioural experiments provide a way of developing and demonstrating self-control through the practice of new skills. Finally, self-control can be promoted using mindfulness, distress tolerance, acceptance, and compassion-based skills. Rather than actively attempting to change feelings or thoughts, a sense of self-control can be promoted by learning to accept what is occurring.

In summary, empowerment promotes increased knowledge, recognition of strengths and skills, and enhanced perceptions of self-efficacy and self-control. The CORE philosophy is therefore positive and empowering, designed to motivate the young person to use their strengths and skills to maintain their well-being and to deal with future challenges.

PRECISE

The therapeutic relationship is collaborative, developmentally sensitive, empathic, creative, empowering, and engaging

CBT occurs within the context of a supportive, open, and non-judgemental relationship. The relationship is a collaborative *partnership* between the clinician, young person, and, as appropriate, their parents/carers. The intervention is pitched at the *right developmental level* to ensure that it is consistent with the young person's cognitive, linguistic, memory, and perspective-taking abilities. The therapeutic relationship is based on *empathy*, which promotes and conveys warmth, genuine concern, and respect. The process is *creative*, with the concepts of CBT being conveyed in ways that match the young person's developmental level, interests, and strengths. Empiricism is promoted through the adoption of a curious, open, and reflective approach in which *investigation* is encouraged. Reflection and the facilitation of self-discovery encourages the development of *self-efficacy*, with attention to *engagement and enjoyment* ensuring that the young person's motivation s maintained.

The therapeutic alliance

The child alliance has been defined by McLeod & Weisz (2005) as the therapist's ability to develop a warm, caring, and empathic relationship and to engage the young person in the therapeutic process. Underpinning this definition is the assumption that specific therapeutic techniques need to be delivered within the context of a warm and supportive therapeutic relationship. This was recognised by Beck (1976), who saw the therapeutic relationship as

A Clinician's Guide to CBT for Children to Young Adults: A Companion to Think Good, Feel Good and Thinking Good, Feeling Better, Second Edition. Paul Stallard.
© 2021 John Wiley & Sons Ltd. Published 2021 by John Wiley & Sons Ltd.
Companion website: www.wiley.com/go/cliniciansguide2e

'an obvious primary component of effective psychotherapy'. This has led some to suggest that the quality of the therapeutic alliance will impact on outcomes and the success of the intervention (Shirk & Karver 2003).

Despite widespread recognition of the importance of the therapeutic alliance, research exploring this is limited and the results are not always consistent. Some researchers have found a modest relationship with treatment outcomes (Karver et al. 2006; Liber et al. 2010; McLeod 2011; Shirk & Karver, 2003;), whereas others have failed to find a relationship or have found only a partial association (Chiu et al. 2009; Chu et al. 2014; Fjermestad et al. 2016; Kendall 1994; Kendall et al. 1997; Marker et al. 2013). Research evaluating which specific aspects of the alliance are particularly important is lacking and is hindered by the absence of consistent terminology and frameworks (Elvins & Green 2008; Fjermestad et al. 2009). Similarly, the therapeutic alliance will fluctuate over time and may be perceived differently by clinician and young people at different stages of the intervention (Elvins & Green 2008). Overall, despite these limitations, meta-reviews suggest a small to medium effect of the therapeutic alliance on outcomes (Karver et al. 2018).

Chu & Kendall (2004) looked at one aspect of the therapeutic relationship, namely child involvement in CBT. The child's willingness to participate in therapeutic activities, engage in self-disclosure, and volunteer and introduce new information into the discussion was associated with better treatment gains. A strong alliance may therefore help to maximise child participation in practical skill-building exercises or exposure tasks (Chu & Kendall 2004; Kendall & Ollendick 2004). Alternatively, and not unexpectedly, a poor therapeutic relationship was a key reason for dropping out of therapy (Garcia & Weisz 2002).

Creed & Kendall (2005) identified collaboration as an important predictor of alliance in CBT with children and young people. This was defined by behaviours suggesting a partnership, with the child and therapist working together as a team, agreeing shared goals, with the therapist actively inviting the young person's participation and involvement. Excessive formality resulting in the therapist talking to the child in an aloof or patronising way and pushing the young person to speak about uncomfortable emotions had a negative effect on the relationship. Russell et al. (2008) found that therapists' responsiveness characterised by warm, positive, and empathic behaviours had a positive effect. The authors noted the importance of establishing these alliance-building behaviours in the first session. Similarly, flexibility or creativity whereby the therapist makes sessions more active, uses different methods to explain ideas such as games, role plays, and involving others, and attempts to match the concepts to the child's interests was positively related to child engagement (Chu & Kendall 2009). Engagement was subsequently associated with positive outcomes, leading the authors to suggest that attention needs to be paid to securing and maintaining engagement with children by making sessions interesting and enjoyable.

Young people are typically referred to psychological services because of concerns identified by others and may not themselves recognise or acknowledge any problems or the need to do anything different (Mcleod & Weisz 2005). It is therefore important to develop self-efficacy through motivational techniques which highlight positive treatment expectancies and challenge pessimism (Russell et al. 2008). A further aspect of the therapeutic process which requires specific attention is that of collaborative inquiry where young people 'become scientific investigators of their own thinking' (Beck & Dozois 2011). The promotion of a reflective and investigative approach requires careful attention when working with children, who are typically used to being provided with information and answers. Finally, the need to adapt CBT to the developmental level of the child or young person has been emphasised by many writers (Friedberg & McClure 2015; Stallard 2002b) and has been reflected in different versions of CBT programmes for young children and adolescents (see FRIENDS; Barrett 2010). This requires the therapist to ensure that CBT is pitched at the right level, consistent with the child's cognitive, emotional, verbal, and reasoning ability.

Partnership

Establishes a collaborative partnership with the young person and their parents/carers

CBT occurs within the context of a partnership based upon collaborative empiricism and shared learning. This is designed to be empowering and to enhance engagement and active participation in the intervention. The partnership involves:

- the young person, parent, and clinician working together to secure a set of agreed goals;

- the young person actively participating in clinical sessions;

- the development of an open and honest process where information is shared in an inclusive way that is understandable to all involved;

- the establishment of a curious process of self-discovery and reflection.

The nature of the active partnership that underpins CBT needs to be discussed during the initial meeting (TGFB p89). Young people are used to adopting a passive relationship with adult authority figures and may expect to be told what their problems are and what they need to do. The nature and expectations of the collaborative partnership should therefore be made clear and explicit at the outset. The active role of the young person and their parents/carers needs to be highlighted and the curious approach, in which they will work to discover why their problems occur and to experiment with different strategies, stressed. The partnership involves the young person, parents/carers, and clinician working together to experiment and discover what happens and what might be helpful.

The power differential between the adults and the young person needs to be acknowledged. It is a reality that cannot be denied or completely removed. However, the importance and expertise of the young person can be promoted by fully and actively encouraging their participation in the process. Young people are 'experts' of their experiences, their thoughts, how they feel, and what they do. They may have interests which can be incorporated into the intervention and can educate the clinician about their favourite music, film, hobbies, or sports team. This process strengthens the partnership, empowers the young person, and highlights that they have useful information to contribute.

The understanding and views of the young person and their parents are elicited

It is important to signal from the outset that the young person is as important as the adults and has useful information and ideas to contribute. It is therefore essential that the young person's personal experience and understanding is obtained, their contributions encouraged, and their views and ideas sought. Discussions therefore need to be inclusive, using language that is pitched at the right level and which is not too complex or technical.

Young people may initially appear reluctant to contribute to discussions. Previous experiences may lead them to believe that their ideas and views may not be valued or to worry that their contributions may not be 'right'. The young person's contributions therefore need to be encouraged and praised and their dichotomous thinking challenged. It should be made explicit that there are no 'right' or 'wrong' answers but that often there are different ways of thinking about events.

Parental views and their understanding of the young person's difficulties need to be identified and it is important to acknowledge that young people and parents/carers might have a different understanding of events or see things differently. This does not imply that one is 'right' and the other is 'wrong'. These different perspectives can coexist and should be welcomed and encouraged with each being validated as important.

Young people may expect their parents/carers to talk for them or parents/carers may dominate discussions resulting in the young person having limited opportunities to directly express their own views. These situations need to be carefully managed and opportunities made to directly hear from the young person.

▶ 'Thanks for telling me that. It would be great to hear what you think Mike.'

▶ 'That is really helpful to hear what you think happens. I would now like to ask you, Mike, to tell me about the situations that make you feel anxious.'

There may be occasions when the young person and/or their parents/carers need separate time to ensure that each has a chance to fully contribute and express their views and understandings.

Encourages and invites the young person to participate in the generation of ideas, option appraisal, and decision making

The central and active role of the young person in the partnership continues throughout the intervention. Their full and active involvement in the generation of ideas, appraisal of options, and decision making increases their ownership of the intervention and their commitment and motivation to experiment with new skills and ways of responding.

The model of learning together needs to be made explicit at the outset. The process is one where the young person, their parents/carers, and the clinician work together to discover helpful ways of responding. The importance of the young person's ideas and experiences is emphasised, and they are encouraged to fully contribute to sessions.

Young people may not necessarily realise that they have useful ideas to contribute. They often respond to questions such as 'What have you found helps you to feel more relaxed?' with short responses such as 'Nothing'. However, young people can be helped to discover useful ideas through the Socratic dialogue, which encourages them to focus and reflect on potentially important information.

▶ 'You told me that you are seldom anxious when you are with your brother. What do you do when you are together?'

▶ 'You have noticed that your mood is worse when you are on your own. What do you do when you are on your own?'

The development of a formulation leads to the consideration of different options for change and the development of new skills. Once again, the young person needs to be fully involved in both the generation and the evaluation of potential options. If they find verbal discussions difficult, then worksheets can provide a helpful way of generating possible ideas (TGFG p211) and appraising options (TGFG p213). Their contributions need to be encouraged and reinforced.

▶ 'This is great. Have you got any other ideas?'

▶ 'Are there any other options that we haven't talked about yet?'

Finally, young people need to be fully involved in decision making. Whilst on many occasions young people and parents/carers will agree, there will be times when they hold different views. The young person may not necessarily be able to verbally express their views, but their non-verbal behaviour may indicate their disagreement. Possible uncertainty and differences in views need to be acknowledged and sensitively responded to.

▶ 'Dad thinks this is a good idea, but you don't seem so sure?'

▶ 'You seem quiet. I wonder if you are feeling unsure about this.'

Involves the young person and parent/carer in goal and target setting, intervention planning, home assignments, and experiments

The use of goals and targets ensures that the intervention remains focused on the outcomes the young person would like to achieve. It is important to ensure that they have ownership of the intervention and that the young person and clinician are working together towards a shared agenda. The achievement of the goals will inform and guide the intervention, the choice of home assignments, and behavioural experiments (Law & Jacob 2013).

The partnership requires the young person to be fully involved in this process and for them to be able to express their views about what they can and cannot do and to identify any help or support that might be required. This needs to be negotiated in an open and honest way. Whilst, for example, it might be preferable to complete a week of self-monitoring, this might be too difficult and a compromise of three days of monitoring agreed.

Similarly, behavioural experiments and home assignments need to be negotiated. This will ensure that the young person has ownership of the task and will increase the likelihood that it will be successfully completed. The role of the parents/carers in supporting home assignments needs to be agreed. With younger children, they will have a more active role in supporting,

encouraging, and enabling completion. With older adolescents, parents/
carers may have a less significant or indeed no role, with responsibility for
assignment completion resting entirely with the young person.

Encourages the young person to provide open and honest feedback about therapy sessions

To ensure that the young person feels fully involved, they can be invited to
provide feedback at the end of each session. Core dimensions of the
therapeutic alliance such as the relationship (felt respected and heard),
session focus (said what I wanted), approach (good fit), and overall
satisfaction (session was right) can be rated on a 1–10 scale (Duncan et al.
2003). This provides a way of tracking whether the child/young person felt
listened too, understood, and provided with opportunities to discuss what
they wanted to and whether the session has given the child/young person
ideas to work on (Law & Wolpert 2014).

Session rating scales such as these tend to be rated highly. Young people tend
to give very favourable ratings, and so ratings should be discussed with an
open and curious approach.

▶ 'What could we do differently next time that would help you feel listened to?'

▶ 'How could we make sure that you are able to say all the things you want
to say?'

▶ 'What would help to make things easier to understand?'

▶ 'How can we make sure that we catch the things that you want to work on?'

Regularly attending to and assessing the partnership provides opportunities
to strengthen the alliance and to identify early, and resolve, any issues that
might result in disengagement.

Right developmental level

Engages with the young person and family in a developmentally sensitive way

Adopting a developmental perspective requires consideration of a range of
issues about the presentation and social context of the young person's
problems as well as their linguistic, memory, and perspective-taking ability.

CBT needs to be pitched at the right developmental level. If pitched too high,
the young person may not be able to fully engage and participate. Similarly, if
pitched too low, the young person may feel patronised and become bored

and disinterested. Important factors in the young person's development that will positively or negatively affect the success of the intervention, including their cognitive and linguistic abilities as well as their interests, need to be carefully considered.

Ensures an optimal balance between cognitive and behavioural techniques

The cognitive capacity of the young person to engage with CBT has been the subject of much attention. The influential cognitive developmental theory of Piaget (1952) suggests that young people cannot begin to engage in abstract thinking until the concrete operational stage (acquired during 7–12 years of age). What is typically assumed to be metacognition or reflective thinking does not develop until what Piaget defined as the formal operations stage (acquired during adolescence). The implication of this model is that pre-adolescent children will be unable to engage in many of the cognitive demands of CBT and thus will derive fewer benefits from this approach (Durlak et al. 1991).

The sequential staged model of cognitive development proposed by Piaget has been challenged and it is now recognised that young people can engage in demanding cognitive tasks if careful consideration is given to the instructions they receive (Thornton 2002). Indeed, many of the cognitive demands of CBT are quite limited and effectively require the young person to reason about concrete issues rather than engaging in highly abstract conceptual cognitive processes (Harrington et al. 1998). It is now accepted that children aged seven years and above can effectively engage in child-focused CBT. With regard to children below this age, there continues to be debate, as highlighted by Piacentini and Bergaman (2001), who suggest that regardless of clinician accommodation, children aged six or less may be precluded from benefiting from many cognitive aspects of treatment. Interventions with children under the age of seven may therefore need to pay less attention to cognitions and focus instead upon behavioural approaches (Bolton 2004). Children aged 7–11 may benefit more from the use of simple, specific, and concrete cognitive techniques such as coping self-talk, whilst adolescents may be able to engage in more sophisticated cognitive techniques in which overarching dysfunctional cognitive assumptions and beliefs are identified and re-evaluated.

If the young person finds it difficult to engage with their cognitions, then a greater emphasis should be placed on behavioural methods (Friedberg & McClure 2015; Stallard 2009). Young people can therefore be helped to understand their cognitions or to develop new skills through practical experiments rather than verbal discussion.

Uses simple, clear, jargon-free language that is respectful and not patronising

Talking therapies rely on language as the medium through which the young person communicates their inner thoughts and feelings. Verbal communications are used to promote self-discovery and efficacy leading to the acquisition of more functional skills. With young people, their language skills are developing, and assumptions about their receptive and expressive language ability should not be made. It is easy to assume a shared level of language when in fact no such understanding exists.

The ability of young people to spontaneously volunteer information in response to open questions may be limited. This may reflect the developing memory capacity of the young person or alternatively a complex question that they are unsure how to answer. Complex, multi-component questions should therefore be avoided. Younger children or those with more limited cognitive ability respond better to specific and direct questions. Possible problems of recall can be addressed by providing specific prompts or by presenting a range of options from which the young person can choose, for example, 'Some young people tell me they feel scared, some angry, and some sad. Do you have any of these feelings?'

The young person's language and the words they use to describe their problems, thoughts, and feelings should be used. However, rather than simply reflecting the young person's words, it is important to fully understand the meaning they ascribe to their descriptors. At the most basic level, professional jargon and theoretical terms should be avoided. Use the young person's terms (e.g. 'head talk') rather than rephrasing using professional language (e.g. 'negative automatic thoughts').

Language should be respectful, with the young person treated as an equal. Young people should not be patronised by talking down to them or by adopting a position of superiority.

▶ Be mindful about making assumptions about the young person.

▶ Respect the views of young people and do not be judgemental.

▶ Talk with young people rather than about them.

▶ Make sure the young person has enough space to express their views.

▶ Avoid being an 'expert' who gives advice, and promote self-discovery.

▶ Don't feel a need to know everything and have all the answers but instead encourage experimentation and learning.

Finally, the young person should be given permission to request further explanations or to correct inaccurate summaries. This should be made explicit so that young people see this as part of the process and understand that they are not being disrespectful or rude by doing so.

> ► 'Sometimes I may not explain things clearly or I may not have fully understood what you have said. If that happens, can you stop me and let me know?'

Uses a variety of verbal (direct and indirect approaches) and non-verbal techniques

Many young people have sufficiently developed verbal skills to engage in a predominantly verbal intervention. They can understand words and their meanings, articulate and express their internal thoughts and emotions, and understand and verbally reason. However, language will need to be matched to the young person's developmental level and their ability to understand, regularly checked by asking them to summarise and explain the concepts that are being discussed.

Whilst they may have sufficient verbal skills, young people may often appear quiet and unforthcoming. In these situations, non-verbal materials should be used as an alternative way of communication or to complement, enhance, or replace verbal discussions. Visual methods provide a permanent record of information and help to overcome the limited verbal memory of some young people. Thought bubbles, magazine pictures of people expressing emotions, simple three-part formulations, quizzes, and drawings are all helpful ways of making some of the key tasks of CBT objective, concrete, visual, and fun. Similarly, complex information such as multiple-component formulations can be built up slowly by looking at connections between two elements (e.g. thoughts and feelings) at a time.

Computers and technology are familiar to young people and some will be motivated and readily able to design their own self-monitoring forms and diary sheets. Emailing and texting is common amongst many adolescents, so the idea of 'downloading one's head' can be an acceptable way of accessing a young person's cognitions. Similarly, phone cameras provide a helpful way of assessing stressful situations which can be used to inform behavioural experiments or exposure tasks.

Appropriately involves parents/carers/others

Parents/carers are important influences for the young person, and their role in the onset and maintenance of the young person's problems needs careful assessment. The initial assessment will provide an understanding of important family beliefs, systemic structure, and context within which the problems present and parental behaviours that may encourage and reinforce the young person's difficulties. This will identify any skills that are lacking, perhaps in parenting or conflict resolution, distorted parental expectations and beliefs about the young person, or any dysfunctional cognitions the parents/carers ascribe to their young person's behaviour or their ability to effect positive change. In turn, this will inform both the focus (e.g. directly working with the young person and/or parent) and the content (e.g. developing new skills for the young person and/or parent) of the intervention.

Parents/carers can be involved in child-focused CBT in different ways, depending upon the purpose of their involvement.

▶ **Facilitator.** This is the most limited role, with parents/carers typically attending two or three parallel sessions. In these sessions, which are psycho-educational, parents/carers are provided with the rationale for using CBT and information about the techniques and strategies the young person will learn. The young person is the direct focus of the intervention and the CBT programme is designed to address their problems.

▶ **Co-clinician.** Parents/carers are more extensively involved in the intervention and attend sessions with the young person. They may be involved in the whole session or join at the end. As co-clinicians, parents/ carers are encouraged to monitor, prompt, and reinforce the young person's use of skills outside of face-to-face sessions. The young person remains the focus of the intervention, with the parents/carers encouraging, supporting, and reinforcing the young person's use of new skills.

▶ **Clinician.** There is evidence that parents/carers can successfully be taught CBT skills which they in turn can use to help their child (Cartwright-Hatton et al. 2011; Creswell et al. 2017). This has primarily been to address anxiety disorders in children under the age of 12. The young person's problems remain the focus of the intervention, with parents/ carers having an active role in teaching them CBT skills.

▶ **Co-client.** This recognises that both the young person and the parents would benefit from a direct intervention. The young person will receive an intervention to address their own problems whilst their parents/carers/ family acquire new skills in order to address family or personal difficulties that contribute to the onset or maintenance of these difficulties. Parent sessions might run alongside and be separate from sessions with the young person and will explore what they can do to help. For example, they might be encouraged to model coping, to motivate and encourage the young person, to be positive and reinforce attempts at change, or to empower the young person to face their problems.

It is rare that parents/carers intentionally set out to harm a young person. When this does occur, appropriate action needs to be taken to ensure that the young person is safe. More often, parents/carers are trying their best but have become trapped in unhelpful interactions or patterns of behaviour. In this situation a 'no-blame' approach should be adopted where parents/

carers are praised for their commitment to help the young person but encouraged to discover and experiment with alternative strategies.

School is another important context where the active involvement of the teaching staff in the intervention should be considered and agreed. Failure to appropriately involve school staff by, for example, assessing their views about the intervention, their commitment to supporting it, and their goals can result in negative outcomes.

Case Study Courtney has anger outbursts

Courtney (15) was referred with problems of persistent rudeness, defiance, and angry outbursts at school. He was in danger of being permanently excluded if he had another outburst and so the immediate focus of the intervention was to help Courtney learn alternative ways to manage his angry feelings. Courtney readily participated in the intervention and he successfully implemented various anger management strategies at school. However, insufficient attention was paid to the school context, where it emerged that their goal was not to support Courtney to manage his temper but rather to remove him from the school. Several teachers were frightened by his angry outbursts and, although he had never physically assaulted any of the teaching staff, some were fearful of their safety. Whilst Courtney did not have any other angry outbursts, he was subsequently permanently suspended for persistent lateness.

Empathy

Promotes empathy through the development of a genuine, warm, and respectful relationship

Empathy means really understanding what the young person is thinking, how they feel, and the meaning they ascribe to events. It is conveyed by adopting a warm, caring, and respectful approach expressed through curiosity, interest, genuineness, and acceptance. Empathy is a key element of the therapeutic partnership and signals to the young person that their experience is important, acknowledged, and understood.

Conveys interest and concern using active listening, reflection, and summaries

Empathy is conveyed by the core counselling skills of active listening, reflection, and summarising. Active listening involves fully focusing attention on what is being said here and now. It is conveyed through eye contact, appropriate facial expressions, and body language such as head nods. These encourage the young person to talk and signal interest in what they have to say.

Although active listening sounds simple, it can be difficult. We are always busy, often juggling many competing work and personal demands, and so it is not uncommon to find our mind wandering. Be mindful of this, and once identified, bring your attention back to the here and now and really focus on what the young person is saying.

To encourage the young person to speak, use open rather than closed questions. Open questions start with, 'How', 'What', 'Where', 'Who', 'Why' and encourage the young person to volunteer information rather than replying 'Yes', 'No', or 'Don't know'.

▶ Instead of asking, 'Have you been feeling down?' ask, 'How have you been feeling?'

▶ Instead of asking, 'Do you notice your heart racing when you become anxious?' ask, 'What body signals do you notice when you become anxious?'

▶ Instead of asking, 'Is it worse when you are school?" ask, 'Where do you feel particularly bad?'

▶ Instead of asking, 'Do your friends know how you feel?" ask, "Who knows how you are feeling?'

▶ Instead of asking, 'Is it because you are worried that you don't try new things?" ask, "Why is it hard to try new things?'

In addition to carefully listening to what the young person says, active listening also involves noticing what they don't say or talk about. This can be brought to the young person's attention with a curious approach.

▶ 'You have told me a lot about how you feel when you become down and that feeling of being frightened and losing control. I wondered what might happen if you did lose control?'

Summaries provide a useful way of showing the young person that they have been heard and involve repeating back to the young person, in their own words, what they said. It is important to establish the meaning of the young person's words since adults may not necessarily be familiar with adolescent slang. Once the meaning is established, their response may be paraphrased but it can be helpful to keep them in the moment by using their own words.

Summaries check that you have heard the young person correctly and provide an opportunity for misunderstandings to be corrected and important parts of the discussion to be highlighted.

► 'Have I got this right? You say that you first noticed feeling anxious when you started your new school.'

Reflections involve repeating back to the young person a single word or phrase they have said. These help to focus the young person's attention on what they have said and encourage them to clarify meanings or explore patterns or connections between different events, thoughts, and feelings in more detail.

► 'Recently I have been very tearful.' – 'Recently?'

► 'I don't know how much longer I can cope with this.' – 'How much longer?'

► 'I always feel worse when I am with my friends.' – 'With your friends?'

They also provide opportunities to connect emotionally and to acknowledge how the young person has been feeling.

► 'It sounds as if you were feeling really frightened.'

► 'You seemed really angry with that teacher.'

► 'You appear very disappointed that your friends let you down.'

Acknowledges and appropriately responds to verbal and non-verbal expressions and emotional responses

Empathy involves connecting with emotions and acknowledging how the young person is feeling. Empathy could be directly expressed verbally.

► 'You have had a lot of house moves, so I hear how anxious you feel starting at a new school.'

► 'Your friends have let you down so many times, I can see how hard it is to trust them again.'

► 'Being successful is so important for you, so I can see how sad you feel when you don't get things right.'

Alternatively, emotion may be conveyed through non-verbal body signals where, for example, the young person appears

► quiet – stops talking, lowers their head, or turns away;

► excited – talking fast, changing the subject, fidgeting, constantly moving around;

► angry – talking loudly, swearing, throwing or crashing things down on the table.

These signals need to be acknowledged and discussed.

- ▶ 'You seem quiet. How are you feeling?'

- ▶ 'You have become excited. What has happened to make you feel so excited?'

- ▶ 'You look really angry. What can you do to calm down?'

It can be hard to establish an empathic relationship with some young people such as those with autistic spectrum disorder (ASD). The use of non-verbal cues such as eye contact, facial expressions, and gestures, intended to convey respect and understanding, may not be recognised or understood. These cues may be less important or may need to be exaggerated.

Demonstrates an open, respectful, non-judgemental, caring approach

Young people might feel embarrassed talking about their problems. They may feel ashamed of what they did, how they thought or behaved. They may worry that they will be judged or criticised or be unsure whether their discussion will be shared with others. These concerns may result in the young person appearing reticent and unforthcoming.

It is important to remain mindful of how hard it may be for the young person to share their experiences or worries. The young person needs to be reassured that although it can be hard to talk about difficult things, it can be helpful to get their worries out of their head. The use of encouragement clearly signals to the young person that you want to hear what they have to say. Simple statements such as 'go on' or 'tell me more about that' and praise such as 'although it has been hard for you to talk about this you are doing really well' can encourage the young person to talk more.

Concerns about the young person becoming upset or distressed might result in important events or experiences being avoided. This implicitly sends a message to the young person that these things are too painful and should not be talked about. In these situations, directly asking for clarification can be a helpful way of signalling that this is OK to talk about and encouraging the young person to talk.

- ▶ 'Can you tell me what happened that was so bad?'

- ▶ 'I appreciate that this is difficult, but it would be helpful to hear more about those thoughts that upset you so much.'

Similarly, it may be important to initiate an open discussion with the young person about what they think will happen if they talk about things.

▶ 'What do you think would happen if we talked about this?'

▶ 'What do you think I would say if you told me?'

If the young person still feels unable to enter onto a discussion, their views should be respected, although the discussion should be revisited in future sessions.

Finally, the extent and limitations of confidentiality need to be made explicit so that the young person is clear when information will be shared and when it will not. In general, what is talked about will not be shared without their permission unless it raises concerns about the young person's safety. If concerns about the young person's safety or that of others are identified, then these will be shared to ensure that everyone is kept safe. Good practice suggests that the young person should be fully involved and understand who will be informed and what will be shared.

Empathises with parents/carers about their own difficulties and the impact of these on their ability to help their child

Parents/carers often feel powerless to help their child and feel confused and unsure what they can do to help. They may have their own problems, which might impact on their child, and feel guilty or blame themselves for their child's difficulties. It is important to establish a 'no blame' culture. Rather than criticising or blaming parents/carers for what has happened, the intervention needs to positively focus on the future and what they can do to bring about positive change.

Sometimes parents/carers try too hard and want to protect their child from any distress. On these occasions, they may need help to clarify their role and they may need 'permission' to step back. For example, instead of trying to protect a young person from feeling anxious, parents/carers might need help to develop problem-solving or anxiety management skills. The young person will still experience anxiety, which the parents/carers may find difficult to tolerate, and this needs to be acknowledged. However, difficult as this may be, parents/ carers can feel reassured that they are helping their child learn to cope.

Similarly, a parent's sense of frustration or powerlessness needs to be acknowledged. This might be particularly strong for parents/carers of adolescents, who may feel frustrated by a young person's apparent lack of interest or motivation to help themselves. Once again, parents/carers need to understand that these feelings are normal and are indications of how much they care about their young person. Learning to accept these feelings can help parents reduce their distress in the knowledge that they are doing all they can to help. Their role is to remain positive and hopeful that the situation can improve whilst the young person begins to accept responsibility for their behaviour and actions.

Any difficulties of the parents/carers that might impede their ability to help their child need to be identified and sensitively acknowledged. A depressed parent may, for example, find it difficult to be positive and to help their child acknowledge their strengths, whilst an anxious parent may find it hard to encourage their child to face anxiety-provoking situations. The extent of parental difficulties needs to be assessed and, where appropriate, parents/carers need to be directed for help. Alternative ways of supporting the young person can be explored so that perhaps a grandparent can help a depressed young person find their strengths or a teacher can help a young person face an anxious situation at school. The parents' desire to help their child needs to be highlighted and their limitations acknowledged, and they should be helped to see the involvement of others as positive, rather than as a sign of their failure. Highlight what parents/carers are doing, rather than focusing on what they have been unable to do.

Creative

Adapts CBT to facilitate the understanding and engagement of the child/young person and their parents/carers

Creativity requires the presentation and adaptation of CBT to match the young person's interests and experiences. This requires an open approach in which CBT is viewed as a unique process in which different methods and media are matched to the developmental level, skills, and interests of the young person. The goal is to engage the young person in a developmentally sensitive therapeutic process where the concepts and tasks are meaningful and are built around their interests.

Creativity can be challenging and requires an ability to think outside of the box. Creativity should therefore be approached in an open way in which different ways of explaining an idea or concept are explored, thereby avoiding the implicit need to get it 'right'. Some ideas will be more helpful than others. This is not a sign of therapeutic failure, but rather part of the inevitable matching of the therapeutic process with the young person that is an intrinsic part of CBT.

Tailors the concepts and methods of CBT around the interests of the young person

CBT is creatively developed to meet the needs and strengths of the young person. The process involves identifying their goals, strengths, interests, and values, which are then integrated into the intervention.

The young person's interests are used to inform the intervention and to help them understand key concepts in the CBT model and develop ways of coping.

▶ If a young person is interested in football, then scenarios involving famous footballers or events can be used to highlight positive or negative thoughts.

▶ If a young person is interested in music, they can be asked to find songs or lyrics that make them feel good or help them to relax.

▶ If a young person enjoys drawing, they could be asked to draw a picture of their future life which can then be discussed to find out what needs to change to help them achieve this.

▶ If a young person enjoys photography, positive and uplifting photographs could be saved in a separate folder on their phone to remind them of the good times when they feel low.

Young people may be unwilling to keep self-monitoring records but may be more motivated if asked to design their own on their computer. Similarly, the identification of important thoughts that accompany hot situations (i.e. when a young person notices a strong emotional reaction) can be captured by asking the young person to download their head onto their phone or into an email message rather than a paper diary (TGFB p110).

The young person's interests can be built upon and incorporated into the intervention. Books and films such as those in the Harry Potter series provide many ideas that can be developed and used. For example, in *Harry Potter and the Prisoner of Azkaban*, Harry learns to beat his fears by thinking about them in a humorous way. The idea of changing an unpleasant emotion such as anxiety or anger to one that is more pleasant and comfortable is a simple technique that is often used in CBT. Similarly, in the film *Shrek*, there is a scene where Shrek rescues the princess from the castle. The resulting dialogue provides a helpful way of discussing the link between positive and helpful thoughts (princess believes that Shrek is the person of her dreams) and critical and unhelpful thoughts (Shrek believes he is ugly and frightening) and their effect on feelings and behaviour.

Uses an appropriate range of verbal and non-verbal methods to facilitate understanding and engagement

Creativity involves using a variety of techniques and methods to engage with the young person and to help them secure their therapeutic goals. It is helpful to have a range of core materials available for each session, such as blackboards/whiteboards, flip charts, drawing materials, worksheets, and tablets, to help maintain interest.

Blackboards and whiteboards provide a helpful way of visually capturing and highlighting information. Important thoughts can be captured and links between events, thoughts, and feelings summarised in case formulations. Printed handouts can provide useful adjuncts to clinical sessions and provide a written record of key issues for future reference. Similarly, pie charts can provide an objective way of identifying, quantifying, and challenging assumptions about the likelihood of events occurring (TGFB p187). Visual rating scales and thermometers are useful to promote and encourage a wider range of dimensionality, thereby challenging the tendency for categorical thinking (TGFG p166).

The process should build upon any issues regarding the young person's abilities. For example, young people with ASD tend to be very concrete and literal in the way they think and understand conversations. Consequently, questions will be more effective if they are descriptive and factual rather than abstract and hypothetical. CBT also needs to be made less abstract and more experiential. Rather than talking about what might happen if the young person behaved in a different way, encourage them to check it out and 'see what happens' by role playing the situation there and then.

Creatively uses a range of methods

Familiar images and examples can provide concrete ways of helping young people to understand some of the ideas and concepts of CBT. The rationale for exposure is 'taking a medicine that tastes "yucky" but makes you feel better' (Freeman et al. 2008). Obsessional thoughts can be described as a song stuck in your head. The image of a tumble drier can explain how thoughts get locked in our heads and keep tumbling round and round, or that of a DVD player to explain repetitive intrusive images. A pair of negative glasses can be used to describe the common cognitive distortion of selective abstraction where only negative things are noticed. Similarly, young people with ASD might find verbal communication difficult and may prefer to engage in a process where texts or emails are used as the primary form of communication.

Metaphors are helpful and effective if they are concrete and relate to items that are familiar to the young person. For example, young people understand that a volcano smokes and smoulders before it erupts and this provides a concrete way of mapping their anger build-up (TGFG p176). Similarly, traffic lights can provide a simple and understandable way to help young people learn a process for problem solving (TGFG p216). Red is to stop and define the problem, amber to prepare and plan a solution, and green to signal that they should go and try their solution.

Abstract concepts and complicated processes need to be made simple and translated into concrete steps and metaphors. A specific step process such as the 4Cs ('catch it, check it, challenge it, change it') provides a simple way to remember the process of thought identification, evaluation, and reappraisal (TGFB p129). The concept of automatic thoughts can be highlighted by asking the young person to participate in a game such as using their non-preferred hand to draw a house or to write their name. Once the task is completed, the young person is asked what thoughts were racing through their head as they undertook this task.

The idea of selective attention can be highlighted by the idea of watching a film. A number of things are noticed first time around, but if the film is watched again then new information is seen. Similarly, a video clip can be used to highlight how we might selectively attend to some information but fail to see something very obvious like a moonwalking bear (https://binged.it/2Lp4RYY). The concept of negative automatic thoughts can be explained to those interested in computers by using the metaphor of computer spam. Turning on the PC and connecting to the Internet (i.e. the young person's brain) results in computer spam suddenly appearing to advertise various products. The spam is not asked for (i.e. automatic), is hard to block (i.e. can't turn them off), most of it is unrecognised (i.e. simply delete without reading), but some messages are read (selectively attend). This metaphor conveys the core features of automatic thoughts in a concrete and understandable way.

Exposure tasks can be adapted in playful ways. Children with separation anxiety could be encouraged to take part in a treasure hunt where they must leave their parent to complete the challenge (Hirshfeld-Becker et al. 2008). Similarly, young people with social anxiety can be encouraged to approach others in order to conduct surveys.

Utilises the preferred media of the young person

Some young people will be happy to sit and talk, whereas others will prefer more non-verbal ways of expressing themselves. Young people may, for example, be unable to volunteer their thoughts or feelings when directly asked but can often convey these through thought bubbles or play. Similarly, situations can be turned into a game in which the young person is asked to guess what someone else might think or feel in their worrying situation. A sorting game can be used to distinguish between thoughts, actions, and feelings, and unfinished sentences as a way of eliciting thoughts related to specific situations or feelings. Young people could be encouraged to create an emotional scrapbook by collecting photographs or pictures of different emotions from magazines. The young person may prefer to draw and can be encouraged to create a film strip about their difficult situation (TGFG p77). Once they have drawn it, the young person can be encouraged to add any emotions or thoughts they can identify.

Increasingly, young people are highly familiar with, and competent in, using computers, the Internet, and smartphones, which can be used in the intervention. The transportability of these devices can help the quick and accurate recording of mood, thoughts, or positive events as they occur. They can provide a way for young people to 'download their heads' when they notice any 'hot thoughts' or strong emotional reactions (TGFB p110). Because young people are often texting and interacting with mobile devices, briefly recording information such as this will not attract peer attention.

Smartphone cameras provide a way of recording difficult or challenging situations. Images can be reviewed to check some of the young person's thoughts or assumptions about what is happening and can help plan how to cope with difficult situations. The young person's photo library can include pictures of their calming place, which can remind them of and help them to create an image of it when required.

The Internet provides a helpful way of researching and normalising common problems such as feeling anxious or low in mood. Celebrities who have suffered such conditions can be found and ways in which these celebrities learned to succeed identified as possible options for the young person to consider (TGFB p54). Websites and apps which provide guidance and instructions on techniques such as mindfulness or relaxation can be accessed to facilitate and guide practice. Similarly, there is a wealth of useful videos of young people talking about their personal experiences of psychological problems and strategies they found helpful. Learning from other young people can be very powerful with video stories and YouTube clips providing helpful ways to bring the perspective of other young people into the meeting.

Investigation

> Adopts an open and curious stance that facilitates guided discovery and reflection

The concept of guided discovery and investigation is a key feature of CBT. It is based upon the premise that thoughts and behaviour will be more readily changed if the rationale for change comes from the young person's and/or carers' own insights. The young person is encouraged to test out and experiment with new skills and ways of thinking to check what happens.

Creates a process of collaborative inquiry in which cognitions, beliefs, and assumptions are subject to objective evaluation

A few concepts have been used to capture this investigative process, including the Private I (Friedberg & McClure 2002), the Social Detective (Spence 1995), and Thought Tracker (Stallard 2002a). The Social Detective, for example, teaches a three-stage process for social problem solving in which the young person detects, investigates, and then solves.

A key element of this investigative process is behavioural experiments, which provide a powerful way of objectively testing beliefs and assumptions and of responding to events in different ways. The investigative process needs to be undertaken with an open mind, and preconceived ideas about outcomes should be suspended. Indeed, experiments should not be undertaken to simply prove an alternative way of thinking or to disprove an unhelpful way of thinking. They should be genuinely open and may indeed confirm the young person's predictions and beliefs. The process of collaborative inquiry therefore helps the young person to objectively test their cognitions and to use this information to discover new or overlooked information. In turn, this can help them to put limits around strong universal beliefs or assumptions.

The process is undertaken in an open manner: 'Shall we try and see what happens?' This approach conveys a number of important messages.

- It builds upon the collaborative process of a partnership working and learning together.

- It conveys a sense of inquisitiveness and openness.

- It highlights that there are often many possible solutions or ways of thinking about events, thereby challenging the dichotomous thinking of many young people.

- It provides an experimental framework that can be applied to other problems.

- It encourages learning from others: 'You told me that Mike never has any problems like this, so can you check out what he does in this situation?'

This objective, scientific approach may appeal to particular groups of young people. Children with ASD, for example, have strengths in both intelligence and logic and may respond well to tasks involving the identification of evidence to support or challenge a particular way of thinking (TGFG p116) or to the creation of responsibility pie charts to visualise the contribution of different factors to events (TGFB p187).

Fully involves young people in the design of experiments

The CORE philosophy of child-focused CBT places the young person at the centre of the intervention. This needs to be emphasised by ensuring that the young person is actively involved in the design of experiments. The design should be approached with curiosity, with young person being invited to suggest answers to the question, 'What could we do to check this out?' The Socratic dialogue can be used to shape the experiment, which should be safe and have a clear aim and an objective way of evaluation. For example, Mike had a strong belief that people didn't like him. Through a curious conversation, Mike identified that if people liked him, they would text or message him. This led to an experiment where Mike recorded how many times over the coming week he received a text or message.

Helps young people and parents/carers to consider alternative explanations about events

Experiments generate new information which the young person will need to assimilate into their cognitive framework. The process is reflective, with the young person being helped to focus on important information and to explore possible explanations for their findings. This inquisitive approach encourages curiosity and cognitive flexibility and challenges the rigid thinking held by many young people.

Many unhelpful beliefs and assumptions tend to be internal, stable, and global. With unhelpful internal explanations, young people assume responsibility and blame themselves for what occurs: 'I am stupid', 'I make people angry'. Explanations such as these are often viewed as stable and enduring, suggesting that they cannot change, thereby generating a sense of helplessness. They also tend to be applied globally to all aspects of life, school, friendships, home, and so on, generating a sense of overwhelming hopelessness.

When developing alternative explanations, the young person should be encouraged to explore possibilities that are external (not personal), unstable (look for exceptions), and specific (put limits around them). To develop external explanations, the young person is encouraged to consider factors other than themselves. For example, instead of 'I am stupid', the young person might be encouraged to consider whether the nature of the work (i.e. new or very hard) may offer an alternative explanation. The development of unstable explanations requires the young person to reflect on whether there are times when their explanation does not fit. Have they, for example, received good marks for different pieces of schoolwork or discovered that their grades improve once they become familiar with the work? Finally, the development of more specific explanations requires the young person to put limits around their global explanations. For example, the young person might find maths hard but get good grades in geography, PE, and art, thereby limiting the belief that they are 'stupid'.

The development of alternative external, unstable, and specific explanations helps to counter feelings of blame, helplessness, and hopelessness. The aim, therefore, is to help the young person generate alternative explanations, not to critically or externally challenge their initial explanation. Different possibilities coexist whilst the young person collects information to support or challenge them.

Encourages reflection

The final task when reviewing the outcome of any experiment or home assignment is that of reflection: 'What have you found out?' or 'What have you discovered?' Young people may have completed a task but not necessarily reflected on what they have learned and how this information can be integrated into their cognitive framework.

This reflection on outcomes will often lead to the discovery of new information, meanings, or skills. For example, reviewing the outcome of self-monitoring tasks may identify new information about situations that trigger strong feelings, common critical thoughts, or unhelpful ways of responding. Experiments can produce new explanations and meanings. For example, a socially anxious young person could be encouraged to drop some of their safety behaviours in a social encounter. Safety behaviours are the things they do, such as talking quietly or avoiding eye contact, to avoid being embarrassed in front of others. The outcome of the experiment might reveal that the young person feels less anxious and self-conscious when they don't engage in their safety behaviours. Similarly, experiments or home assignments might involve trying new skills, such as mindfulness or self-compassion. Focusing on the outcome with questions such as whether it helped or influenced how they felt or whether they encountered any difficulties can help to promote insight and encourage ongoing usage.

Self-efficacy

Develops strengths and promotes positive attempts at change

The concept of self-efficacy highlights the positive, empowering nature of child-focused CBT. The aim is to help the young person find and build upon their strengths and skills. Maintaining this positive and enabling focus is important since there is a danger within any therapy, but particularly one that is concerned with identifying dysfunctional cognitive processes, that the model can become deficit driven. Whilst dysfunctional processes need to be addressed, the young person's skills and strengths need to be highlighted and, where possible, built upon and used to promote more adaptive and functional processes.

Identifies and highlights strengths and personal resources

It is often easier to identify what we are not good at than find our strengths. Young people often overlook their strengths and may appear tentative, unconvinced, or embarrassed when these are reflected to them. This may indicate a lack of confidence or a belief that because their skills do not work on every occasion that they are ineffective. Alternatively, they may be embarrassed, particularly if they have low self-esteem or strong critical core beliefs. To acknowledge that they have positive strengths and skills will be inconsistent with their beliefs.

Diaries can be useful for young people who find it difficult to identify or acknowledge their strengths (TGFB p52) or who feel that the world is against them (TGFB p67; TGFG p48). These encourage the young person to actively seek and find their strengths and skills and the kind things that happen that they often overlook. This can be empowering and helps them to challenge critical beliefs about themselves, their performance, and the world in which they live.

When identifying skills and strengths, the young person should be encouraged to consider multiple domains, including:

▶ school – academic skills, contributions to class discussions, completion of assignments;

▶ work – reliable, hard-working, willing to help;

▶ leisure activities – playing an instrument, skilled at gaming, caring for animals;

▶ relationships – loyal friend, good listener, trustworthy, supportive;

▶ personal skills – organised, thoughtful, caring, practical;

▶ specific achievements – member of a sports team, acted in a play, performed well in a competition.

Young people who struggle to find anything positive can be encouraged to ask others or think from a third-party perspective.

▶ 'What would your best friend say or someone who is important to you?'

▶ 'Why do your friends want to spend time with you?'

It is often easier to identify strengths by thinking from a third-party perspective rather than identifying them oneself.

Encourages identification of helpful skills and strategies

An important part of developing self-efficacy is helping young people to identify the skills and strengths they already possess that have shown some success. The belief that a strategy always needs to work to be successful needs to be challenged. Single strategies will not always work, but if they help on some occasions, they are useful. The idea is therefore to develop not a single skill but a toolbox of skills that can be drawn upon and used in different situations.

Young people should be helped to focus on successful experiences. Often, clinical discussions focus on problems or times when the young person has not coped, resulting in successful experiences being overlooked. To counter this, the young person should be encouraged to highlight positive experiences and to reflect on how they coped, what they found helpful, and what they did.

▶ 'What did you do that helped you to cope with that situation?'

▶ 'What sort of things have you found helpful?'

▶ 'There are times when it hasn't been too bad. What did you do differently that helped?'

Adopting a positive, coping focus can be very empowering and clearly signals to the young person that they possess skills and ideas that can be helpful.

Develops personal coping strategies

Once strengths and coping skills are identified, the young person can be helped to consider how they could be applied to different situations. Once again, the conversation is curious and open as the young person is helped to reflect on how particular skills and strengths could be used.

▶ Could the way the young person developed their gaming skills help them to approach their problems. Do they need to practise, watch someone, or ask for help?

▶ Could their personal quality of strong mindedness help them face a challenging situation they have avoided? Can this help them to develop positive and coping self-talk?

▶ Could their personal organisation skills help them create a self-monitoring diary?

▶ Could their sense of humour help to reduce the negative impact of something going wrong? Learn to laugh and move on rather than ruminate?

A young person may have an idea which could be shaped into a helpful coping strategy.

▶ A young person may comment that counting to 10 helps them to relax. This could be developed by encouraging them to focus on their breathing as they count, as they breathe out to say 'relax' and visualise their tension being released.

At other times, coping strategies can be identified by learning from others, by asking or watching someone who is successful (TGFG p212). What do they do and how do they cope with those situations the young person finds difficult?

Finally, once identified, the young person needs to discover how they can integrate these skills into their everyday life. For example, self-compassion can be enhanced through the development of a kinder inner voice (TGFB p66), which is practised each day as the young person speaks their compassionate voice whilst looking into a mirror. For younger children, they can be encouraged to identify and practise their positive (TGFG p144) and coping (TGFG p145) self-talk. These are short empowering statements that motivate and help the young person to face and cope with challenging situations.

Reinforces use of new skills

The application of new skills and practice should be noticed, acknowledged, and celebrated. This is important and counters any negative or critical biases that might result in positive experiences, successes, or coping being overlooked.

In the early stages, it is important to reward the use of skills rather than the outcome. For problems like low mood, it might take a little time for new skills such as behavioural activation or mindfulness to have a positive effect. Similarly, the adoption of new and helpful parenting behaviours should be noticed, acknowledged, and celebrated. Parents/carers should be encouraged to reward themselves for implementing new approaches.

Some young people are embarrassed to receive praise or to have their positive attempts at change acknowledged. This can feel difficult and runs counter to the strongly entrenched critical and negative self-beliefs of some young people. At these times, there is a danger of colluding with this by ignoring or playing down the young person's use of new skills. Their discomfort should be acknowledged, the importance of attending to their attempts to change highlighted, and a way of acknowledging these agreed.

Enjoyable and engaging

Sessions are interesting and absorbing

Young people are often referred due to concerns identified by others and, as such, their commitment and interest in change may be limited. In order to maintain engagement and motivation, it is important for CBT to be enjoyable and to continue to capture the young person's interests and maintain their motivation.

Uses an appropriate mix of materials, activities, humour

There are a number of ways in which the young person's engagement and enjoyment can be enhanced. As already described, a variety of materials should be used to maintain the young person's interest. A session exploring the link between thoughts and feelings could start with a brief verbal introduction. This could be followed by completing a worksheet (TGFG p158) and then a game in which the young person sorts thought, feeling, and behaviour cards into separate piles.

The young person should be involved in agenda setting and prioritising tasks. Clinical sessions should be more active and may involve moving around or going out of the clinic room. The young person could be involved in drawing the formulation or in drawing or completing a worksheet. Sessions should not be too long. For many children, a 50–60-minute session may result in them becoming bored or losing interest, so make the sessions shorter.

Humour can be used effectively within the therapeutic relationship to draw attention to issues. For example, a young person's comment that they 'always get things wrong' prompted a clinician to rush for their camera saying that they had never ever met anyone before who 'always' got things wrong and so wanted to take a picture. This swift intervention drew the young person's attention, in a humorous way, to the thinking trap they often fell into.

Maintains an appropriate balance between task and relationship-strengthening activities

Although CBT is a structured and focused approach, it needs to be flexible and sensitive to the needs of the young person. There may be times when the young person is agitated, unfocused, upset, or disinterested. Rather than continuing with the session as planned, there needs to be some flexibility and a balance between task-focused activities and relationship- or rapport-building activities. This may result in the planned session being modified as the focus shifts towards relationship-building activities, aimed at securing and maintaining the young person's engagement for future work.

Non-task activities strengthen the relationship and often focus on the young person's interests, hobbies, and pastimes. There will be a greater focus on non-task activities during the initial sessions, where the young person may be unsure about attending sessions or reluctant to talk about personal issues.

Subsequent sessions will also involve time for relationship-strengthening activities, although this needs to be carefully monitored to ensure that sufficient time is allocated for task-/goal-based activities.

Depending on the age of the young person, non-task relationship-strengthening activities could involve the following.

▶ Games and quizzes such as 'What I like'. A series of statements can be written on cards, which the young person and clinician take it in turns to choose and answer. Statements could include: 'What I like to do on my own'; 'What I like to do with my friends'; 'What I like to watch on TV'; 'What I like to do at school'; 'What I like to do with my family'; 'What I like to do online'; 'What I like to listen to'.

▶ Online surfing to discover the young person's interests and favourite sites. These might include YouTube videos; blogger sites; sport or music sites; funny video clips; links to causes that are important to them, such as climate change or animal welfare.

▶ Asking the young person to bring examples of what they enjoy to sessions. Young people who enjoy art, writing, poems, or music could be asked to bring examples of work they are pleased with.

▶ Sharing photographs of events that the young person has attended or enjoyed.

▶ Moving out of the clinical setting by going for a walk or to a café.

Attends to the young person's interests and incorporates them into the intervention

Advances in digital technology provide new opportunities for making CBT fun and engaging. Digital interventions may be particularly appealing for adolescents who are early adopters and regular users of new technology (Johnson et al. 2015). However, digital interventions are costly to develop, and to date relatively few have been evaluated (Grist et al. 2017; Hollis et al. 2017).

The structured nature of CBT readily allows it to be transferred into a format that can be delivered via a computer or the Internet. Reviews have demonstrated that, although research is limited, computerised CBT is effective (Pennant et al. 2015; Richardson et al. 2010). For example, *Stressbusters*, a computerised CBT programme, has been found to be effective for the treatment of depression (Smith et al. 2015; Wright et al. 2017). Similarly, for anxiety, computerised programmes such as *BRAVE-Online* (Spence et al. 2011), *Camp Cope-A-Lot* (Khanna & Kendall 2010), and *Cool Teens* have demonstrated encouraging results (Wuthrich et al. 2012). A few

CBT-based games have been developed. For example, *SPARX*, a computerised CBT game, proved effective as both a depression intervention and a depression prevention programme (Merry, Stasiak, et al. 2012; Perry et al. 2017).

Finally, smartphones provide an opportunity to support or deliver interventions for children and young people. However, despite the thousands of apps available, few have been developed for children and young people with mental health problems or subject to any evaluation (Grist et al. 2017).

Presents as positive and hopeful

The presentation of the clinician during child-focused CBT is important and will have an important motivational role for the young person. The clinician needs to present in an honest and open way whilst remaining positive, hopeful, and confident. They need to acknowledge that they do not know whether CBT will help the young person or which ideas or techniques will be useful. However, they also need to remain positive and hopeful by drawing on research data and their experience to highlight that many young people with similar problems have found CBT helpful and have been able to make some important changes to their lives.

This positive and hopeful stance is important in terms of engaging the young person, maintaining their commitment, and reassuring and motivating them when undertaking important but demanding tasks such as exposure.

PRECISE in practice

Case Study Ella's obsessional thoughts

Ella (seven) had many obsessive thoughts related to the safety of her family and engaged in a range of compulsive safety-checking behaviours. Before she went to bed, she would check that the windows in their flat were shut and that the doors were locked. She would check that all the electrical appliances were unplugged and that the cooker was turned off. Once in bed, Ella would continue to have these obsessive thoughts and it would take her approximately two hours before she could fall asleep. Ella would typically wake two or three times each night, and on each occasion, she would go around the house and engage in her compulsive safety-checking behaviour.

Ella engaged in CBT to address these problems, but during one meeting Ella was particularly troubled by her obsessive thoughts and wanted to stop them. When asked what Ella would like to do with her thoughts at bedtime, she replied, 'I'd like to lock them away so they can't get at me.' This was discussed in more detail, and Ella's idea of how things could be safely locked away developed into a prison. Ella saw a prison as a place where bad people go and are kept locked up so that they can't get out. The idea of locking her bad (i.e. worrying) thoughts somewhere safe so that they couldn't get out seemed a helpful metaphor. Ella was helped to develop an image of herself writing her worrying thoughts across the chest of a prisoner and locking them away in a cell each night. Ella was encouraged to describe this image in detail and to visualise herself writing her worries and then locking them away so that they could not trouble her. Ella became quite excited by this idea and was keen to try it at home.

This brief summary highlights the key aspects of the PRECISE process. The *partnership* with Ella encouraged her to voice her ideas. Ella was helped to create a *developmentally appropriate* concrete metaphor of locking her worries away somewhere safe so that they couldn't trouble her. The clinician conveyed *empathy* by really listening to what Ella had to say and by reflecting and highlighting what she had said. The idea for helping Ella to control her thoughts was *creative* and encouraged Ella to *investigate* whether change was possible and whether her idea could help. The process was empowering and, by building upon Ella's suggestion, promoted *self-efficacy*. Finally, the process was *enjoyable* and engaging for Ella, who was highly motivated to try her ideas at night-time.

Case Study Joshua's negative thinking

Joshua was aged nine and presented with low mood, panic attacks, and generalised anxiety, problems that were particularly noticeable at school. During the assessment, it became clear that Joshua had several unhelpful cognitions. Joshua misinterpreted ambiguous events as threatening, expected bad things to happen, focused on negative events, and failed to recognise his successes. A major aim was to help Joshua recognise his negative bias and to check to see whether there was information that he was overlooking.

Joshua was a keen Harry Potter fan. He had read the books many times and was very interested by the idea of magic. During one session, we explored some of the ideas from the books that could be used to help Joshua test his thoughts and check whether he was seeing the whole picture or just noticing the negative things. Joshua talked about the mirror of ERISED, in which Harry Potter could look and see everything he ever desired. We explored and developed this idea so that Joshua could look into a mirror and find the positive things that he overlooked. Joshua became very interested by this idea and went home and made his own mirror. Upon returning home from school he would tell his mother what had happened and would then be encouraged to look into his mirror and 'take another look'. This time, Joshua would find the positive things he had overlooked. This countered his initial negative cognitions and provided a more balanced view of events. Each day, Joshua would use his mirror to check out what had happened. He began to recognise his negative biases and started to challenge his thoughts and develop a more balanced way of thinking.

Once again, the *partnership* with Joshua helped him to express his ideas. The process of thought testing was undertaken in a *developmentally appropriate* way that made the idea of 'looking again' concrete using a magic mirror. *Empathy* was used to encourage Joshua to express his ideas and to understand his interest in Harry Potter. The intervention was imaginative and *creative*, and Joshua was motivated to *investigate* whether he was overlooking important information. The idea for the mirror came from Joshua and so built upon the idea of *self-efficacy*. The intervention was both effective and *enjoyable* and provided Joshua and his mother with a very practical way of challenging Joshua's biased thinking.

CHAPTER THREE

A: Assessment and goals

Establishes clear goals for the intervention and appropriately uses diaries, questionnaires, and rating scales for assessment

The aim of the initial assessment is to establish the extent and nature of the young person's difficulties and their expectations, readiness to change, suitability for a CBT intervention, and goals. The assessment will involve, as appropriate, information gathered during a clinical interview, through direct observation, and by standardised outcome measures and idiographic (goal-based) assessments. It will also involve, as necessary, information from the young person, their parents/carers, and any other relevant adults (e.g. teachers) who may observe the young person in different settings.

Undertakes a full assessment of the presenting problem involving, as appropriate, reports from others

The assessment will collect the information required to develop an initial understanding of the presenting problems (Creed et al. 2011). The assessment is dynamic and will inform the intervention plan, modify it in response to changes, and determine when treatment should end (Weisz et al. 2004). The assessment therefore needs to include information about the child, their family, and context as well as information about the nature, development, and maintenance of their specific problems.

In terms of the family and wider context, the assessment should provide a brief overview of:

▶ family structure, relationships, and a basic understanding of family dynamics;

▶ education, including academic performance, relationships, attendance, and behaviour;

▶ work, including performance, attendance, and relationship issues;

▶ significant events such as trauma, bereavement, health issues, or developmental problems;

▶ parental/family issues such as relationship difficulties, financial worries, mental and physical health issues, or work problems;

▶ the young person's friendships, interests, social life, and personal strengths.

The second part of the assessment should focus on the young person's presenting problems and should include:

▶ a clear description of each problem, including onset, frequency, severity, and impact on everyday functioning;

▶ the young person's and their parents/carers' understanding of why these problems have occurred;

▶ assessment of any triggering events or situations;

▶ identification of strong, distressing, and dominant unpleasant emotions and how these are dealt with;

▶ any common patterns of thinking that might be associated with their problems;

▶ how the young person and/or their parents are dealing with these problems;

▶ what has previously been tried and what was helpful or unhelpful;

▶ young person and parent/carer expectations about what CBT might achieve and possible goals;

▶ young person and parent/carer readiness to change and motivation to engage with a CBT intervention.

Young people may initially appear anxious, reticent, or unforthcoming and will often be unsure about the purpose of the assessment meeting. The aim of the assessment needs to be clarified and the young person's active participation emphasised. The views of the young person and their parents/carers are encouraged, and it is made clear that they may see things differently. Questions should be directed towards the young person and they should be given regular opportunities to agree or disagree with the reports and accounts of others.

Verbal communication may not be the preferred method of many younger children and so a variety of non-verbal assessment materials should be available. A younger child may, for example, be asked to draw a picture or make a film strip (TGFG p77) of what happens in a situation they feel worried about. They can draw what happens before, during, and immediately after a particularly difficult situation and can add any feelings or thoughts they might notice.

The assessment needs to be structured and actively managed to ensure that everyone has an opportunity to contribute. This may involve making separate time within the assessment for young people or their parents/carers to discuss anything they might find difficult to talk about together. The rules of confidentiality need to be agreed at the outset so that young people and parents are aware of what is and is not shared, and under what circumstances sharing of information would occur.

The assessment may identify differences in the way that the young person and their parents understand the problems. For example, parents might attribute a young person's reluctance to go out as an indication that they are not motivated to help themselves. However, the young person may feel worried and unsure how to cope with social situations and may be dealing with this by avoiding them. The assessment will therefore clarify different understandings and meanings so that a shared formulation can be developed, and goals agreed. In this case, the young person needs to systematically engage with social situations and not avoid them by staying at home.

The assessment is typically the first contact with the young person. This is the first opportunity for engagement and to educate the young person about the CBT model (TGFB p89). It provides an opportunity to model the child-centred, outcome-focused, reflective, and empowering philosophy and to establish the PRECISE process. The assessment interview will also provide an indication of the young person's verbal and non-verbal skills, cognitive awareness, and emotional literacy. It will provide an opportunity to observe family communication styles and to hear different family members' perspectives and understandings about events. It will also confirm whether CBT is an appropriate intervention.

Complements assessment with routine outcome measures (ROMs)

The assessment interview should be augmented by routine outcome measures (ROMs). These are short standardised measures used at different times during an intervention to assess changes in symptoms and clinical outcomes (Hall et al. 2013). ROMs provide opportunities for young people to report their symptoms and monitor progress and for this information to inform and guide the intervention. The use of ROMs has been shown to facilitate faster psychological improvement (Bickman et al. 2011; Knaup et al. 2009; Lambert & Archer 2006), better patient–clinician communication (Carlier et al. 2012), and improved early identification of those cases who are not responding as expected (Lambert & Shimokawa 2011).

In the UK, the successful Improving Access to Psychological Therapies (IAPT) programme requires ROMs to be completed at each appointment (Clark et al. 2018). Extension of this programme to children and young people (CYP-IAPT) has resulted in the widespread use of ROMs in the UK. Session-by-session comparisons provide an indication of the direction of any change in symptomatology whilst pre-post comparisons determine change and recovery. ROMs are popular with young people and, because they are short and quick to complete, can readily be completed at the start of each session.

There are many ROMs that can be used to assess clinical outcomes, depending upon the age of the young person and the nature of the presenting problems. Examples of ROMs can be found on the Child Outcomes Research Consortium (CORC) website (www.corc.uk.net/). Some of the most commonly used ROMs in the United Kingdom include:

▶ **Revised Child Anxiety and Depression Scale (RCADS).** A 47-item self-reported measure with versions available for completion by parents and young people (8–18 years). The RCADS is based around the Spence Children's Anxiety Scale (1997), with items corresponding to *Diagnostic and Statistical Manual of Mental Disorders, Fourth Edition* (DSM-IV) criteria for anxiety in the areas of social phobia, separation anxiety, obsessive-compulsive disorder, panic disorder, generalised anxiety disorder, and for major depressive disorder. Each item is rated on a four-point Likert scale of frequency, and these are then summed to produce total sub-scale and total anxiety scores. Relevant sub-scales can be completed at each session to track changes in symptoms (Chorpita et al. 2005).

▶ **Generalised Anxiety Disorder Assessment (GAD-7).** A short seven-item self-report questionnaire assessing generalised anxiety, for completion by young people aged 16 years and upwards (Spitzer et al. 2006). The severity of each symptom over the past week is rated on a four-point scale, with individual scores being summed to calculate a total score.

▶ **Mood and Feelings Questionnaire (MFQ).** A 33-item self-report measure for completion by young people aged 6–17 years of age and by parents. Each item is rated as either 'true' (scores 2), 'sometimes true' (scores 1), or 'not true' (scores 0), with items summed to provide a total score (Wood et al. 1995).

▶ **_Patient Health Questionnaire (PHQ-9)._** A 9-item self-report measure for use with young people aged 13 and above (Kroenke et al. 2001). It is widely used and assesses each of the nine DSM-IV criteria for depression on a scale from 0 (not at all) to 3 (nearly every day).

▶ **_Strengths and Difficulties Questionnaire (SDQ)._** A widely used behavioural screening questionnaire consisting of 25 items assessing emotional symptoms, conduct problems, hyperactivity and/or inattention, peer relationship problems, and pro-social behaviour. Versions are available for child self-report (age 11–17) and parent (3–17 years) and teacher (3–17 years) report (Goodman 1997).

▶ **_Child Revised Impact of Events Scale (CRIES)._** This brief measure is widely used to screen children aged eight and above for post-traumatic stress disorder (Perrin et al. 2005). The eight-item version assesses symptoms of trauma-related intrusion and avoidance. The 13-item version incudes an additional sub-scale assessing arousal. Each item is rated on a four-point scale scored from 0 (not at all) to 5 (often).

The regular use of ROMs provides an indication of individual change over time and ensures that the young person's view of progress is assessed.

Negotiates goals and the dates when progress will be reviewed

Idiographic, goal-based measures (TGFB p91) complement standardised ROMs and provide helpful information to inform treatment decisions. These are the personal goals the young person would like to achieve and are rated at each session on a 1–10 or 1–100 scale to indicate progress. The use of goal-based outcomes ensures that the intervention remains clearly focused on what the young person wants to achieve and informs and shapes the agenda (Weisz et al. 2011). Session-by-session ratings provide timely information that can be used to adjust the intervention and to inform when the intervention is complete.

Idiographic measures may be more acceptable and relevant for young people (Bromley & Westwood 2013; Edbrooke-Childs et al. 2015). They provide an opportunity for the young person to think about the future and identify what they want to achieve. They may measure domains, such as coping, impact on daily life, or personal growth, that are not captured by standardised symptom-focused measures (Bradley et al. 2013). A young person may, for example, present with similar levels of symptomatology as measured by ROMs but find that they are better able to cope and to engage with everyday life and activities.

An agreed set of goals should be negotiated and progress towards their achievement regularly reviewed. Vague, negatively phrased general goals such as 'to feel less sad' or 'not to worry so much' should be avoided. These are hard to measure, difficult to know when they have been achieved, and do not positively describe what the young person needs to do. Goals should follow the SMART mnemonic.

▶ Specific – clearly and positively define what the young person will do;

▶ Measurable – ensure that progress can be readily assessed;

▶ Achievable – be realistic and achievable;

▶ Relevant – be important and motivating for the young person;

▶ Timely – be achievable within a reasonable time frame.

Ambitious goals that may be unachievable run the risk of demotivating the young person and strengthening unhelpful beliefs about failure and lack of self-efficacy. Large goals should be broken down into a series of smaller steps. This increases the likelihood of success, promotes confidence and beliefs about self-efficacy, and creates a positive sense of momentum.

Identification of goals

Young people may find it difficult to identify goals. Their thinking may be fixed on their problems and they may be unable to think how their life would be different without them. On these occasions, the Miracle Question (TGFB p90), drawn from brief solution-focused therapy pioneered by Steve de Shazer, may be helpful.

To help the young person think differently, the miracle question is future orientated. By orientating it in this way, attention is shifted away from the young person's past and current problems towards a future free of problems. The young person is asked to imagine that a miracle has happened overnight as they slept.

▶ 'Imagine that overnight, as you slept, a miracle happened. When you wake in the morning, you find that all your problems have gone.'

The miracle question is then followed with a series or prompts to help the young person focus on what would be different.

▶ 'How would you feel – for example, would you be noticing that you were calmer, happier, or more relaxed?'

▶ 'What would you be doing – would you be doing something different, going somewhere new, or behaving differently?'

▶ 'Would you be thinking differently – would you, for example, be noticing but not engaging with your thoughts or being kinder in the way you were thinking about yourself?'

If the young person is still finding it difficult to identify what might be different, encourage them to adopt a third-party perspective.

▶ 'How would other people, like your mum or best friend, know that your problems had gone? What would they notice?'

Prioritisation of goals

Young people may identify a few SMART goals, which will then need to be prioritised. Rather than attempting to work on too many goals at the same time, it is best to maintain a more limited focus on up to three goals (TGFB p91). These will be the goals that are the most important for the young person (Weisz et al. 2011) and can be identified by asking the young person to consider the impact of each on their life.

▶ 'You have identified a number of goals. If we were to select one to work on, which would make the biggest difference to your life?'

The most important goals may be the hardest to achieve. Initially, to secure some success and to motivate the young person, it may be better to choose a less demanding goal that can quickly be achieved. This can be empowering and enabling for the young person and demonstrates that they can be successful.

Whose goals?

Young people, their parents/carers, and other adults such as teachers will inevitably have their own goals and expectations about what the intervention should focus upon. Often, they will agree, but sometimes their goals and priorities or the way the goals are achieved may differ.

▶ A young person who has not been attending school may prioritise a goal 'to make a new friend'. Walking to school with a friend may help them to feel less anxious and make it easier to attend school.

▶ Their parents may prioritise a goal of 'attending school full-time', believing that the young person needs to be in school quickly to ensure that they do not fall too far behind with their work.

▶ Their teacher may prioritise focusing on a specific subject such as 'to catch up with maths coursework', feeling that this is the most important subject to work on.

In this example, everyone shares the overall goal (e.g. of regularly attending school), but each has a different idea about how this can be achieved.

- The young person wants to establish friendships to support their attendance at school.

- The parents want a quick return to full-time attendance.

- The teacher wants the academic pressure to be reduced by catching up on one subject.

Discussing each option and highlighting how they can lead to the successful achievement of the overall shared goal can be reassuring. The differing goals need to be acknowledged and written down so that they can be reviewed in future meetings. However, in order to maximise engagement and to secure the young person's commitment and motivation, it is often helpful to select one of their goals to work on first. The goals of the parents and teachers are not ignored or lost but are 'parked'. Once the young person has successfully accomplished their target, the 'parked' goals are revisited, discussed, and the next one negotiated.

Inappropriate goals

Finally, there will be times when a young person's goals are inappropriate or unrealistic.

- A young person with an eating disorder may want to prioritise a goal of maintaining their current, dangerously low, body weight.

- A young person who has been bullied may want a goal to become physically stronger so that they are able to assault the bullies.

- A young person who is depressed may choose a goal 'to be happy every day'.

The young person's goal needs to be heard but it also needs to be challenged with a clear message that such goals are not appropriate or are unrealistic. The difficulty the young person may have in changing their eating needs to be acknowledged whilst being explicit that no change is not an option. Their frustration at being bullied needs to be heard whilst the potential danger of assaulting the bullies needs to be highlighted and alternative goals explored. Similarly, to be happy every day is unlikely, and so the young person needs to be encouraged to develop a more realistic goal.

Uses diaries, tick charts, thought bubbles, and rating scales to identify and assess symptoms, emotions, thoughts, and behaviour

Diaries can be used as part of the assessment and can collect data for many different purposes. They can capture information to clarify common emotions and bodily symptoms (TGFB p151, p152), ways of thinking (TGFG p87, p88: TGFB p108; p109, p110), particular patterns of responding, strengths (TGFB p52), positive events (TGFG p143; TGFB p53), or acts of kindness (TGFG p48: TGFB p67). In all instances, the purpose of the diary needs to be clearly explained, the information to be collected specified, and the length of recording or number of episodes to be monitored agreed. Good practice suggests that the diary should not be onerous to complete and that it should capture the minimum amount of information required to be informative. The process is collaborative, with diary content, method, and recording period being discussed, negotiated, and agreed. In terms of method, some young people prefer to keep paper diaries, others electronic or a record on their phone. The recording period will depend on the frequency of the target behaviour but will also be determined by what the young person can realistically manage.

Case Study Sarah feels faint

Sarah (16) had 'funny turns' during which she would feel faint but did not think there was any pattern or trigger for these episodes. Sarah was worried by these funny turns and agreed it would be helpful to find out more. Sarah thought she had at least two episodes a week and agreed to keep a diary for one week. She agreed to record when and where these occurred to see if there were any common events that triggered them (Table 3.1). She also agreed to capture how she was thinking and what she did when she felt faint.

Sarah's diary had three events. The day and time of these episodes varied and, although they were triggered by different events, there was a common theme. They all occurred when Sarah was in large groups of people. As she felt faint, Sarah recalled thinking that she could not cope and needed to leave the situation. This simple diary helped Sarah to discover that there was a pattern and that these events were not as random as she first thought.

Table 3.1 Sarah's diary.

Day and time	What was happening?	How did you feel?	What were you thinking?	What did you do?
Monday morning	School assembly	Faint, nervous	I can't breathe. I need to get out of here.	Went out and sat in the nurse office
Saturday afternoon	In town with friends	Shaking, faint, felt hot	There are so many people about. I need to go home. I can't handle this.	Phoned mum and she picked me up
Tuesday afternoon	Dance class	Sweating, faint	I am not feeling well and so will have to leave early and go home.	Told instructor I wasn't well and phoned mum

Tick charts

Tick charts provide a simple and quick way of recording how often a behaviour, feeling, or thought occurs. Once the recording target is agreed, the young person or their parents simply make a tick or a mark to record every time it occurs. The recording demands (make a mark) are limited and, for this reason, tick charts provide a useful way of quantifying high-frequency behaviours.

▶ Dan had frequent intrusive thoughts that he might hurt someone and so kept a record on his phone to quantify how often these occurred.

▶ Sue had generalised anxiety disorder and was often seeking reassurance from her parents. Her parents kept a tick chart to quantify how often this occurred and used this as a way of monitoring whether Sue's reassurance seeking was changing.

▶ Abdul wasn't very good at noticing when acts of kindness occurred and so kept a tick chart on his phone whenever he noticed that someone was being kind.

Thought bubbles

The assessment needs to gain an initial understanding of whether the young person can access and communicate their thoughts and the type and content of those that are causing distress. Direct attempts to assess cognitions with questions such, as 'What were you thinking?' or 'What thoughts did you notice racing through your mind?' can be helpful. If a young person can engage in such a dialogue, a direct discussion offers a useful way of identifying common thoughts and thinking traps.

Sometimes, direct attempts such as these are greeted with a shrug of the shoulders or a short statement such as 'don't know' or 'nothing'. When this occurs, alternative, non-verbal ways of assessing cognitions should be considered. Cartoons and thought bubbles offer a helpful non-verbal alternative. Children as young as three can, with some preliminary training, understand that thought bubbles represent what a person may think (Wellman et al. 1996). Similarly, studies have highlighted how children under the age of seven can distinguish between thoughts, feelings, and actions, and can acknowledge that thoughts are subjective and that two people can have different thoughts about the same event (Quakley et al. 2004; Wellman et al. 1996). In terms of self-awareness, Flavell et al. (2001) suggest that children can recognise their own inner speech by approximately six years of age. Thus, the concept of talking to oneself, and thus the use of positive self-talk that forms a key part of many interventions, is both accessible and familiar to young children.

Worksheets involving cartoon figures and thought bubbles can be used during the assessment. For example, a young person can complete the thought bubble of a figure or cartoon character (TGFG p94) to introduce them to the idea that thought bubbles communicate what we think. Thought bubbles can be applied to the young person through worksheets on which they can draw or write common thoughts about themselves (TGFG p91), their future (TGFG p92), and their performance (TGFG p93). Similarly, they can be asked to use thought bubbles to communicate what they think in their problematic situations.

▶ 'Write or draw what you would put in your thought bubble when you have to talk to someone new.'

▶ 'Complete your thought bubble when your friends forget to invite you out.'

▶ 'What would you put in your thought bubble when your dad tells you off?'

Visualisation

Visualisation is another method that can be used to assess whether the young person is able to identify feelings and cognitions. For example, important or high-profile sporting events can provide the content for creating images which can prompt the identification of cognitions and emotions.

▶ A young person interested in football could be asked to create an image of their favourite footballer taking a penalty. They could imagine the footballer standing in front of the goal facing the goalkeeper. The ball is on the penalty spot and the footballer looks at the goal. The young person is asked to describe what the footballer may be feeling or thinking as they run forwards to kick the ball. The image can continue with the young person being asked to consider what the footballer might think and feel after scoring or missing the penalty.

Stories

Assessment stories can be created around the young person's problems. Stories are created jointly and provide opportunities to ask questions that directly assess what the young person might think or feel or how they might behave. For example, Zara, an unhappy child who was bullied at school, was invited to tell a story about a little bear who was scared to go to school.

PS: Can you tell me a story about a little bear who had just moved to a new school?

ZARA: If you like.

PS: What would you like to call the bear?

ZARA: Boo.

PS: So, where does Boo live and what is she like?

ZARA: Boo lives in a hole under a small tree with her mum and brother. Boo isn't very good at sports and games and doesn't talk much with the other bears.

PS: Does Boo have any friends?

ZARA: No, she's new to the area and so she hasn't made any friends yet.

PS: Does Boo go to school?

ZARA: Yes, and today is her first day.

PS: Wow, her first day, I wonder what will happen.

ZARA: Well, Boo will be taken to school by her mum. She will be really scared, will start to cry, and won't want her mum to leave her.

PS: I wonder what Boo is scared about.

ZARA: I told you. She doesn't know anyone at school, and she isn't very good at making friends.

PS: So, what does Boo think will happen when she goes into school?

ZARA: Oh, the usual stuff.

PS: The usual stuff?

ZARA: Yes, the other bears will want to know where she moved from, why she hasn't got a dad, and will laugh at her because she talks with such a quiet voice.

The story highlighted some of Zara's past experiences and worries. Zara's father was a drug addict who regularly broke into houses in the local neighbourhood and terrorised her mother for money to fund his addiction. This resulted in the family frequently having to move to a new house and Zara having to settle into a number of different schools. On each occasion she would be asked by the other children about her family and father, questions Zara found very difficult to answer. She became increasingly reluctant to attend school and became upset each morning when she had to leave for school.

Rating scales

A core feature of CBT is quantification. This involves the young person rating various aspects of their behaviour, strength of feelings, or beliefs. Quantification is an important part of the assessment since it:

- provides an objective way of rating internal cognitive processes and emotions;

- challenges the dichotomous thinking that is common during adolescence by highlighting the graduations between two anchor points;

- highlights change within the session (e.g. during exposure);

- demonstrates the potential effectiveness of specific techniques (e.g. relaxation);

- highlights longer-term progress.

Many of the emotions that are the focus of CBT interventions, such as sadness, anger, or anxiety, are normal emotions. The problem is that the emotion has become very intense or severe and is adversely affecting the young person's ability to engage in everyday life. The aim of CBT is not to completely remove the emotion, but to reduce its severity and thus minimise the adverse impact upon the young person. Similarly, the young person will continue to be aware of unhelpful cognitions. Cognitive challenging and restructuring may reduce the frequency of these unhelpful cognitions, but they will continue to occur. However, as with mindfulness, the goal may not be to reduce the frequency of cognitions, but to reduce the distress they generate.

Simple rating scales provide a helpful way of quantifying severity and documenting small, but important, changes. Scale can be 1–10 or 1–100 and can assess different dimensions such as frequency, strength of feelings, or beliefs (TGFG p166).

Pie charts

Pie charts can be used during assessment to visually quantify the specific contribution of various factors.

Case Study Theo's washing

Theo had many compulsive behaviours and engaged in regular hand washing in which he felt a need to wash his hands four times before he thought his hands were clean. The pie chart in Figure 3.1 was constructed with Theo to assess and quantify how much each of the four washes contributed to his hands becoming clean.

This exercise helped Theo to recognise that the fourth wash added comparatively little to his sense of cleanliness. This motivated him to undertake an experiment where he limited his washing and prevented himself from engaging with the fourth wash.

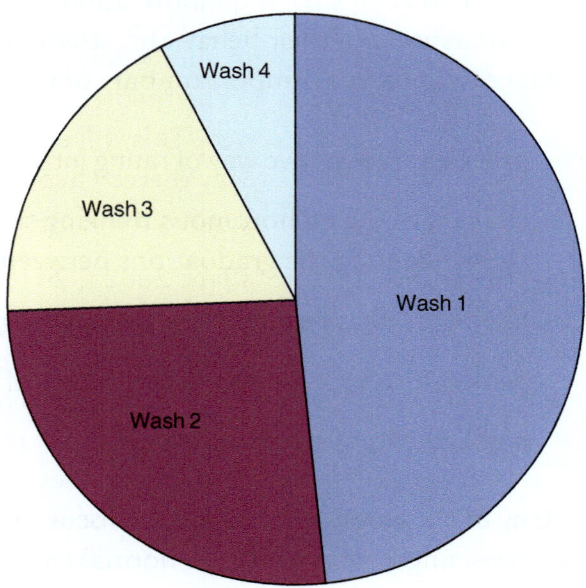

Figure 3.1   Theo's washing.

Assesses motivation and readiness to change

To engage in an active process of change requires the young person to acknowledge that:

- there is a difficulty or problem;
- this problem could be changed;
- the form of help offered could bring about this change;
- the clinician can help the young person develop the skills they require to secure this change.

The assessment should consider the young person's motivation and readiness to change. A useful framework for considering readiness for actively participating in therapy is provided in the Stages of Change model (Prochaska et al. 1992) that has been extensively used in the drug and alcohol field. The model highlights how readiness to change is a process that develops gradually, varies over time, and is not simply a dichotomous decision. The assumption implicit in the model is that the clinician's behaviour needs to reflect where the young person is in the change cycle. The model therefore provides a framework that can guide and pitch the focus of the therapeutic process at the most appropriate level.

The framework conceptualises individuals as moving from being unwilling or unmotivated to make any change through to considering possible targets and then deciding and preparing to make some small change. More determined and significant changes follow, with these new skills being incorporated into everyday life and maintained over time. Inevitably, this will be followed by some degree of relapse. At this stage, confidence may need to be rebuilt, and so reflection upon past experiences and helpful strategies is encouraged.

Understanding the young person's readiness to change and where they are in the cycle can help to determine the type and focus of the intervention. As highlighted in Figure 3.2, in the initial stages, the focus is on securing and increasing the young person's commitment to change using motivational interviewing techniques. It is only in the latter stages, after the young person has identified the change they would like to secure, that an active process of cognitive behaviour therapy can begin.

Pre-contemplation

This is the stage at which many young people have their first contact with the clinician. Often, they attend appointments due to pressure from others and have little or no ownership of the presenting problem, and they will usually not have considered the need for, or indeed the possibility of, change.

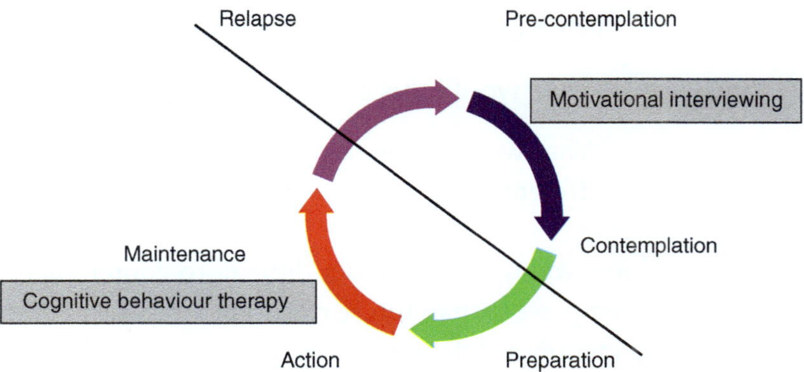

Figure 3.2   The Stages of Change model and primary therapeutic focus.

The young person may appear angry or in denial, stating that 'I don't have a problem' or 'There is nothing wrong with me'. They may appear disinterested, 'I don't need to be here', or resigned to the current situation, 'I have always felt like this'. Alternatively, they may appear unmotivated, feeling that they have no control over what happens, 'There is nothing I can do about this'. This indicates that the young person has not identified a problem, has no possible agenda for change, or does not believe that the current situation could be different.

In this situation, the task is to elicit from the young person their views about potential targets and the possibility of change. This may require careful assessment of the young person's knowledge in order to assess whether their apparent passivity is due to a lack of information. Putting the young person's difficulties in context and highlighting how the situation could possibly be different may provide the young person with new information upon which they could consider possible goals and the need to change.

▶ 'A number of young people struggle with written schoolwork, but sometimes they can be helped to get their ideas down by using computers.'

▶ 'Young people often worry about their parents, but many can be helped to control these worries so that they can do things like sleeping over at a friend's house.'

▶ 'I hear that you think your teacher picks on you, and this is her problem. But you told me that you are the only one in the class she picks on. Is there something you do that means she notices you more than the others?'

Identifying possible gaps in the young person's knowledge by providing new information may help them to reconsider the need for, and possibility of, change.

Questions during the pre-contemplation stage should aim to identify discrepancies between where the young person is now and where they would like to be in the future. They should clarify the young person's views.

▶ 'Is there anything at home or school that you would like to be different?'

▶ 'What are the biggest worries for you at the moment?'

▶ 'When would this become a worry or problem for you?'

▶ 'What would have to happen for you to want things to change and be different?'

Some young people find it difficult to contemplate future change, tending to be more present than future orientated in their outlook. They may find it difficult to identify a different future or the potential benefits of engaging in any intervention, which might take time to secure (Piacentini & Bergman 2001).

If the young person continues to be unable to identify any potential goals, then this should be acknowledged. The clinician remains optimistic about the possibility of change but acknowledges that the time may not be right to engage in a programme of active change.

Contemplation

By this stage the young person has begun to identify some potential areas that they would like to change but may appear unsure about the possibility that this can be achieved. They may appear ambivalent and will often follow any positive statements with a number of obstacles and barriers as to why this could not be pursued or achieved.

▶ 'I suppose it would be good … but … it will take too much time.'

▶ 'It would be nice if this was different … but … I can't be bothered.'

▶ 'It would create less hassle … but … it just won't work.'

A full exploration of the potential benefits and barriers to change should be undertaken before any experiments are considered. Thoroughly working through these issues provides opportunities to highlight and acknowledge uncertainties, discuss any ambivalence, and prepare the young person for any potential problems, thereby increasing the likelihood of success.

Questions that might help the young person to articulate their ambivalence and to begin to identify potential solutions include:

▶ 'What might stop you from trying this?'

▶ 'What might go wrong?'

▶ 'What might help you to give this a try?'

▶ 'What has helped in the past?'

Preparation

By this stage, the young person is ready to make some small change. They will have identified potential targets, worked through their ambivalence, discussed potential barriers, and are prepared to experiment. The young person may not, however, feel very confident about the likelihood of success and may focus upon and recount previous episodes where they have tried and failed.

The aim is to continue to build upon the young person's growing motivation and confidence to maximise the possibility of a successful experience. This will involve drawing upon previous successes and focusing the young person's attention upon some of the skills, thoughts, and behaviours that have been important and helpful in the past. The approach is positive, focusing on the young person's strengths whilst highlighting potential pitfalls that need to be addressed.

Action

During this stage, the young person is ready to fully engage in therapy and to secure significant change. The young person is now ready to actively participate in CBT and to build upon their early successes.

Maintenance

During the maintenance stage, the young person is encouraged to generalise their new skills to different situations and to monitor and reflect upon their practice. The aim is to encourage integration of these skills into the young person's everyday life so that positive skills are sustained. In addition, the young person is helped to consider and expect future difficulties and to develop problem-solving skills that can be used to plan and cope with any future relapses.

Relapse

Inevitably, the young person will experience future problems and setbacks and encounter situations when their old patterns and difficulties return. At these times, the young person may question the usefulness and effectiveness of their new skills. The aim is to maintain the young person's confidence and to encourage reflection about how they coped with previous situations and to consider what they found helpful. It is also important to challenge any beliefs about the permanency of the setback and to emphasise that, whilst the situation is difficult, the young person has been able to positively change it in the past and probably can do so again. The young person is encouraged to remain hopeful and optimistic and to attend to information and use skills that have proven to be useful.

The Stages of Change model provides a way of understanding the young person's readiness to change, which in turn informs the main therapeutic focus. The young person is better able to benefit from CBT during the preparation, action, and maintenance stages. By these stages, the young person will have identified possible goals and will be sufficiently motivated to secure their achievement. However, in the relapse, pre-contemplation, and contemplation stages, the intervention will primarily be concerned with increasing the young person's motivation using motivational interviewing.

CHAPTER FOUR

B: Behavioural

Demonstrates use of a variety of behavioural techniques to facilitate therapeutic change

The behavioural domain is one of the core systems of cognitive behavioural therapy. It offers a range of techniques based on classical and operant conditioning theory to promote and support positive and helpful behaviours. The process of systematic desensitisation helps the young person to confront and cope with feared events and situations. Through the construction of a fear hierarchy, the young person is gradually exposed to their feared event. Response prevention and exposure help young people with obsessive-compulsive disorder (OCD) overcome their repetitive compulsive behaviours as they face their feared situation whilst not engaging in their habits. Activity scheduling involves planning mood-lifting activities into the day, particularly at those times when the young person is feeling low or anxious. Behavioural activation encourages the young person to become more active and to participate in more rewarding activities. Reward charts and contingency plans help to focus on behaviours that are to be developed, encouraged, and celebrated, whilst the development of problem-solving skills helps to overcome problems and increase interpersonal effectiveness.

A Clinician's Guide to CBT for Children to Young Adults: A Companion to Think Good, Feel Good and Thinking Good, Feeling Better, Second Edition. Paul Stallard.
© 2021 John Wiley & Sons Ltd. Published 2021 by John Wiley & Sons Ltd.
Companion website: www.wiley.com/go/cliniciansguide2e

Uses behavioural techniques such as developing hierarchies, graded exposure, and response prevention

Developing hierarchies

CBT helps young people to develop skills to face and overcome situations or events that they have been avoiding through a process of graduated exposure. In order to increase the likelihood of success, challenges and fears are broken into smaller steps. If the challenge is too large or ambitious it increases the possibility of failure and will strengthen unhelpful negative beliefs about a lack of self-efficacy or the impossibility of change.

The process of breaking down challenges or fears involves generating a list of the small steps that will take the young person towards their goal of overcoming their fear or challenge (TGFB p195; TGFG p196). If fearful, the young person can be encouraged to identify all the situations, places, or objects their fear makes them avoid (TGFB p194).

▶ If a young person is anxious in crowded situations they might avoid going into town, the local shop, the cinema, school assemblies, or travelling on public transport.

▶ If a young person is worried about germs, they might avoid using public toilets, touching door handles, using a shared computer, or drinking from certain cups.

▶ A young person might worry about going somewhere new and has a particular challenge in continuing their studies at a new college.

Once the challenge or avoided events or situations are identified, the young person is encouraged to select a specific goal that they will work towards.

▶ If anxious in crowded situations, their goal might be to go for a coffee with a friend.

▶ If worried about germs, their goal might be to watch a film and be able to use the public toilets if needed.

▶ If facing a challenge of going to college, the young person might have a goal of attending college and signing up for their course.

The young person is then asked to identify the small steps that will help them to face their fear and achieve their goal. When generating steps, it can be useful to write each one down on a sticky post-it note. As the young person arranges these to develop their hierarchy and build their ladder to success, new steps can be added. At the top of the ladder, the young person is encouraged to write their goal, for example, 'to go for a coffee with my friend', 'to go to the cinema', or 'to sign up for a course at college'. They then arrange their steps in order of difficulty, starting at the bottom with the easiest and progressing up the ladder to the hardest (TGFB p175). To help with this process, each step can be rated from 1 to 100 for difficulty or anxiety.

Achieving the goal of going with a friend for a coffee might involve the following steps:

Goal:	To go for a coffee on a Monday morning with my friend Sophie	
Step	Stay and have a coffee with sister on Monday morning	Anxiety 90
Step	Stay and have a coffee with mum on Monday morning	Anxiety 80
Step	Go to coffee shop on Saturday morning and buy a takeaway	Anxiety 70
Step	Go to the coffee shop on a Monday and buy a takeaway	Anxiety 60
Step	Walk to the coffee shop on a Monday morning when quiet	Anxiety 30

Achieving the goal of using the toilets at the cinema might involve the following steps:

Goal:	Going to the cinema and able to use the toilets	
Step	Use the toilet at school	Anxiety 90
Step	Use the toilet at a shopping mall	Anxiety 75
Step	Use the toilet at my friend's house	Anxiety 48
Step	Use the toilet at aunty's house	Anxiety 35
Step	Use the toilet at gran's house	Anxiety 15

Achieving the challenge of signing up for a course at college might involve the following steps:

Goal:	Meet the Head of Studies and sign up for the course	
Step	Visit college, get a map, and find right room	Anxiety 90
Step	Visit college and get the application form	Anxiety 65
Step	Phone and ask for an appointment with the Head of studies	Anxiety 25
Step	Find out which buses go to college and their timetable	Anxiety 10

A fear hierarchy does not need a set number of steps. The number required will be guided by the young person and their parents and the degree of difficulty involved in each step. In order to maintain motivation and self-efficacy, it is important that each step feels achievable. If a step feels too large, consider inserting another intermediate step.

The process of hierarchy development can also be used with young people with OCD. In OCD, repetitive behaviours or habits are undertaken as a way of providing temporary relief from unpleasant feelings such as anxiety which are typically caused by obsessive thoughts about unpleasant things happening. Often these thoughts are catastrophic in content, with the young person assuming responsibility for people being harmed or dying, which they prevent from happening by engaging in their habits. Interventions involve exposure and response prevention, where the young person faces their fears and obsessive thoughts without undertaking their habits. The process involves identifying all of the young person's different habits and then arranging them on a habit ladder in order of difficulty (TGFG p197). Those that are more difficult to stop are placed at the top of the ladder and those that are easier to stop at the bottom.

Graded exposure

Once the fear or habit hierarchy has been developed, the final stage is exposure, where the young person faces their fears (TGFB p196; TGFG p198). The first step on the fear hierarchy or habit ladder is selected and a plan agreed for when the young person will face their fear. For OCD, the young person is encouraged to attend to their thoughts (exposure) without engaging in their habit (response prevention). The exposure provides new information for the young person that they are able to cope with their anxiety or worrying thoughts without avoiding situations or engaging in their habits. Once successful, the next step up the ladder is undertaken until the young person has completed all the steps and reclaimed their life.

When planning exposure, it is important that the young person understands the rationale for facing their fear.

- ▶ Refer to the formulation and highlight that the young person is managing their anxiety by avoiding the things that make them anxious or by engaging in repetitive behaviours.

- ▶ Highlight that whilst avoidance may provide short-term relief, it does not help the young person to cope with their anxious feelings. The anxious feelings return.

- ▶ Emphasise that the young person needs to try a different approach to reclaim their life by facing their fears.

- Acknowledge that they will feel anxious when they face their fears. However, instead of their anxious feelings stopping them from doing things, they are going to take their anxiety with them.

- Through this process, the young person will discover that they can tolerate their unpleasant feelings and that their anxiety will reduce.

The following explanation could be used to explain exposure to a young person.

- 'Because you have been feeling anxious, you have avoided doing those things that trigger these unpleasant feelings. These unpleasant feelings have stopped you from doing what you want to do. This may make you feel better in the short term, but you never discover that you can cope. We are going to help you to face your fears. You will probably feel anxious, but you will discover that you can take your anxiety with you and be successful.'

Young people may sometimes want to be flexible about when they face their fear, saying they will do it when they 'feel OK'. This may indicate that they are apprehensive, and so explaining the rationale and exploring how they can cope may be helpful. Similarly, it could indicate that the step is too large, and the young person is concerned that they may be unsuccessful. The step can be reviewed and, if required, a smaller step agreed. Finally, it should be acknowledged that it is normal to feel anxious as fears are confronted. Waiting until the young person feels relaxed to face their fear is unlikely to happen. Specifying a day and time regardless of how they are feeling can help to address this problem as the young person learns to take their anxiety with them.

During exposure, ratings can be a useful way of quantifying anxiety and how it might change over time. The young person can rate their anxiety on a 1–10 or a 1–100 scale before, during, and after they face their fear (TGFG p166). These ratings inform the exposure process, since it is important that the young person stays in the situation long enough for their anxiety to decline. Previously they would be bailing out or avoiding situations as soon as they became aware of their anxiety increasing. Exposure helps the young person discover that their anxiety will decline if they stay in the situation, so it is important that the length of the exposure is long enough for this to occur.

Afterwards, the young person should be encouraged to reflect on what they have discovered. They might discover that whilst they felt anxious these feelings reduced or that they are able to cope with them. This success needs to be acknowledged and celebrated and the next step agreed.

Exposure needs to be repeated a number of times before the young person feels less anxious. For example, a young person with anxiety about talking to others may need to practise saying 'hello' several times before they feel less anxious doing this.

Response prevention

With OCD, young people engage in repetitive and compulsive behaviours as way of preventing bad things from happening. These 'safety behaviours' can take many forms, including:

- cleaning – washing hands, cups, and plates, changing and washing clothes;

- checking – that doors are locked, electrical plugs unplugged, taps turned off;

- counting – repeating things a set number to times or arranging things in a particular order.

Typically, these bring short-term relief from anxiety, but this does not last. The worrying thoughts return, and the repetitive behaviours are repeated again and again. Treatment for OCD involves facing the fear (exposure) whilst not engaging in any compulsive behaviours (response prevention).

- A young person may repeatedly wash their hands because they fear that they will be contaminated with germs if they touch things. Response prevention might involve touching a toilet seat whilst refraining from hand washing.

- A young person may worry that the bathroom tap will be left on and flood the house unless they repeatedly check that it is turned off. Response prevention might involve washing their hands but only turning the tap off once.

- A young person may worry that something bad will happen if they do not keep their books arranged in a particular order. Response prevention might involve disrupting this order by putting a book back but not in the right order.

As with exposure, response prevention will create anxiety and so the young person needs a clear rationale why this will be helpful. This will relate to the formulation and will highlight that

- 'You use your habits to reduce your anxious feelings and to prevent or stop bad things from happening. Your habits may make you feel better for a little while, but your worrying thoughts return, and you have to repeat your habits over and over again. We are going to help you to dump your habits and to discover that you do not have to engage in these habits when you notice your worrying thoughts.'

Case Study John is worried about germs

John (13) was worried that he would pass germs on to the people in his family who he loved and that they would die. This started when his grandmother was being treated with chemotherapy for cancer. John was told that her immune system and ability to fight infections would be weak, so it was important for him to be very clean when he visited her. John worried about passing on germs and engaged in many behaviours (hand washing, not touching doors or door handles, changing his clothes, etc.) to minimise the risk of contamination. John decided to dump his habits.

▶ John made a habit ladder and put touching the door handle in the bathroom without washing as the first step.

▶ He planned how he would cope with the anxiety when he prevented himself from washing his hands. John developed some coping self-talk (TGFG p145) where he redefined his thoughts about germs. He relabelled his thoughts 'my hands aren't dirty, I am having a worrying thought that they are' and re-attributed his thoughts 'it is my OCD that is making me think that my hands are dirty'. He externalised his thoughts as OCD bossing him around and planned how he would not engage and listen to this bully (his thoughts) and practised mindfulness (TGFB p78; TGFG p63).

▶ John then touched the bathroom door handle and prevented himself from washing his hands. He rated his anxiety and observed it coming down over time without having to engage in his hand washing.

Problems when undertaking exposure

Young person avoidance

Exposure is designed to induce anxiety as the young person is encouraged to face their fears. This will inevitably be distressing for the young person, who may then become hesitant or reluctant to engage with an exposure task. In effect, they are continuing with their pattern of avoidance.

In these situations, a firm, encouraging, and supportive approach is required. The rationale for exposure should be reviewed and the costs of avoidance emphasised. This will highlight that the young person will need to change what they are currently doing if they are to achieve their goals and reclaim their life. The young person's strengths and the skills they have acquired should be highlighted and the young person's attention drawn to past achievements that might help with the current task.

If it is not possible to resolve the young person's ambivalence, then it may be necessary to abandon the planned task. However, rather than avoid any exposure, an alternative exposure task should be agreed.

▶ 'It is important to face your fears and to show yourself that you can cope with your anxiety. It sounds as if this task is too difficult at the moment, so what task are you able to tackle today?'

Clinician avoidance

Exposure can be difficult for clinicians who need to encourage young people to do something which will make them feel uncomfortable. Clinicians therefore need to be positive and reassuring and confidently able to tolerate the young person's distress. Uncertainty may result in them unconsciously colluding with the young person and inadvertently avoiding anxiety-generating exposure. This can occur when real-life exposure is avoided as imaginal exposure tasks are practised time and time again. Whilst imaginal exposure is helpful, the process addresses anticipated worries or beliefs rather than real-life exposure which provides powerful learning about what actually happens. Remaining focused on the fear hierarchy and the need to progress to more demanding real-life exposures can be a helpful way of identifying this pitfall.

A second sign of possible avoidance is procrastination, where exposure tasks are discussed but are never undertaken. Any ambivalence on the part of the young person is perceived as evidence that they are not yet ready to undertake exposure rather than the natural anxiety that they will experience when this is undertaken. It may be useful to address this during personal supervision, where the clinician's worries can be explored and a plan developed.

Anxiety does not come down

When undertaking exposure, it is important that the young person learns that their anxiety will come down and that they can cope. If this does not occur, the young person's beliefs that their anxiety is unbearable and that they are unable to cope will be strengthened. It is therefore important that the exposure task is of sufficient length for the anxiety to decline. If undertaking an exposure task during a session, additional time may be required to ensure that the reduction in anxiety occurs. This can be monitored through the use of rating scales and the exposure should be maintained until the anxiety rating has declined.

Is the young person focusing on their anxiety?

Some techniques such as distraction or mind games (TGFG p133) can provide helpful short-term relief to cope with anticipatory anxiety thereby allowing the young person to be able to confront their feared situation.

▶ Distraction helped a young person who was worried about going to school to cope with the journey by attending to neutral external stimuli rather than focusing on their internal anxiety symptoms. The parent encouraged them to engage in a number of sequential puzzles, such as 'finding three red cars', 'one bicycle with a shopping basket', 'one brown dog', 'one post box', until they successfully arrived at school.

However, during the process of exposure, distraction should be discouraged. The young person needs to fully experience and tolerate their anxiety rather than distracting themselves from these feelings and thoughts. Instead, the young person can be encouraged to repeat their positive or coping self-talk (TGFG p144, p145).

Are parents/carers appropriately involved?

With exposure tasks, it is important to consider who should be involved and available to support the young person. Parents/carers may, for example, be unconsciously colluding with the young person's avoidance or may be unable to tolerate their distress as they face their fears. In this situation, there is a need to ensure that parents fully understand the rationale for exposure and that by understanding the rationale they are helping the young person reclaim their life. It needs to be acknowledged that the young person will be distressed as they face their fears and that this is a normal response as they learn that they can cope.

It is also helpful to engage in an open discussion about who is best placed to support the young person. If a parent finds it very difficult to cope with their child's distress then explore whether there is someone else who can cope (e.g. other parent, uncle, or grandparent) and could be involved.

Uses behavioural techniques such as activity rescheduling and behavioural activation

Activity rescheduling

This simple technique involves building mood-lifting activities into the daily routine at those times when the young person may feel particularly low or stressed. The idea is to counter unpleasant feelings by doing something that evokes the opposite emotional response of enjoyment or relaxation.

The process starts by mood monitoring to identify problematic times. The young person keeps a diary to record what they were doing, how they felt, and the strength of their emotion (TGFB p204; TGFG p192). They may prefer to do this every hour for a couple of days or less frequently for a longer time period. The aim is to identify times or events associated with strong unpleasant feelings. Once these have been identified, the young person is encouraged to explore whether they can change what they do at those times to help themselves feel better.

Case Study Alison feels down

Alison (17) felt constantly low in her mood and agreed to keep a diary for a week to see if there were any patterns (Table 4.1). She didn't think she would remember to monitor her mood every hour but agreed that she would break her day into six time periods and for each would rate the strength of her low mood. Alison found it difficult to keep the diary. She recorded less towards the end of the week, saying that there was 'no point, it's all the same'.

The diary confirmed that Alison's mood was very low and that these feelings were strong, never less than 7/10. However, the diary showed that there was some slight variation throughout the day, with her feelings being strongest in the morning when she awoke and after school. This led to a conversation about whether it was possible to do things differently.

▶ Alison tended to wake in the morning and immediately started to worry about what might happen that day, focusing on all the things that might go wrong. Activity rescheduling involved finding a different activity to engage with when she woke so that she didn't listen to her unhelpful thoughts. Alison enjoyed music and so agreed to put her radio on as soon as she woke up. This helped her to focus her attention away from her worrying thoughts on to something more pleasurable.

▶ The other time that was difficult for Alison was after school. She returned to an empty house, which gave her time to ruminate about what had happened and how bad her day had been. Alison enjoyed running but had stopped this since she became depressed. We discussed whether Alison could start running again and whether she could build in a brief run after school instead of sitting in an empty house listening to her unhelpful thoughts.

Table 4.1   Alison's diary.

Day	When you woke	Mid-morning	Lunch time	After school	Tea time	Bedtime
Mon	10	8	9	9	7	9
Tues	10	7		9		9
Weds	10		7	10	7	10
Thurs	10		9	10	7	9
Fri	10	8	8	8	8	
Sat	9	7	7		8	
Sun	9		7		8	10
Mon						9
Tues	10			9		

Behavioural activation

A useful first step for helping young people with low mood and depression is behavioural activation. This is based on the observation that as people become depressed, they do less and spend more time on their own listening to their negative thoughts. They have fewer opportunities to engage in the things they used to enjoy, they socialise less, and they undertake fewer activities that create a sense of purpose and achievement. Behavioural activation helps the young person to become busier and to engage with rewarding activities.

It is important to explain the rationale and that the initial goal is to become more active not to feel better. Changes in mood will come later. The young person therefore needs to push themselves to become busier and to reward their efforts and not to be despondent as their mood may initially show little improvement.

After providing a rationale, the process starts by helping the young person to identify what they can do to have more fun. This may involve identifying activities that make them feel good (TGFG p193), activities they use to enjoy but stopped, those they enjoy but don't do very often, or those they would like to do (TGFB p205; TGFG p195).

It is not unusual for young people to find this apparently simple task challenging, and so it is helpful to guide them through different activities.

▶ **Social activities.** These are activities undertaken with other people, like going shopping with your sister, eating with your family, or doing homework with a friend.

▶ **Physical activities.** These activities involve some form of physical exertion such as running, attending a dance class, walking, or cycling.

▶ **Enjoyable activities.** These activities create personal pleasure, like baking biscuits, gaming, drawing, or listening to music.

▶ **Achievement activities.** These activities create a sense of pride or accomplishment, such as fixing your bike, painting or drawing, sorting out your clothes, helping someone with a chore.

Once a list has been generated, the idea is to plan more fun by choosing one or two activities to build into the weekly schedule (TGFB p206). When considering the activities, it is helpful to select those that are important, meaningful, and value based. For example, a young person may:

▶ be committed to environmental issues, so that a task of sorting out the weekly recycling may be personally important and motivating;

▶ have strong values about living a healthy life, so that tasks relating to getting fit may be very relevant and consistent with their values;

▶ feel that it is personally important to help and care for others, so that volunteering at a care home may be rewarding.

When selecting activities, it is important not to be too ambitious and to take it slowly. It is probable that the young person will not have been very busy for a while, so select small tasks to maximise the likelihood of success. Encourage the young person to start as soon as possible, since putting this off will make it harder to get started. Do not wait until they say they are feeling better. Being busier will ultimately help to improve their mood, but it is unlikely that they will feel better before they start. Finally, the young person should be encouraged to acknowledge and celebrate their achievements. Reviewing the activities they have undertaken can be motivating and provides a way of objectively identifying the progress they have made.

Problems when undertaking behavioural activation

I didn't feel like doing it

The most common problem with behavioural activation is motivation. Often young people are feeling down in their mood and may report that they 'didn't feel like doing it' or 'I'll do it when I feel better'. This lack of motivation is part of their problem and a core reason why they are feeling as they do. When they are less active, they spend more time listening to their critical and unhelpful thoughts and the worse they become.

It is important to be supportive and to acknowledge how they are feeling whilst being motivating and encouraging. The consequence of their inactivity needs to be discussed and the need to push through this emphasised. The young person should be discouraged from using how they are feeling as a criterion for undertaking behavioural activation. The reality is that they need to become more active in order to feel better and need to push on regardless of how they are feeling. Use of the structured worksheets to plan more fun (TGFB p206) can help to schedule tasks for days.

I did it, but I don't feel any better

It should be made very clear to the young person that the initial goal is to become more active rather than feeling better. Behavioural activation therefore involves pushing through their lack of motivation and undertaking the task regardless of how they are feeling. Changes in mood will occur later.

Undertaking the task signals important messages. It challenges beliefs about perceived hopelessness and promotes a sense of self-empowerment where the young person is able to do something to help themselves. It also challenges beliefs about helplessness by promoting self-efficacy and the belief that the young person can do things to make themselves feel better.

I did it, but so what?

When people feel down, they often overlook or dismiss their achievements as unimportant. It is common for young people to fail to acknowledge what they have achieved as they make comparisons with their past. They may comment, 'I read a page of this book, but I used to read a book in a week' or 'I kicked a football in the garden, but it's not important. I used to train and play for our football team all the time.' In these situations, the young person should be encouraged to focus on the here and now and not make comparisons with the past.

▶ They may have read a book a week, but they haven't even picked up a book for the past six months.

▶ They may have played football for the local team, but they haven't even gone outside and kicked a football for the past year.

It's not important

Behavioural activation aims to increase the number of pleasurable and rewarding activities that the young person engages with. It is therefore important that identified activities are personally meaningful and valued by the young person. Activities that they think they 'should be doing' or which they think other people 'expect them to do' should be avoided. Inevitably, these will not be personally motivating or rewarding to the young person, resulting in achievements being dismissed as unimportant. Instead, the young person should be helped to identify what they want to do, the activities that fit with their personal values and which are intrinsically more motivating.

Provides a clear rationale for using behavioural strategies

Providing the young person and their parents with a clear explanation about the methods that can help them overcome their problems is a fundamental aspect of CBT. It strengthens the underlying collaborative approach, motivates and empowers the young person to try new ideas, and progresses them towards the ultimate goal of becoming their own therapist or life guide.

As already mentioned, one behavioural technique which particularly requires a clear rationale is that of exposure, where the young person actively confronts their fears. Exposure is a core element of the treatment of anxiety and will be in direct contrast to the avoidant way the young person has been dealing with their fears or unpleasant emotions. However, by its very nature, the process of exposure can be very frightening. Young people are in effect being asked to stop avoiding the things they fear and to confront them. It therefore needs to be clear that exposure tasks will be collaboratively agreed. The young person is therefore reassured that they are in control of what happens. The approach is firm, gently challenging the young person's ambivalence or procrastination.

Finally, it is important to be open and honest. It needs to be acknowledged that the young person will feel anxious when they face their fear. This is normal, but the difference is that the young person will have developed some new cognitive and emotional skills they can use to help them tolerate their anxiety.

Identifies and implements reward and contingency plans

It is common for young people with psychological problems to ignore or overlook their achievements. Success and effort are not acknowledged or celebrated as the young person remains focused on their failures and perceived inadequacies. This failure to reward effort can reduce motivation as small but important changes and successes are overlooked or ignored.

Contingency management is based on the principle that behaviour is shaped by the consequences that follow it. Positive consequences are likely to increase the likelihood of a behaviour occurring whilst negative consequences will reduce the probability.

- A child with anxiety may spend considerable time talking with their parents about their worries and how they are unable to do things. The time and attention from their parents may reinforce anxiety-talk and not coping.

- The parents may decide to reinforce their child for being brave and focus their time and attention on courageous coping. Talk about dealing with their anxiety is now reinforced whilst anxiety-talk is ignored or extinguished.

Reward charts are a useful way of highlighting behaviours to be encouraged and how they will be reinforced. Rewards need to reflect the developmental level of the young person. Young children may prefer tangible or concrete rewards such as sticker charts, certificates, or small gifts, whilst adolescents may prefer intrinsic rewards such as saying well done to themselves. It may also be important to involve parents so that they can celebrate and reward their child's efforts to change. Rewards can take many different forms (TGFG p200). They do not need to involve money or special gifts and can include small, naturally occurring rewards such as:

- self-praise and positive self-statements;

- praise from others, including positive comments, attention, hugs, or cuddles;

- extra time doing something the young person enjoys, like staying up later or an extra half an hour playing computer games;

- special treats, like watching an episode of a favourite box set, baking a cake, deciding on what to eat for tea;

- pampering activities, like a long bath with candles, painting nails, or making a hot chocolate;

- social activities, like going on a bike ride with dad, shopping with a favourite aunt, playing a game with mum, or hanging out with a friend.

For younger children, a structured approach helps to explicitly define the target behaviours to be encouraged and the rewards that will be provided. This can be made into a reward chart, a visual way of motivating the child to behave in a different way. The reward chart can be displayed somewhere visible so that everyone can be involved to prompt and praise the child.

There are a few steps involved in setting up a reward chart.

▶ *Clarify the target behaviour*

The first step is to be clear about the target behaviour, which should be specific and positively defined. Avoid general targets that are open to interpretation, such as 'being good', or negatively defined targets that do not emphasise the behaviour to be encouraged, such as 'stop fighting with your brother'. Instead be specific, for example, 'stay seated at the table at mealtimes', and be positive, 'share your toys with your brother'.

▶ *Agree the reward*

Decide on the reward so that the young person knows exactly what they are working towards. As mentioned above, rewards do not need to be large or cost money. What is important is that the reward is motivating and meaningful for the young person. Regardless of whether a tangible reward is provided, it is important that the parent praises the young person.

▶ *Agree how many times the target needs to be achieved*

If using tangible rewards, it is important that the reward can be earned in a realistic time frame. If it takes too long, the young person may feel that the reward is unobtainable and lose motivation. Similarly, this needs to reflect how often the target behaviour can be demonstrated. For example, a target of 'getting ready for bed on time' can only be earned once per day, whilst a target of 'sharing toys' could be earned several times per day.

▶ *Be consistent*

Once the reward has been agreed, it is important to stick with it. The reward system will continue to be motivating if parents are positive and enthusiastic and continue to praise and reward the target behaviour. If parents forget to reward or lose interest, then the young person's motivation will similarly decrease.

Consistency also means sticking to the rules. The rewards are earned only for the target behaviour. The reward is earned once the agreed level has been reached, and rewards, ticks, or stars cannot be taken away for other misbehaviour.

▶ *Make it important*

A reward chart helps to focus attention on the target behaviour so that everyone can monitor and praise progress. Ensure that the target behaviour is made important and provide plenty of praise and attention.

If the young person had a difficult day and found it hard to demonstrate their target behaviour, ensure that they are reminded at the start of the next day to try hard and see what they can achieve.

Parents may find that their child rejects their positive statements and may be tempted to give up because 'it is not working'. It they stop praising their child, they will be sending a message that positive behaviour is not important and will be ignored. It is not so much what the young person says but what the parents do that is important, so even though their praise is rejected, it needs to be provided. This may require an adjustment in the way this is provided to a shorter statement, 'that's another star well done', or the addition of a brief statement, 'I know you don't like me saying these things, but I want to let you know when you have achieved your target.'

Models, uses role play, structured problem-solving approaches, or skills training

Model how to cope

Parents have a key role in modelling, coaching, and reinforcing the development of new coping skills. Young people learn by watching others and will pick up on how their parents are feeling and how they behave. If parents regularly talk about their fears, worries, or anxious feelings, they may unconsciously be teaching their child that the world is a scary place which they will be unable to cope with.

Parents will have their own fears and worries and will have times when they find it hard to cope. This should not be denied. However, instead of modelling how they can't cope and how they avoid situations, they can use some of the skills their child is learning to model how they can face, cope with, and overcome their anxiety. In effect, the parent becomes a positive role model for their child and shows them that although it may be hard, there are helpful things they can do.

Reward the child for facing their challenge

No parent likes to see their child distressed, and they will do what they can to reduce this. Sometimes this might result in unintended consequences.

▶ 'There is no point getting worked up about that birthday party. Stay here and we will find something nice to do instead.'

Whilst this may make the young person feel better, it doesn't help them learn how to cope with their unpleasant emotions. It encourages them to avoid the things that make them feel unpleasant. Instead, parents can reward and model coping behaviour where the young person is encouraged to face their challenges and take their unpleasant feelings with them.

Be positive and encouraging

Parents are keen to help their children. To help them be successful, parents may coach and encourage them to practise making their performance perfect. The unintended consequence of this is that parents may be overly critical and focus on what their child is not able to do rather than what they are doing well. This will confirm the young person's thoughts that they can't be successful and won't be able to cope.

Attending to, and rewarding, what the young person can do focuses on their skills and strengths. It doesn't matter if they are not perfect. Focusing on the positive will encourage them to try.

Learn to tolerate unpleasant emotions

Parents want to prevent their child experiencing any distress and may find ways to stop this from happening. If a young person becomes anxious in busy spaces, it may be easier to avoid taking them shopping so they don't become upset. Whilst this will reduce the potentially stressful situations the young person is exposed to, they never learn how to cope with and tolerate their strong emotions. Instead of trying to protect the young person from their emotions, parents need to encourage them to face their fears and challenges and learn how to tolerate them.

Encourage and reward independence

It can sometimes be quicker and easier to do things for a young person rather than helping them to do it themselves. For example, a young person may want to go on a school trip but is worried about asking their teacher questions. Their parent may contact the teacher and find the answer to their questions. This can be helpful, although, if it becomes a repeated pattern, the young person may be relying on their parents to sort out their problems.

To encourage independence, parents can help the young person to find and implement solutions to their problems. The young person could be encouraged to problem solve and to write down the questions they want their teacher to answer. The parent could then role play how they will go about asking their teacher these questions.

Learn from others

In addition to learning from parents, young people learn by watching other successful role models. The young person can be helped to identify successful role models with whom they can discuss their problems or whom they can observe to see how they cope (TGFG p212).

▶ A socially anxious young person who doesn't know what to talk about could ask or observe their talkative aunt.

▶ A young person who worries about giving a wrong answer to a question in class could observe what happens if someone gets a question wrong.

Role play

Role play is a powerful technique that can be used to bring past events into the clinical session ('Show me what happened') or to safely expose a young person to a difficult situation to practise new coping skills ('Show me what you will do'). Whilst discussing this with a young person might be helpful, role play provides an opportunity for active learning and for the young person to show what happened or how they will behave.

Past events can be acted in role plays to demonstrate what happened and to catch any accompanying thoughts and feelings. They provide opportunities for reflection ('What would you do differently next time?') or challenge ('You said that everyone was laughing, but it looks as if this was only Yara').

Practice role plays are constructed around specific events (i.e. giving a presentation to the class, asking for their choice of food from the dinner lady, or calling a friend to ask them to meet up). Role plays can vary in difficulty and provide opportunities for the young person to develop their confidence and prepare for different scenarios. The aim is not to develop one perfect or fixed way of responding, but to help the young person to practise and demonstrate that they can use their skills to cope with different outcomes.

▶ If giving a presentation, how do they cope with anticipatory anxiety, or what will they do if they forget what they want to say?

▶ If asking for their lunch, what will they do if the dinner lady ignores them, or what if she doesn't hear what has been asked for?

▶ What will they do if their friend does not answer the phone or is busy today?

Role plays provide opportunities for different levels of challenge to be experienced and practised. Role plays can be videoed and reviewed, with the young person being encouraged to identify what they did well and what they might do differently and then to repeat the role play.

If the young person freezes or struggles, the role play should be stopped and the opportunity taken to identify the automatic thoughts racing through their head. The young person can then be actively coached through how they can challenge or stand back from these unhelpful thoughts and the role play practised again.

Problem solving

Young people sometimes lack the skills to think through and solve problems. This may be because the problem is complex and there is no easy solution, resulting in decisions being put off or avoided. Sometimes emotions take over and emotive decisions are made rather than reasoned choices. Alternatively, it could be that the young person cannot think of possible options and so reverts to previous, unsuccessful approaches.

Problem solving provides a structured way of approaching challenges that involves the generation and appraisal of alternative options and reflection on outcomes. For younger children, this might involve a simple three-step traffic light process (TGFG p216).

▶ RED is to stop, to stand back, and to clearly define what the problem is.

▶ AMBER is to think and explore possible solutions. A simple process involving repeatedly prompting further suggestions with the word 'or' can be used to generate alternatives (TGFG p211). Each option can then be appraised, with the positive and negative consequences being assessed and a decision made on which to try (TGFG p213).

▶ GREEN is for go and to implement the chosen solution. Any help or support can be identified, with the young person being encouraged to reflect afterwards whether this was a good solution and one they would use again.

For adolescents and young adults, a five-step process can be used (TGFB p174).

Step 1: Clearly define the problem or decision to be made. Taking time out to think about this stops decisions being made hastily or when the young person is feeling very emotional. It also helps the young person to really consider what their problem is. For example, a young person may describe how their social life is limited: 'I can't go to the football game on Saturday', 'I can't meet my friends in town tomorrow',

'I can't go out at the weekend'. However, the reason they can't do these things may be because they don't have any money. The problem they need to address is how they can earn money so that they can socialise with their friends.

Step 2: Be open-minded and generate a list of choices. This encourages creative thinking. Judgement should be suspended as the aim is to think of as many different solutions as possible. If the young person is struggling to think of options, they can be encouraged to ask friends or family to help.

Step 3: Appraise the options and their consequences. This can help with complicated problems where there is no straightforward or clear solution. The consequences of each should be assessed in both the short and longer term and for the young person and others who might be involved. For example, hitting back at a bully may make the young person feel good in the short term but may result in them being suspended from school. Similarly, whilst joining a new peer group may help the young person find a wider friendship group, what will be the effect on their current friend?

Step 4: Evaluate the options and decide what, on balance, is the best solution. Often there is not a clear or an ideal solution and so the choices need to be weighed up and a choice made to ensure that decisions are not put off or avoided. The decision is then implemented.

Step 5: The final step is reflection and evaluation and to consider whether it worked and what, if anything, the young person would do differently next time.

Skills training

Problems arise for some young people because they lack effective interpersonal skills. Most commonly, these relate to deficient social, communication, or assertion skills.

- Poor social skills, such as a lack of eye contact, speaking in a quiet voice, or inappropriate facial expressions, may lead to young people finding it hard to make friendships.

- Young people may find it difficult to clearly and effectively communicate their ideas, resulting in their views being ignored and their ability to negotiate being compromised.

- A lack of effective assertive skills may lead to young people being coerced or bullied.

Sessions may focus on developing interpersonal skills. The aim is to help the young person more effectively communicate and express their ideas so that potential misunderstandings or upset are minimised. This may involve videoing and reviewing role plays of difficult situations to:

- improve social competence by identifying and developing specific social skills such as eye contact, voice volume, or question asking;

- reduce conflict by developing more effective negotiation skills in which other views are heard and acknowledged but a compromise, reflecting the young person's views, is sought;

- enhance assertiveness by learning to calmly, politely, and firmly assert a point of view.

CHAPTER FIVE

C: Cognitions

Demonstrates use of a variety of cognitive techniques to facilitate
therapeutic change

In the cognitive domain, the young person is helped to identify and
understand how they think and the effect of this on how they feel and
what they do. Unhelpful ways of thinking are identified, and the young
person is helped to recognise biased and critical cognitive distortions or
thinking traps. Once identified, traditional CBT (often called second
wave CBT) attempts to directly challenge and change these critical and
biased ways of thinking and to develop more helpful and balanced
cognitions. The young person is encouraged to catch, check, challenge,
and change their unhelpful ways of thinking. They are helped to put their
thoughts on trial to check the evidence to support or disprove them and
to take different perspectives to develop alternative, more balanced ways
of thinking. Alternatively, they can use techniques from third wave CBT
to develop a different relationship with their thoughts. Rather than
attempting to directly change these cognitions, the young person learns
to observe and accept their thoughts as passing mental activity, rather
than evidence of reality, through mindfulness and self-compassion.
Regardless of the approach, the overall goal is to increase cognitive
awareness in order to reduce emotional distress and enhance
functioning.

A Clinician's Guide to CBT for Children to Young Adults: A Companion to Think Good, Feel Good and Thinking Good, Feeling Better, Second Edition. Paul Stallard.
© 2021 John Wiley & Sons Ltd. Published 2021 by John Wiley & Sons Ltd.
Companion website: www.wiley.com/go/cliniciansguide2e

Facilitates cognitive awareness

Cognitive content

CBT assumes that dysfunctional, critical, and biased ways of thinking are associated with strong unpleasant emotions and unhelpful behaviours.
For example:

▶ Aggressive young people are biased towards aggressive intent: they are more likely to perceive ambiguous situations as threatening, hostile, and provocative and to choose aggressive solutions (Lansford et al. 2006; Yaros et al. 2014).

▶ Anxious adolescents are biased towards threat: they attend to more threat cues, interpret ambiguous situations as threatening, and anticipate that they will be unable to cope (Barrett, Rapee, et al. 1996; Bögels & Zigterman 2000; Waite et al. 2015).

▶ Depressed adolescents are biased towards personal failure: they have negative views and expectations of themselves, ignore or overlook any positives, generalise failure in one area to other areas, and attribute positive events to external rather than internal causes (Curry & Craighead 1990; Kendall et al. 1990; Shirk et al. 2003).

Levels of cognitions

The cognitive model proposed by Beck (1976) identifies three different types of cognitions:

▶ core beliefs/cognitive schemas;

▶ predictions (assumptions about life);

▶ automatic thoughts.

Core beliefs/cognitive schemas

Core beliefs and schemas are deep-seated, fixed, and rigid ways of thinking. Models developed with adults hypothesise that unhelpful core beliefs or self-protecting but dysfunctional schemas develop during childhood and are assumed to underpin many psychological problems (Beck 1976; Young 1990). Research with children and adolescents is limited, although there is evidence that strong, rigid beliefs and schemas are present in children (Rijkeboer & de Boo 2010; Stallard & Rayner 2005). Furthermore, these maladaptive schemas are associated with psychological problems (Stallard 2007; van Vlierberghe et al. 2010), including depression (Lumley & Harkness 2007), obesity (van Vlierberghe & Brate 2007), and aggression (Rijkeboer & de Boo 2010). The stage during childhood where these schemas and beliefs develop and the process by which they become fixed and enduring is not known.

Identifying core beliefs/cognitive schemas: the downward arrow

Core beliefs/schemas tend to be absolute statements, such as 'I am a failure', 'no one loves me', 'I am a bad person', but are often not directly voiced during interview. The downward arrow technique (Burns 1981) can be a useful way of identifying them (TGFB p 139; TGFG p 124). After identifying one of the young person's common or powerful thoughts, the young person is repeatedly asked, 'So what (if this was true) does this mean?' until the underlying core belief emerges.

Case Study Freya worries about making a fool of herself

Freya has social anxiety and often describes how she worries that she will make a fool of herself in social situations. The downward arrow technique (Figure 5.1) was used to identify the core belief that was underlying this thought.

Identifying this belief helped Freya understand her behaviour and why she avoided social situations. If in a group, she didn't talk very much and carefully checked what she said for fear of being rejected.

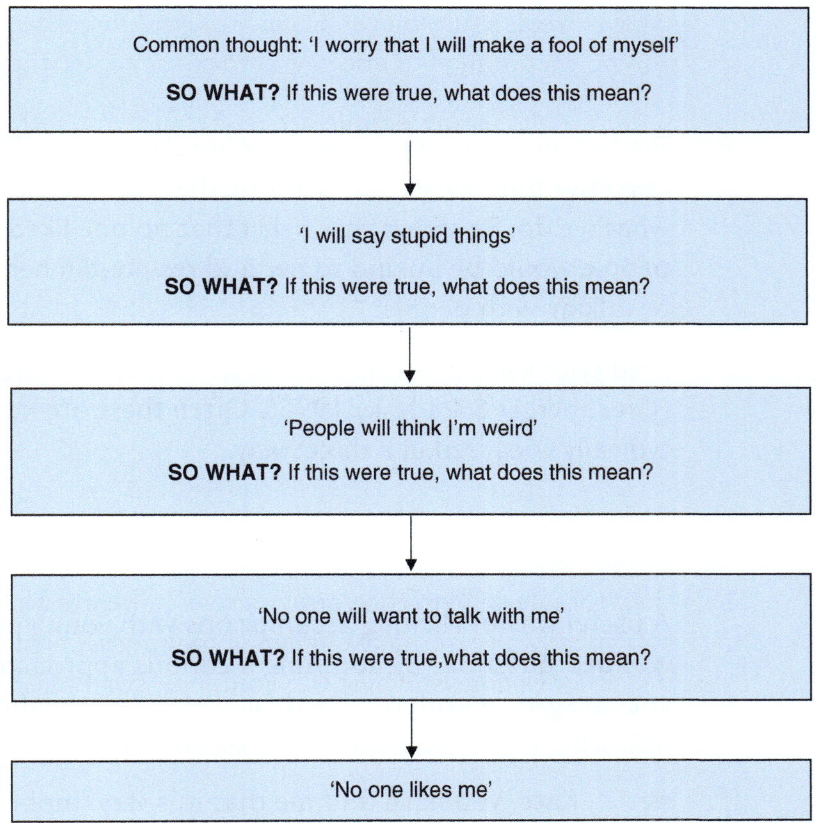

Figure 5.1 Freya's downward arrow.

Identifying core beliefs/cognitive schemas: questionnaires

Another way of identifying core beliefs is to supplement information obtained during the clinical interview with questionnaires. These provide an indication of the beliefs and schemas that might potentially be important for the young person and which can be explored further during subsequent discussions.

The Schema Questionnaire for Children (Stallard & Rayner 2005) was designed to assess the 15 early maladaptive schemas identified by Young (1990) (TGFB p141; TGFG p 126). Each schema is captured by a single statement, for example, 'no one understands me' (social isolation), 'bad things happen to me' (vulnerability), 'I must not show my feelings to others' (emotional inhibition). Each statement is rated on a visual 10-point scale ranging from 'I don't really believe it at all' (1) to 'very strongly believe' (10).

The Schema Inventory for Children (Rijkeboer & de Boo 2010) is also based on the original schemas identified by Young. It consists of 40 items, assessing 11 schemas, for example, 'I think I should always get my own way' (entitlement), 'you can never trust someone else' (mistrust/abuse), 'I am always trying to please others' (self-sacrifice). Each item is rated on a four-point Likert scale from 'not true' to 'yes, definitely'.

Predictions

Predictions or assumptions are our rules for life. They operationalise the cognitive framework and describe the relationship between how we think and what we do. For Freya, her belief that no one liked her led her to predict that people would be unkind to her and resulted in her avoiding social situations or talking with people.

Predictions are often referred to as 'if/then' or 'should/must' statements (Greenberger & Padesky 1995). Often these are not apparent and are not typically vocalised in a direct way.

'I wonder what happens'

A useful way of eliciting assumptions with young people is to use the 'I wonder' question. By adopting a curious approach, the young person can be encouraged to explore how their core beliefs might lead them to behave. The following highlights how Kate's assumptions became clear.

PS:	Kate, you have told me that it is very important that everything you do has to be right. So, I wonder what happens when you have to do a piece of homework for school?

KATE: I get really worried and it seems to take me ages to finish it.

PS: Is that because you work slowly?

KATE: No, not really.

PS: So why does it take so long?

KATE: Well it never seems good enough. I must keep going over it, checking and changing, and it takes me ages.

PS: Have you tried doing it one night and then handing it in the next day?

KATE: No. That wouldn't work. It wouldn't be good enough.

PS: What would be wrong with that?

KATE: Well, I probably wouldn't have done enough work.

PS: So does that mean that if you spend lots of time on your work then you will get better marks?

KATE: Yes. That's why I have to keep doing it again and again.

Kate's assumptions were now becoming clear. For her it was important to get everything right. This led her to assume that **if** she spent a lot of time on her work **then** she would be more likely to be successful.

The if/then quiz

Another way of identifying the young person's assumptions or predictions is through the use of a quiz (TGFG p78). The young person is asked to play a game where they are provided with an 'if' statement and asked to complete the sentence by saying what they expect will happen. Specific questions can be generated to assess assumptions that are suspected to be particularly important for the young person.

▶ IF I get things wrong THEN ... 'people will be angry'.

▶ IF I am successful THEN ... 'I'm lucky'.

▶ IF people like me THEN ... 'they are just being kind'.

What if assumptions aren't clear

There will be times when it is not possible to identify the young person's assumptions or beliefs. At these times, it can be useful to acknowledge this. The use of question marks in formulations can be helpful. This signals that there are some things that are not fully understood and that can be checked again in later sessions to see if the operational relationship has become clearer.

Automatic thoughts

Automatic thoughts are the most accessible level of cognitions. They tumble through our heads and provide a running commentary about what is going on. These thoughts are:

- automatic: they just happen, and we don't actively need to generate them;

- continuous: they are there all the time, but there are times when we are more aware of them;

- reasonable: we hear them so often they seem reasonable and we accept them as true without challenging or questioning them;

- private: we seldom share these thoughts with others; they are private and keep tumbling around our heads.

Automatic thoughts can be positive and helpful or negative and unhelpful. In clinical settings, the primary interest is in those unhelpful automatic thoughts that accompany uncomfortable feelings (e.g. make the young person feel sad, anxious, or angry) and have an unhelpful effect on the young person's behaviour (e.g. are demotivating, make the young person avoid situations or behave inappropriately).

Uses thought records and bubbles

Direct questions

Direct attempts to elicit automatic thoughts can be made by asking questions such as, 'What were you thinking when that happened?' Direct questions may be successful and, if so, should be pursued. Friedberg and McClure (2002) suggest some alternative ways of phrasing this question:

- 'What raced through your head?'

- 'What did you say to yourself?'

- 'What popped into your mind?'

Indirect approaches
The thought catcher

There are occasions when direct questions are met with a shrug of the shoulders or a simple 'nothing' or 'I don't know' response. When direct questions result in the young person appearing uncomfortable or unable to access any thoughts, then an indirect approach should be adopted.

Young people volunteer a great deal of information about their thoughts during conversation. Adopting the role of the 'thought catcher', where the young person is encouraged to talk whilst any thoughts they volunteer are caught, can be helpful. To avoid disrupting the flow of conversation, these can be noted and reflected to the young person at a more appropriate time.

▶ 'Last time we meet, I heard you say ...'

▶ 'You told me that when that happened you remembered thinking ...'

When catching thoughts, it is important to record exactly what the young person says, rather than paraphrasing or summarising. Using the young person's own words ensures that the meaning they attribute to events is accurately captured. The use of their own words strengthens the therapeutic relationship and helps to maximise understanding.

The young person can be asked to start this process outside of the clinical session with exercises such as 'downloading their head' (TGFB p110). When they notice a strong emotional reaction, they are encouraged to write down what happened, who was there, what was said, and how they felt in as much detail as possible. This can be reviewed during their next meeting and any important thoughts identified.

Thought bubbles

Cartoons and thought bubbles are particularly useful with younger children as an entertaining and fun way of assessing specific cognitions and cognitive processes. They offer a visual way of communicating about thoughts and of demonstrating that there is more than one way to think about an event. A range of worksheets can be used to:

▶ introduce the young person to the idea of describing their thoughts (TGFG p94);

▶ help them identify common thoughts about themselves (TGFG p91), their performance (TGFG p93), and their future (TGFG p92);

▶ highlight how there are different ways of thinking about the same event (TGFG 95);

▶ emphasise how thoughts are associated with feelings (TGFB p109).

Children aged seven can readily understand that a thought bubble represents what a person is thinking. Once understood, the idea of a thought bubble can then be applied to the young person's problem situations, thereby providing a means through which their thoughts can be communicated.

Thought diaries

Thought records or diaries provide a way of identifying common thoughts. These could focus on identifying 'hot thoughts', the thoughts racing through the young person's head when they notice a strong emotional reaction (TGFB p108; TGFG p 88).

Self-monitoring and completing diaries are often not popular with young people. It is therefore important that they be provided with a clear rationale for why keeping a diary might be helpful.

▶ 'I can't be with you 24/7, so it would be really helpful if you could keep a diary to help us understand what happens and some of your common thoughts.'

The nature and extent of the diary needs to be agreed.

▶ Is the purpose of the diary or record clear?

▶ Will the young person set up their own diary or would they prefer a worksheet?

▶ Would they like to use some headings to structure the record or would a more informal approach such as 'downloading their head' be preferable?

▶ How would they want to keep their record – paper, laptop, phone, etc?

▶ How long can they realistically keep the diary?

▶ How many events would it be useful to capture?

Some young people will prefer to design their own computer record, capture their thoughts on their phone, or send an email after any difficult situations. If a young person is unwilling or unable to keep any form of diary or record, then their thoughts can still be assessed during the next clinical session. Difficult situations can be discussed in detail and any strong accompanying thoughts identified.

Identifies cognitions that are functional and helpful and those that are dysfunctional or unhelpful

Once able to identify their cognitions, the young person is helped to discover how these affect how they feel and what they do. This introduces the idea of helpful and unhelpful thoughts.

Unhelpful thoughts

Unhelpful thoughts are demotivating and disempowering and stop us from doing what we would really like to do. Unhelpful thoughts are negative, critical of ourselves, focus on the things that go wrong, and/or tell us that we will be unable to cope or be successful.

- 'There will be lots of people in town and I won't be able to cope.'

- 'I will get this work wrong, so there is no point in trying.'

- 'I am always ill when I sleep over at my friend's house. I might as well say I can't go.'

Thinking in these unhelpful ways increases unpleasant feelings and the likelihood that challenges will be put off or avoided.

For younger children, the analogy of a traffic light can explain the effect of these thoughts on their behaviour. These unhelpful thoughts are 'red' or 'stop thoughts'; they get in the way and prevent them from doing the things they would really like to do (TGFG p89).

Helpful thoughts

Helpful thoughts are motivating and empowering and encourage us to face our challenges. They are more balanced and positive, acknowledge our strengths and successes, focus on our achievements, and tell us that we will be able to cope and be successful.

- 'There will be lots of people in town, but I have done this before.'

- 'This work is hard, but I can only try my best.'

- 'It will be good to sleep over, and I can call home if I need to.'

Thinking in these helpful ways increases pleasant feelings and the likelihood that challenges will be faced. These helpful thoughts are the 'green' or 'go' thoughts, which motivate and encourage us to face our challenges (TGFG p 90).

Identifies important dysfunctional cognitions and common cognitive biases ('thinking traps')

Unhelpful ways of thinking are dysfunctional and biased, and for young people can be described as 'thinking traps'. Learning to understand the way they think can help young people to stop falling into their thinking traps and to challenge these unhelpful, critical, and biased ways of thinking. There are five main types of thinking traps (TGFG p103), which include 11 common biased ways of thinking (TGFB p117).

The negative filter

With this trap, anything positive is filtered out by our negative filter and remains unrecognised or ignored. This happens in two main ways, with the first being the 'negative glasses' or selective abstraction. The young person is looking at their world through a pair of negative glasses which only allow them to see the negative things that happen.

> ▶ Muhammad had a good day at school; he got a good mark for an assignment, scored a goal during football training, and hung out with friends at lunchtime, but he forgot to take his sports kit home. He found himself wearing his negative glasses as he focused on this one event: 'This is rubbish. If Miss Smith hadn't wanted to see me, I would have remembered to take my bag.'

The second is 'positive doesn't count' or disqualifying the positive, where anything positive that happens is dismissed as unimportant or irrelevant.

> ▶ Charlie didn't think he was very good at art, but he got a good grade for his latest assignment. He dismissed this as unimportant, 'everyone got a good mark', as he continued to convince himself that he was not good at art.

Blowing things up

This trap involves blowing up the negative things that happen to something larger or more important than they really are. This can happen in three main ways.

'Magnifying the negative' (magnification) is where the importance attached to small events is inflated.

> ▶ Mia was late for her dance class. As she walked into the gym, she noticed one person looking at her and thought 'everyone is staring at me and thinking I am stupid'.

'All-or-nothing' (dichotomous) thinking is where thinking is polarised into two extremes and there is nothing in between. It is either boiling hot or freezing cold.

> ▶ Lily had an argument with her best friend and found herself thinking 'she'll never talk to me again'.

'Disaster thinking' (catastrophising) is where small events lead the person to expect the worst possible outcome.

▶ Freddie was feeling quite anxious and noticed his heart was racing fast. He found himself thinking 'I am going to have a heart attack'.

Predicting failure

This is where we predict what will happen and often reach our conclusions based on little or no evidence (arbitrary inference). Our predictions tend to assume the worst, and this happens in two ways.

The 'mind reader' assumes they know what others are thinking about them, and it is usually the worst.

▶ 'Martha and Josie looked at me and smiled. I bet they think my hair is a mess.'

Similarly, the 'fortune-teller' knows what is going to happen and often predicts that they will fail or be unsuccessful.

▶ 'No point in doing any work. I'm going to do rubbish in that test tomorrow.'

Being down on yourself

This is where we are overly critical of ourselves and take responsibility for the things that go wrong.

'Dustbin labels' (labelling) is where we assign a negative personal label to all aspects of our life:

▶ 'I'm a loser' or 'I'm a failure'.

The second way this occurs is with 'blame me' (personalisation), where the young person assumes responsibility for the things that go wrong.

▶ Your best friend may have fallen over and hurt her knee and you end up thinking, 'If only I had been with her, this wouldn't have happened.'

Setting yourself up to fail

The final thinking trap is where we set ourselves up to fail (unrealistic expectations). We expect too much of ourselves and, because our standards are so high, we never achieve them.

Sometimes we don't think about or acknowledge what we have achieved but instead focus on what we haven't. 'Should and must' thinking makes us aware of our failings and our thoughts as we think that we 'should' or 'must' do something else.

▶ 'I should do more work.'

▶ 'I must get an A grade.'

▶ 'I should be able to cope.'

This also happens in 'expecting to be perfect', where we set ourselves unachievable standards which we can never hope to meet.

▶ Sienna wanted to do well with her schoolwork but became upset and angry when she didn't get an A grade.

Facilitates the generation of alternative balanced cognitions by thought challenging and alternative perspective taking

Once unhelpful and dysfunctional patterns of thinking are identified, the young person can be encouraged to question and challenge them. The process involves helping the young person attend to information that their thinking traps are leading them to dismiss or ignore and helping them to discover new information and meanings that they have overlooked. Through this, the young person is helped to develop alternative, more balanced ways of thinking that better fit the evidence.

Balanced thinking is not about trying to make everything positive. Bad things happen, people will be unkind, and we are not always successful. It is about acknowledging this whilst looking at the whole picture and recognising any important positive and helpful information that has been ignored or dismissed.

What is the evidence?

This provides a series of steps to help the young person check that they have considered all the evidence that supports or disproves their way of thinking (TGFG p116). In effect, the young person puts their unhelpful thoughts on trial and works through the following steps before making a balanced judgement.

▶ What evidence is there to support this way of thinking?

▶ What evidence is there to question this way of thinking?

▶ What would your best friend (first witness) say if they heard you thinking like this?

▶ What would your parent, teacher, cousin, etc. (second witness) say if they heard you thinking like this?

▶ Examine the evidence – are you caught in a thinking trap?

▶ What is your verdict? Is there another, more balanced way of thinking which better fits the evidence?

The 4Cs

This offers a four-step process to guide the young person through the process of thought identification and challenging through to the final stage of cognitive restructuring (TGFB p129; TGFG p117).

▶ The first step is to 'Catch' the unhelpful thoughts that are making the young person feel unpleasant or that get in the way and stop them from doing things.

▶ Once caught, the second step is to 'Check' whether they have fallen into a thinking trap where they are making things out to be worse than they really are. This will involve checking for the *blowing things up*, *predicting failure*, or *being down on themselves* thinking traps.

▶ The third step is to 'Challenge' their unhelpful thoughts by actively looking for evidence that questions them. Looking for the *negative filter* and *unrealistic expectations* thinking traps can help to identify new or important information that has been overlooked.

▶ The final step is reflecting on what has been discovered to 'Change' their way of thinking to something that is more balanced and helpful and better fits the evidence.

What would someone else say?

Young people may find it difficult to challenge their own negative automatic thoughts. They may have heard them so often that they simply accept them as true. On these occasions, it may be easier to challenge these thoughts by adopting another perspective. This alternative perspective is introduced in 'What is the evidence?', where important people are called as witnesses. The third-party perspective can also be used on other occasions to help young people generate alternative thoughts and meanings (TGFB p 130; TGFG p118). The young person is encouraged to think what someone important to them would say if they heard the way they were thinking. Alternatively, the young person can be asked what they would say to their best friend or someone they care about if they heard them thinking the way they do.

Case Study Jaz falls out with her friend

Jaz had an argument with her friend Ruby and found herself with negative thoughts going around in her head: 'I am always falling out with people, no one likes me.' She decided to think from another perspective and imagine what her best friend Sophie would say if she heard her thinking like this. She would probably say, 'Ruby seems very sensitive at the moment. She is always arguing with people.' This helped Jaz to put this in perspective. She had fallen into the *blame me* thinking trap where she was talking responsibility for this fallout. She also had her *negative glasses* on and had overlooked how Ruby was also arguing with her other friends.

Facilitates continuum work using rating scales

Core beliefs are powerful and enduring and are often resistant to challenge and change. Many of these are all-or-nothing beliefs such as 'I am a failure'. In these situations, it can be helpful to adopt a continuum approach to highlight and quantify small, but important, changes.

The young person's dysfunctional core belief can be identified (e.g. 'I am worthless') and the degree to which they believe it rated on a 1–100 scale. With core beliefs, it can be helpful to develop an alternative, more functional belief (e.g. 'I am important') that can coexist alongside their negative belief. This will inevitably be at variance with their dysfunctional belief and will be one which they will not believe and will give a low rating.

Rating scales can be used to explore what effect events might have on their beliefs.

▶ 'What would happen to reduce your belief that you are worthless from 96 to 90?'

▶ 'What might a friend do to show that you are important?'

▶ 'How can a parent show that they care?'

Experiences can be used to reassess the strength of these beliefs.

▶ 'What effect does your teacher offering to help you with your maths have on your belief that you are worthless?'

▶ 'Last week three people messaged you. How does that affect your belief that you are worthless or the belief that you are important?'

The continuum approach allows two or more beliefs to coexist. It challenges the dichotomous tendency to assume that a dysfunctional belief ('I am worthless') cannot coexist alongside a functional ('I am important') belief. It acknowledges that the dysfunctional belief will continue to exist, with the use of ratings providing a way of quantifying change. Over time, this will highlight that the strength of dysfunctional beliefs may reduce whilst the strength of functional beliefs may increase.

Uses techniques such as mindfulness, acceptance, and compassion

Mindfulness

Some young people do not find the process of actively challenging and reappraising cognitions easy. They may go through the steps, but it becomes a detached, academic process which does not result in any important or enduring changes.

An alternative approach to challenging the content of unhelpful cognitions involves changing the nature of our relationship with our thoughts. This has stimulated considerable interest in the use of mindfulness, the practice of 'paying attention in a particular way: on purpose, in the present moment and nonjudgmentally' (Kabat-Zinn 2005). Mindfulness develops an attitude of openness, acceptance, and curiosity (Bishop et al. 2004). Research is growing, with meta reviews demonstrating the positive effects of mindfulness on attention and psychological functioning, including anxiety and depression (Dunning et al. 2019; Klingbeil et al. 2017; Maynard et al. 2017; Zenner et al. 2014; Zoogman et al. 2015), and how it is associated with increased self-compassion and pro-social behaviour (Cheang et al. 2019).

Mindfulness provides a way of reconnecting with the present moment and the thoughts and emotions that are experienced here and now. We often spend considerable time in our heads, listening to our worries, arguing with our thoughts, rehearsing what has happened, and worrying about what will happen. This focus on the past leads us to ruminate and dwell on the negative things that have happened whilst the focus on the future leads us to worry and expect the worst, leading to much unhappiness, anger, and stress.

With mindfulness, cognitions and emotions are accepted as passing activity rather than evidence of a reality that we must engage with or attempt to change. Instead, cognitions and emotions are embraced and observed in a curious, non-judgemental way. By so doing, we learn to notice our thoughts and feelings and to step back from them and let them pass.

With children and young people, it is important to keep explanations simple. Mindfulness can be explained to young people as focusing on the here and now.

> 'We spend a lot of our time going over what has happened or worrying about what will happen and seldom notice what is happening here and now. By focusing our mind on the here and now, we can be less bothered by the negative clutter that goes around our heads.'

The aim of mindfulness is to notice and curiously observe what is happening, not to stop or change the way we think. Rather than reacting to passing thoughts or emotions, the young person is encouraged to make space to observe and understand what is happening.

FOCUS

To help young people understand the steps involved in mindfulness, the acronym FOCUS can be used (TGFG p61).

> **F**ocus your attention.

> **O**bserve what is happening.

> Be **C**urious.

> **U**se all your senses.

> **S**tay with it and suspend judgement.

The first step is to learn to focus attention on the here and now. We often don't fully notice what is happening as our minds wander off and inevitably find negative things to rehearse or worry about. Focusing involves becoming aware of what is happening and, when attention wanders, pulling it back to the here and now.

The process of focusing can be encouraged by observation. Young people are helped to observe what is happening by imagining they are looking through a zoom lens. Initially, they will see lots of things, but as they zoom in, their attention becomes more focused. They observe less but notice things in much greater detail. Observation can be enhanced by encouraging the young person to describe what they see to someone else and to find at least one thing they have never noticed before.

The young person can be encouraged to observe by using all their senses. If, for example, mindfully eating:

> What does the food **look** like?

> What does it **smell** like?

▶ What does it **feel** like in your mouth?

▶ What does it **taste** like?

▶ What do you **hear** as you eat?

Finally, the young person is encouraged to stay with it. If they notice their attention wandering, they are encouraged to steer it back to the here and now. If they notice they are engaging with or reacting to their thoughts, they are encouraged to stand back, observe, and suspend judgement.

Mindful activities

Mindfulness doesn't have to take long. Short mindfulness sessions of a couple of minutes, repeated at different times of the day, can be helpful. The young person can set the timer on their phone for two minutes to signal the end. Building short mindfulness sessions into the daily routine can prompt and encourage regular use, for example, whilst washing, walking to school/college, whilst eating, before bedtime.

Mindfulness can be undertaken at any time and in any place, and could involve focusing on eating (TGFG p60), breathing (TGFB p77; TGFG p59), everyday objects (TGFB p79; TGFG p61), thoughts (TGFB p78; TGFG p63), or feelings (TGFG p64).

Like all skills, mindfulness takes time to learn and improves with practice.

Compassion

A great deal of distress arises from our critical thoughts and the way that our inner critic tears us apart. A compassionate approach can be helpful for young people who are very self-critical and find it difficult to self-soothe or generate feelings of kindness. Instead of being so critical, a more compassionate approach can help the young person to feel more comfortable with who they are and to recognise and acknowledge their strengths.

Compassion is concerned with developing awareness of and sensitivity to suffering or distress in self and others (Gilbert 2013). With adults, low self-compassion has been found to be associated with higher levels of psychological problems, whilst higher self-compassion was associated with lower levels of mental health (Macbeth & Gumley 2012).

Self-compassion can be developed through helpful habits, where young people are encouraged to experiment with, and develop, a less critical and more compassionate approach to life that embraces the elements of self-compassion, acceptance, and kindness.

Treat yourself like a friend

The critical negative thoughts that tumble around in our heads are seldom shared. Because they are private, we are often harder on ourselves than we would be on someone else. To counter this critical inner voice, young people can be encouraged to treat themselves as they would treat a friend. When they become aware of their critical inner voice, they can be prompted to ask, 'What would I say to my best friend if I heard them thinking and saying these things?' Inevitably, the young person will be less harsh and will adopt a kinder, more encouraging approach. Once the young person has identified this critical inner voice and how to deal with it, they are encouraged to apply this to themselves as they learn to treat themselves like a friend (TGFB p 64; TGFG p 44).

Speak kindly to yourself

The young person can be helped to develop a kinder, less critical inner voice by learning to speak kindly to themselves (TGFB p66; TGFG p47). Our critical inner voice can be very harsh, and many young people find it embarrassing or are ashamed to say their thoughts out loud. To counter these thoughts, young people can be encouraged to develop a kinder inner voice. This involves developing one or two short statements that acknowledge how they are feeling, that they are not alone, and that they need to be kind to themselves.

- ▶ 'I am feeling really down. Lots of people feel like me. I need to look after myself.'

- ▶ 'I am feeling really anxious. Everyone gets anxious at some time. It is OK if you get things wrong.'

It can be helpful to practise saying these short statements out aloud at the start of each day or when the critical inner voice is noticed. Repeating this with conviction whilst standing in front of a mirror can help to develop confidence and strengthen belief in these more compassionate statements.

Look after yourself

Self-compassion can be promoted by encouraging the young person to care for themselves when they are feeling down (TGFB p65; TGFG p46). Instead of kicking, criticising, or blaming themselves, young people are encouraged to look after themselves. They are encouraged to stop beating themselves up for feeling so bad and to do something to help themselves feel better. This could be a long relaxing bath, watching an episode of a favourite box set, or making a drink of hot chocolate.

Acceptance

A great deal of time is spent focusing on our faults, our imperfections, and how we would like to be different. This personal dissatisfaction generates anxiety, makes us feel down, and can reduce our confidence to do things. We beat ourselves up and tear ourselves apart as we:

▶ are never satisfied with what we do or achieve;

▶ blame ourselves for the things that go wrong;

▶ focus on our imperfections and failures;

▶ never acknowledge our strengths or success.

An alternative approach is to learn to accept that:

▶ things do go wrong;

▶ no one is perfect;

▶ we all make mistakes;

▶ unkind things happen.

Instead of striving to be somebody else, young people can be helped to accept and value who they are (TGFG p45). An important step involves discovering and acknowledging personal strengths.

▶ If a young person doesn't like themselves, encourage them to find their positive qualities – are they patient, determined, hard-working, reliable, or kind?

▶ If a young person doesn't think people like them, encourage them to find their positive relationship skills – are they a good listener, loyal, supportive, caring, or good at cheering people up?

▶ If a young person doesn't like how they look, find those aspects of their appearance that they do like – are they well proportioned, have nice hair, nails, hands, or voice?

▶ If a young person thinks they are a failure at everything, encourage them to find their skills – are they good at sport, art, music, cooking, being creative?

Instead of them focusing on the things they would like to change, remind them that they are special and encourage them to accept themselves for who they are.

Focus on strengths and achievements

The young person's inner critic can be challenged by helping them to notice and accept what they achieve rather than focusing on what they have failed to do.

▶ They frequently compare themselves to others and often choose the most successful person, resulting in feelings of inadequacy or dissatisfaction.

▶ They often fail to recognise and accept what they have achieved as they constantly think about what they 'must' or 'should' do better.

▶ They don't always celebrate effort as they remain focused on outcomes.

Encourage the young person to focus on their strengths and achievements (TGFB p52) and to accept that whilst they cannot always be the best, they have many personal skills and qualities.

Kindness

When people feel down, anxious, or angry, it often seems that everyone is picking on them, the world is out to get them, and that everyone is unkind. This becomes a self-perpetuating process, where the expectations of unkind things inevitably lead to their discovery.

To develop a kinder, more balanced perspective, young people can be encouraged to notice times when someone has been caring or considerate (TGFG p46; TGFB p67). By shifting their focus, they learn to assume the best in people and notice and enjoy acts of kindness, no matter how small. For example, when someone:

▶ makes time to say hello and talk;

▶ says something nice, for example, 'your hair looks good' or 'I like your jumper';

▶ shares a text, picture, or message;

▶ says 'thank you' to a friend, bus driver, or teacher;

▶ offers to help with a chore or task;

▶ shows concern or says something kind or funny.

After discovering how good acts of kindness make them feel, young people can be encouraged to be kind to someone else. Small acts of kindness, such as giving a compliment, smiling, offering to help, or making time to listen to someone, are important and show that people do care and are kind to each other.

CHAPTER SIX

D: Discovery

Uses a variety of methods to facilitate self-discovery and understanding

The process of CBT is designed to promote self-discovery. This involves the young person discovering their strengths and skills and finding new information or meanings about the events that occur. These insights are facilitated using the Socratic dialogue, a curious conversation that helps the young person to attend to new or overlooked information that is inconsistent with and challenges their biased and critical cognitions. The discovery process is open, inquisitive, and objective, with behavioural experiments being used to objectively 'check out' the accuracy of beliefs and predictions. The young person is encouraged to reflect on the outcomes of these experiments and to integrate this new information into their cognitive framework. A more balanced cognitive framework is developed as the young person learns to establish appropriate limits around their beliefs and assumptions.

Facilitates self-discovery and reflection through use of the Socratic dialogue

A common misapprehension amongst those inexperienced in CBT is that this process of cognitive restructuring is achieved by encouraging the young person to simply think in rational or logical ways. Inevitably, such a naive approach involves the use of a series of 'clever' questions designed to challenge, disprove, or discredit the young person's cognitions. The clinician therefore has a preconceived, closed idea about the outcome they would like

A Clinician's Guide to CBT for Children to Young Adults: A Companion to Think Good, Feel Good and Thinking Good, Feeling Better, Second Edition. Paul Stallard.
© 2021 John Wiley & Sons Ltd. Published 2021 by John Wiley & Sons Ltd.
Companion website: www.wiley.com/go/cliniciansguide2e

the young person to achieve and uses questions to guide the young person to this conclusion. The process is neither empowering nor collaborative and simply serves to highlight the irrationality of the young person's thoughts and to prove them wrong. This becomes a negative, abstract, and intellectual exercise in which the young person has no ownership of the process or outcome. Adolescents will find such an approach particularly unhelpful and it will typically result in the clinician becoming locked into an increasingly adversarial relationship as the adolescent is forced to maintain and defend their beliefs and assumptions in the face of this external challenge.

In contrast, the Socratic dialogue helps the young person to discover, assess, and reappraise their cognitions. The process is positive, enabling, and supportive and is based upon genuine openness. This sense of curiosity encourages the identification of the universal definitions, the cognitive generalisations, the young person applies to their life. Important thoughts, beliefs, assumptions, and experiences are made explicit as the meaning the young person attributes to them is clarified. The young person is encouraged to suspend their preconceived ideas and to keep an open mind as they test and evaluate their beliefs and assumptions. The young person's cognitions are therefore viewed as hypotheses that are open for empirical validation rather than established facts. Through the Socratic dialogue, the young person is encouraged to draw upon their past knowledge and empowered to discover new information that can help them re-evaluate and reappraise their cognitions. The young person is helped to become their own therapist and to learn a process that can be applied to future problems in order to foster more adaptive and functional ways of thinking and behaving.

The Socratic dialogue is approached in a collaborative and non-judgemental way where each partner is aware of their own assumptions and preconceived ideas. The young person's thoughts are not automatically assumed to be dysfunctional, with the Socratic dialogue being used to understand the young person's way of thinking. Once understood, a gentle and curious approach is adopted where questions and prompts help the young person reappraise and test their thoughts. Questions help the young person attend to and consider information that they had previously overlooked or considered unimportant. Attending to this new information helps the young person to consider a broader range of factors and possibilities. It highlights how there may be a variety of different ways of explaining events and that the young person's universal definitions may have limits. Once again, the philosophy of self-discovery is important. Questions designed to directly criticise or challenge the young person's thoughts (e.g. 'I think you've got that wrong' or 'No, it isn't really like that') should be avoided. Similarly, the clinician should avoid imposing their own preconceived ideas (e.g. 'I think it may be more like this').

The process by which the young person is helped to explore and analyse similarities and differences between events is that of inductive reasoning. This helps to identify and test any overgeneralisations, selection biases, or dichotomous thinking that result in general beliefs (e.g. 'I am stupid') being widely and inappropriately applied. Overgeneralisation involves the extrapolation of specific beliefs to a wide range of different situations. Subtle but important differences go unnoticed as the universal definition is uncritically applied. This practice is common and, indeed, many of the cognitive biases encountered in CBT are based upon inaccurate overgeneralisations (Ellis 1977). Typically, these overgeneralisations become self-perpetuating as the young person seeks and attends to confirmatory information whilst negating or ignoring information that would challenge or contradict their views. This may result in the young person developing extreme and polarised dichotomous beliefs in which events are considered from two mutually exclusive positions whilst overlooking any intermediate graduations. The Socratic process encourages inductive reasoning and helps young people attend to new or overlooked information that allows them to reconsider and revise their generalisations and biases.

The Socratic dialogue

Overholser (1993b) describes a Socratic process based upon the three steps of identification, evaluation, and redefinition. During the identification stage, the focus is on eliciting important 'universal definitions'. These are the cognitive generalisations and biases the young person uses to filter, interpret, guide, and predict what happens in their life. Once identified, these universal definitions are clarified so that the meaning the young person ascribes to them is unambiguously defined. Inevitably, this starts to highlight some degree of confusion and leads to the second stage, that of evaluation. The evaluation stage is concerned with testing the definition and in identifying any exceptions or limitations. Universal definitions need to be stable and consistent over time and account for all eventualities. Establishing exceptions or inconsistencies helps the young person to establish limits around their universal and global definitions, which leads to the final stage of the Socratic process. This is the stage of redefinition, where the new information that has been discovered is integrated and assimilated within the young person's cognitive framework. This promotes a new definition or set of more balanced and helpful cognitions.

Overholser (1993a) identified seven types of questions, each with different functions, that can be used at various stages of the Socratic dialogue to facilitate the process of self-discovery, understanding, appraisal, and re-evaluation.

Memory questions

The first, and perhaps the easiest for the young person to engage with, are descriptive memory questions. These are concerned with clarifying facts or details and are designed to help the young person focus upon and recall information relevant to the present discussion. Overholser (1993a) highlights that memory questions provide an insight into the young person's experiences, feelings, and thoughts and facilitate the development of a shared understanding. Memory questions have a factual and descriptive focus such as:

- ▶ 'When did this start?'
- ▶ 'What do you do when you feel like this?'
- ▶ 'How often does this happen?'

Translation questions

The next level of questioning uses translation questions to discover the meaning the young person attributes to these events. Reflection encourages the young person to explore what they have said.

- ▶ 'What do you make of this?'
- ▶ 'Any idea why you get those funny feelings?'
- ▶ 'Does this only happen to you?'

Translation questions start to identify some of the attributions and assumptions the young person makes. They provide an insight into the young person's cognitive framework and begin to highlight important biases that might need further evaluation.

Interpretation questions

Interpretation questions logically follow and are used to explore possible relationships or connections between events. They are designed to help the young person identify possible patterns and similarities. Typically, this involves bringing together two or more events and asking the young person to consider whether there are any similarities or connections between them.

- ▶ 'Is the feeling you get when you go into school the same as the one you get when you meet up with your friends in town?'
- ▶ 'Have you noticed a link between those negative thoughts and how you feel?'
- ▶ 'Is it after you have an argument with your friend that you cut yourself?'

Application questions

At the fourth level are application questions, which are designed to draw upon the young person's previous knowledge or skills. These questions are used to identify relevant or important information that may have been overlooked or forgotten.

- ▶ 'What have you done in the past when you have felt like this?'

- ▶ 'You said that the last time this happened it didn't seem so bad. Was there anything you did differently that may have helped?'

- ▶ 'You don't seem to have these worrying thoughts at school. Is there anything different at school that helps you to ignore these thoughts?'

Analysis questions

These are designed to help the young person systematically and logically think through their problems, thoughts, and coping strategies. This is the process of rational analysis or inductive reasoning. Analysis questions are designed to foster logical conclusions by promoting objectivity and the use of inductive reasoning to critically evaluate and challenge beliefs, assumptions, and inferences. Inductive reasoning helps the young person to consider and attend to new or overlooked information or to systematically test the assumed relationship between events.

- ▶ 'When you think like that, what is the evidence that supports your thoughts?'

- ▶ 'Is there any evidence that you have overlooked?'

- ▶ 'What would your best friend say if they heard you thinking this way?'

Similarly, gentle questioning can help the young person to test the assumed causal relationship between events.

- ▶ 'Are there any times when this hasn't happened?'

- ▶ 'Are there times when it did happen, but it was due to something else?'

Synthesis questions

Synthesis questions take the discussion to a higher level and encourage the young person to think 'outside of the box' in order to identify new or alternative explanations and solutions. Overholser (1993a) stresses the needs to retain an open mind during this process and not to have a single preconceived idea about what the young person will 'discover'.

- ► 'Let's list all the different ways we could cope with this, even if some might sound a little odd or silly.'
- ► 'What do you think your best friend would do?'
- ► 'Are there any other ways we could explain what has happened?'

Evaluation questions

The completion of the Socratic process is achieved using evaluation questions. The initial thoughts, beliefs, and assumptions are now reappraised and modified in the light of the discussion.

- ► 'So, what sense do you make of this now?'
- ► 'Do you still see yourself as a failure?'
- ► 'Is there another way of thinking about this?'

The prime focus of the questions will depend upon the stage of the Socratic dialogue. Memory and translation questions are used more often to gather information and establish meaning. Interpretation and application questions are used to help the young person focus on overlooked information and to explore the connection between events. Analysis questions facilitate inductive reasoning, with synthesis and evaluation questions integrating this information as the young person considers the new information and reappraises their thoughts.

What makes a good Socratic question?

Clear and specific

Evaluating and reappraising thoughts can be an abstract process, especially for younger children, and so it is important to make Socratic questions as clear and specific as possible. The initial stages of the Socratic dialogue are concerned with establishing facts, and so simple, specific, and concrete questions are useful. Questions that are helpful tend to be:

- ► 'What' questions – 'What did you do?' 'What did he say?'
- ► 'How' questions – 'How did you feel?' 'How did he do that?'
- ► 'Where' questions – 'Where did you go?' 'Where does this happen most?'
- ► 'When' questions – 'When does this happen?'

Answerable

The Socratic dialogue is designed to be empowering by highlighting how the young person already possesses useful knowledge or could discover helpful information. It is then essential to ensure that questions are answerable and that they do not seem to the young person to be impossible to address. In particular, 'why' questions, which require the young person to make some interpretation or judgement rather than recounting factual details' are important, but their use should be carefully monitored. Similarly, complex and multiple-component questions should be avoided, whilst abstract and hypothetical questions should be used with care.

Uses the young person's language

Questions need to be phrased in the young person's language and be consistent with their developmental level. This involves carefully listening to what the young person says and the words or metaphors they use so that these can be incorporated into the Socratic dialogue. This validates the young person's use of language and constructs a dialogue based upon their words and meaning.

Attends to overlooked information

The young person's unhelpful thoughts will arise from some bias in cognitive processing. The young person may, for example, be selectively attending to information that supports their thoughts whilst overlooking that which might provide a different perspective. The Socratic dialogue brings to the young person's attention relevant information that is currently being overlooked. By being helped to attend to this new information, the young person is provided with new opportunities to question and reappraise their beliefs.

Remains focused

In many instances, the young person will be in possession of a great deal of information that could be used to reappraise and challenge their thoughts. Often the young person will be unaware of this and will not have made the relevant links that will help them to piece this together in a coherent and helpful way. The Socratic dialogue helps the young person to remain focused upon relevant information that will enable them to make the links and connections that will allow them to systematically evaluate their thoughts. It is all too easy to allow the dialogue to meander across subjects or to become distracted by interesting but non-relevant information.

Case Study Mike is worried about his cat

Mike was 12 years of age and had many obsessive behaviours and thoughts. His current preoccupation was with the safety of the family cat, which resulted in him insisting that the cat be locked in the house each night. This preoccupation was based upon his assumption that if the cat were to go out at night then she would be knocked down by a car. This was discussed during our next meeting, with the Socratic dialogue helping Mike to discover, evaluate, and reappraise this assumption.

PS: Mike, mum tells me that you are very worried about your cat.

MIKE: Yes. I am. I don't like her going outside.

PS: **When** do you most worry about her going out?

MIKE: At night-time when it is dark.

PS: Ok, so **what** do you think will happen if she is out at night?

MIKE: She'll have an accident.

PS: **What** type of accident do you think she could have?

MIKE: Don't know. Knocked down by a car and killed, I suppose.

PS: I remember you telling me about how things always seem to go wrong and that you expect bad things to happen to you and your family.

MIKE: Yeah, that's right.

PS: So now you are worried that something bad will happen to your cat. How do you cope with this worry? **What** do you do each night when your cat wants to go out?

MIKE: I must go and find her and lock her in the house.

PS: **What** time do you usually shut her in?

MIKE: When I get home from school, usually.

PS: Does she mind being locked in?

MIKE: Yeah, she hates it. She scratches me and tries to get out again.

PS: So **how** does it make you feel when she is locked in?

MIKE: Relieved I suppose. I know she is safe.

PS: Let me check that I've got this right. You worry that if your cat goes out at night she will get knocked over by a car. It seems to you that bad things often happen to your family. To make sure this doesn't happen, you keep her locked in where you know she is safe. She doesn't like this and wants to be outside, but locking her in makes you feel better.

MIKE: Yes, that's right.

PS: **What** happens during the daytime?

MIKE: What do you mean?

PS: Well, I wondered whether you had to lock her in during the daytime?

MIKE: No. She goes out.

PS: **How** do you feel about her being out during the daytime?

MIKE: It doesn't bother me.

PS: Is your road not so busy during the daytime?

MIKE: Oh yes, it is still quite busy.

PS: **When** is it busier, during the day or at night-time?

MIKE: Daytime, I suppose. Lots of people drive up and down to school and there is that big office block at the top of our road.

PS: But you aren't so worried about your cat going out in the daytime even though the road is busier?

MIKE: No, I'm not so worried during the daytime.

PS: **When** would she be more likely to be hit by a car?

MIKE: Don't know. I hadn't really thought about it.

PS: Yeah, I know, sometimes we just end up with an idea in our heads. But now we are thinking about this, when would she be most likely to be hit by a car?

MIKE: I suppose it would be during the daytime when there are more cars about.

PS: I think I am a bit confused Mike. It sounds as if your cat is more likely to be knocked over during the daytime and yet you keep her locked in at night. Is there something else we need to think about, or can you help me make sense of this?

MIKE: Well there isn't anything else I am worried about, but this doesn't really make sense. I hadn't thought about the road being busier during the daytime before.

PS: Now we know that, does it help you to think about this differently?

MIKE: It tells me that if she is safe being out during the daytime, then I suppose she should also be safe at night-time.

This example highlights how the Socratic dialogue helped Mike to evaluate and reappraise his assumption that 'if I lock my cat in at night then she won't get knocked down by a car'. This assumption was based upon the premise that night-time was more dangerous than during the day. The questioning process used clear and specific 'what', 'when', and 'how' questions which Mike was readily able to answer. The questions remained focused upon helping Mike to attend to new information that highlighted how his cat would be more likely to be hit by a car during the day rather than at night. In turn, this helped him to challenge his assumption that he needed to lock his cat in at night and to reassess his behavior.

In terms of process, the interview progressed through the first stage of identifying Mike's assumption and the feelings and behaviours associated with it. Using emphatic listening and summarising, Mike's understanding of events was checked and he was helped to consider new information that he had overlooked. Finally, he was helped to synthesise this new information and to reappraise his assumption.

Common difficulties

It becomes an unpleasant question-and-answer inquisition

A Socratic dialogue is constructed around many clinician-initiated questions. If not undertaken sensitively, it can feel like a question-and-answer session, with the clinician acting as an inquisitor, firing question after question for the young person to answer. With younger children, this form of questioning may be associated with past situations where they have done something wrong, or with adolescents, where they have needed to justify themselves. The inevitable outcome of such a process will be to alienate the child or young person and to make them become increasingly defensive and passive. Adolescents may, for example, appear irritated and refuse to talk; they may lose interest, become bored, and stop participating in the dialogue. Younger children may become worried, concerned about whether they are providing the 'right' answer.

It is important that this potentially unpleasant situation be avoided. A gentle, curious approach can reduce the possibility of an inquisition. Summarising provides a useful break from questions and can take the form of a fun activity where the conversation can be drawn or written on a blackboard/whiteboard or a piece of paper. Similarly, the Socratic dialogue could be conducted over more than one session. If the process feels uncomfortable, then stop and break it up.

If these problems continue, then this needs to be directly raised and discussed with the young person. The need to ask questions to understand how the young person views events and experiences should be highlighted. Clarifying that there is no right answer and that there are many ways of looking at and understanding events might be reassuring. The emotional reactions of the young person should be acknowledged and lead into a discussion about how the process can be made more comfortable. Finally, if the Socratic dialogue results in the young person continuing to appear angry, bored, or worried, then examine the way therapy is being undertaken. Consider whether it remains collaborative, fun, and relaxed and whether it is being undertaken at an appropriate speed. Pacing is an important consideration so that the potentially unpleasant quickfire question-and-answer cycle is avoided.

The young person can't understand or answer the questions

The aim of the Socratic dialogue is to help the young person discover and explore their thoughts, feelings, and behaviour. There will, however, be times during any interview when the young person seems unable to find or access the information to answer questions. If this becomes a repeated problem, it may be useful to reflect upon the dialogue and whether the young person has the information or knowledge to answer the questions. This is particularly important with younger children, who may find complex, more abstract or open questions difficult. At these times, it may be better to experiment with more concrete and narrowly defined questions. These may help to ground the child and place your question in a context to which they can relate. Thus, instead of asking a very general question such as 'How would you like things to be different?', you may want to ask a series of more defined questions such as, 'What would you like to start doing?', 'Would you like to go to any new clubs?', 'What would change at school?', 'How would mum be different?'

If the young person still finds it hard to answer, then try to be even more specific, 'Would you like to have more friends, see your friends more often, or play outside more?' This presents the young person with firm options whilst highlighting that there can be more than one answer. It also gives them opportunities to say 'No, this does not apply to me.' Alternatively, consider actively involving a parent or other family member in the discussion and ask them to suggest some ideas. However, this needs to be carefully monitored to ensure that the young person has genuine opportunities to express their own views rather than simply agreeing with the options that are being provided by others.

Can't synthesise new information

Some young people may engage in the Socratic dialogue, but it becomes a detached rationale exercise that does not lead them to the final step of reflection and reappraisal. New and challenging information is identified but is viewed as somewhat separate and is not synthesised into the young person's cognitive construction of their world.

Persistence and patience are required as the young person is helped to discover more information and their attention is brought back to what they have overlooked. Reviews and summaries are useful to capture new information and to reflect on what has been discovered. Non-verbal summaries can be included in each session and provide a powerful and objective way of highlighting important information. They should be followed by a discussion in which the young person is encouraged to reflect on this information. Regularly asking the young person to reconsider their cognitions in light of this new knowledge provides opportunities for the old and new information to be integrated and cognitions to be reappraised.

Facilitates self-discovery through alternative perspective taking and attending to new or overlooked information

Perspective taking

To counter the inherent self-selection and subjective bias that underpins many generalisations, young people can be helped to consider their cognitions from a different perspective. The introduction of a third-party perspective promotes objectivity and helps the young person to distance themselves from the emotional component of their cognitions whilst allowing them to recognise and acknowledge alternative and possibly conflicting views. For example:

▶ A young person who regularly describes themselves as a 'failure' may be asked to consider whether their best friend would see them in this way (TGFB p130). What might they say if they heard them using such a statement?

If the young person was unable to consider this from a different perspective, they could be encouraged to 'check it out' as the task is developed into a behavioural experiment (TGFB p185; TGFG p141). In the above example, the young person could ask those people they value and feel safe talking with to identify what they thought the young person was good at. The positive focus upon success is a direct challenge to the belief of being a 'failure' and will help the young person to recognise that their negative generalisation may have limitations. This may help the young person to put limits around their universal definitions and to define their 'failure' more specifically, for example, 'I often fail my maths test at school.' This allows them to develop alternative cognitions about different events, for example, 'I often win races with the local swimming team.'

Responsibility pies

In addition to providing a means of assessment, 'responsibility pies' (TGFB p 187) also provide a visual way of exploring different perspectives of the same event. Each person can be asked to identify all the factors that might have contributed to an event and then to consider how much each contributed to the overall outcome. If a factor is considered to have a major effect upon the outcome, then it is assigned a large slice of the responsibility pie, whereas more minor factors will have smaller slices.

Case Study Joshua's accident

Joshua's was recently involved in a car accident and drew a responsibility pie for what had happened (Figure 6.1). The pie clearly highlighted how Joshua saw himself as the major reason for the accident. From Joshua's perspective, he thought that the accident would have been unlikely if he had been ready for school on time and hadn't been arguing with his mother.

Once Joshua's attributions about the accident had been identified, it was possible to compare his understanding with that of his mother, who was driving (Figure 6.2). Joshua's mother attributed the accident to the other

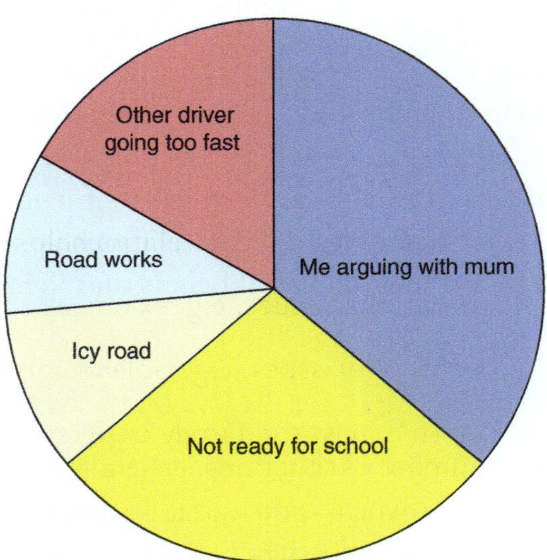

Figure 6.1   Joshua's responsibility pie for the car crash.

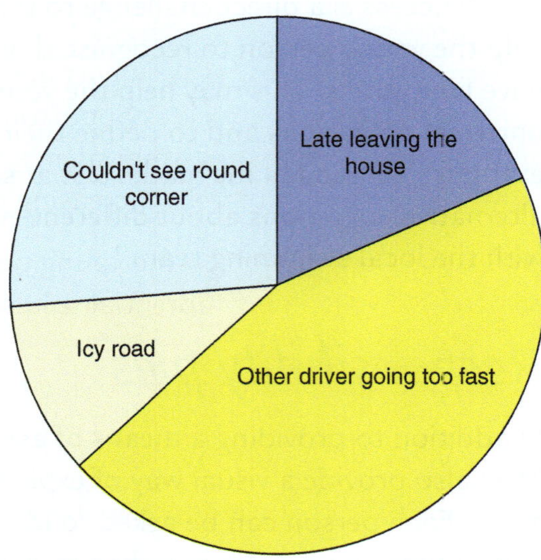

Figure 6.2   Joshua's mother's responsibility pie for the car crash.

driver going too fast around a corner on an icy road. Although she also recognised that she was late leaving the house, she did not identify the argument with her son as a contributing factor. Joshua's mother described that she was late because she was collecting the washing so that she could set the washing machine running before they left. This provided a visual and objective way of testing Joshua's attributions and of helping him to reappraise his understanding and to reduce his personal responsibility for the accident.

Attends to overlooked information

A second way of limit setting is to help the young person attend to new information, past experiences, or events that they may have overlooked. A young person who believes that people are unkind and want to hurt them may be helped to consider previous times when this has occurred. This may help them to discover that the bullying they experienced was confined to a small and specific group of children. Similarly, exploration of current events might highlight examples where friendships have developed, and kind acts have occurred (TGFB p67). This helps to establish some appropriate limits around their universal beliefs that 'people are unkind'.

Analogical comparisons

In a number of situations, generalisations are made based on one observed similarity, which is then used to assume the presence of other factors that have not been identified. For example, a young person may have experienced some episodes of bullying that led them to believe that people are unkind. This belief is then generalised to other situations where they encounter other young people.

Analogical comparisons help the young person attend to a broader range of information. They help them to identify important differences between events by mapping the conceptual structure of the young person's ideas on to another set of ideas taken from a different domain. These two events or situations are then compared on several relevant but not immediately obvious variables. Thus, young people can be helped in a concrete manner to develop new and wider perspectives by looking beyond single or surface similarities (e.g. all other young people) in order to identify and understand some of the other factors that may result in them being unkind (e.g. familiarity, gender, age, nature of their relationship, etc.).

Analogical comparisons can be developed using metaphors. For example, the young person who assumes that others are unkind could be helped to think about cars. Whilst most cars share several observable similarities, it is only once the door and bonnet are opened that the differences become clear. Young people may therefore look similar, but it is only once you get to know them (get inside or lift the bonnet) that you discover that some are nicer or better than others. Metaphors such as this can be used to broaden the young person's perspective and to challenge universal definitions.

Systematically testing the assumed relationship

Young people make assumptions about the relationship between events, where one event is assumed to be the cause of another. A young person with obsessive-compulsive disorder (OCD) may, for example, assume that they will cause their parents to be involved in an accident if they do not repeat a set of words or carry out some form of compulsive behaviour to prevent this happening. In these situations, it can be useful to systematically test this assumed relationship. This can be achieved through causal reasoning, which involves a logical analysis of these assumptions by either confirming or disproving the assumed relationship. For the young person with OCD, confirmation would involve exploring both aspects of the assumed relationship, that is, firstly, whether performing the ritual prevented accidents, and, secondly, whether failure to perform them resulted in accidents happening. This could be undertaken as a behavioural experiment, where the young person checked whether:

▶ performing the rituals made the parents safe. The young person might predict that their parents would not have had any accidents since they started their compulsive behaviour. Is this the case?

▶ not performing the rituals results in accidents. The young person might predict that accidents would occur if they did not engage in their rituals. Have the parents been involved in an accident when the young person forgot or did not engage in their rituals?

Disconfirmation would involve an exploration of the range of factors that could cause an accident that are independent of whether the ritual was undertaken.

This can be undertaken by detailing the multiple steps that would need to occur before the young person's prediction could possibly come true. A useful visual way of undertaking this is through an exercise such as the Chain of Events, which details all the links in the chain that need to be in place before the event could possibly happen. If one of the many links is missing, the chain is broken.

Case Study Marla worries she will pass germs to others

Marla (11) had OCD and feared that she would be responsible for infecting other people and that they would die. She engaged in a variety of compulsive behaviours in order to neutralise these thoughts. Inductive reasoning was undertaken using the Chain of Events to highlight some of the many steps that would be involved before this could possibly happen. Figure 6.3 is the Chain of Events that was constructed with Marla.

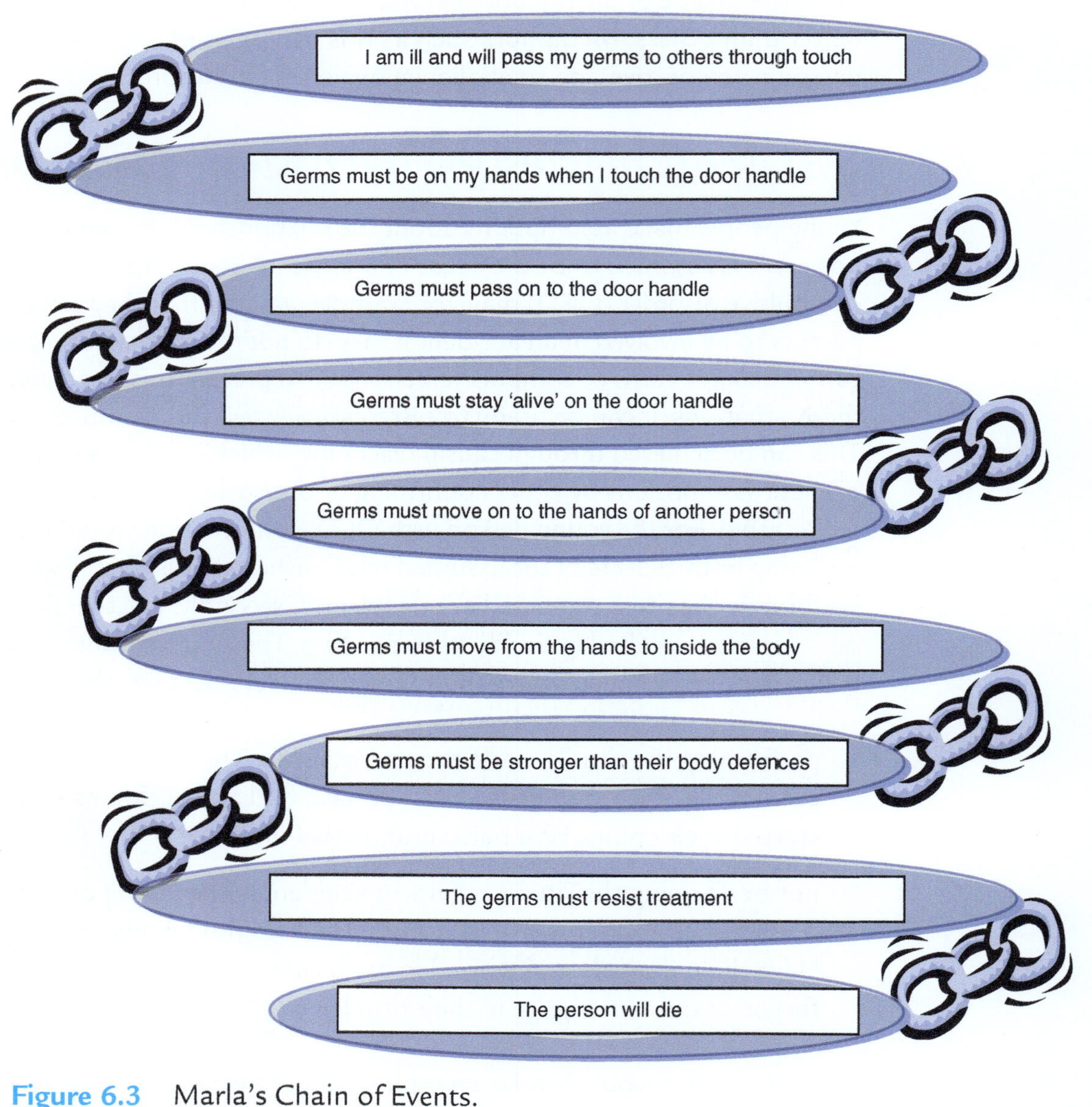

Figure 6.3 Marla's Chain of Events.

Evaluates beliefs, assumptions, and cognitions through behavioural experiments or prediction testing

An objective way of evaluating cognitions is to 'check them out' through behavioural experiments. Experiments are powerful ways of objectively seeking new information. Younger children can be encouraged to act as a scientist, Private I (Friedberg & McClure 2002), Social Detective (Spence 1995), or Thought Tracker (Stallard 2002a) who sets out to discover information to test their cognitions.

Behavioural experiments are practical ways to test whether beliefs and assumptions are always true, to discover alternative explanations for events or what might happen if things were done differently. Experiments can therefore help to put limits around overarching general definitions or to provide new information to assimilate into the cognitive framework. Bennett-Levy et al. (2004) identified different types of behavioural experiments.

Cognition- and prediction-testing experiments

These are monitoring or observational experiments to check out a young person's beliefs, predictions, or thoughts. For example, a young person who has a belief that they 'have no friends' could be asked to monitor any telephone calls, texts, or WhatsApp or Instagram messages they receive over the course of a week. If they had no friends, they would predict receiving no messages.

Experiments to test what happens if they behave differently

Experiments can test a young person's beliefs or assumptions by investigation of what happens if they behave differently. For example, a young person could experiment by running on the spot to test whether an increase in their heart rate is a sign of exercise rather than a signal that they 'are having a heart attack'. Similarly, a young person with social anxiety may be asked to drop their 'safety behaviour' of not looking at someone to discover what happens if they behave differently.

Information-gathering experiments

These experiments generate new information to check out a young person's beliefs or assumptions. These could involve actively searching for information that questions their core beliefs (TGFB p140) or Internet searches or surveys to gather new information (TGFB p150, p186).

Planning a behavioural experiment

When planning a behavioural experiment, it is important to adopt a curious approach and to keep an open mind. The aim is to 'check out what happens', not to consciously set out to disprove a young person's beliefs. Indeed, there will be occasions when the experiment supports and validates the belief. Information from the experiment, whatever the outcome, is helpful and can be used to inform what action may be required.

▶ The experiment of a young person with a belief that they have no friends may reveal that they have not been contacted by anyone over the course of the week. Waiting for other young people to contact them is therefore unlikely to help them develop friendships. The approach may therefore shift towards being more proactive and may involve an experiment to see what happens if the young person takes the initiative and reaches out to contact others.

Experiments need to be safe and to minimise the possibility of any harm coming to the young person.

▶ It may be helpful for a young person who has been verbally teased to experiment with being more assertive and being better at standing up for themselves. However, the possible adverse consequences of this need careful exploration before implementation.

Similarly, experiments with very unpredictable outcomes need to be carefully planned.

▶ It may be helpful for a young person to experiment with behaving differently in social situations. However, rather than experimenting in a large social group, a smaller, more predictable situation should be identified.

Finally, before embarking upon an experiment, it is important to check what support the young person may require and that all relevant parties are aware of and support the experiment. Without this support, the experiment may inadvertently be undermined.

When planning behavioural experiments, they should have a clear rationale and follow the following steps (TGFB p185).

▶ The cognition to be tested should be clearly specified and the strength of belief rated.

▶ The experiment should be clearly defined, and possible obstacles explored.

▶ The predicted outcome is identified.

▶ The actual outcome of the experiment is described.

▶ The young person is encouraged to reflect on what they have discovered and how this information might affect and change their cognitions.

Case Study Prediction-testing experiments: Caleb thinks he is a failure

Caleb (19) was feeling very depressed and had a strong belief that he was a failure. He generalised this belief to all aspects of his life, which resulted in him feeling unmotivated and reluctant to do things.

What thought or belief do you want to test?

▶ Caleb agreed to check out his belief that he 'is a failure', which he strongly believed, scoring it as 92 on a 1–100 scale.

What experiment could you undertake to test this?

▶ Possible experiments were explored, any obstacles identified, and it was agreed to focus on his work at college. Caleb agreed that he would keep a diary of the marks he was assigned for his next five pieces of college work.

What do you think will happen?

▶ Caleb thought that he was a failure and so wouldn't get a good grade for any of his work. He didn't think he would get a grade higher than a D.

What happened?

▶ Caleb failed two pieces of work (both maths). He was awarded two D grades (English and History) and a B grade in his sports assessment.

What have you found out?

▶ Caleb was encouraged to reflect on his results and to consider whether he was predicting things to be worse than they really were; whether there were times when he was not a failure and how he made sense of what happened. He was encouraged to think about whether there were some limits to his global belief of being a failure, for example, 'I struggle with my lessons but do well with sport.'

Has this changed your thought or belief?

▶ In the light of what happened, Caleb rated his belief again. He rated it as still very strong (90), arguing that what happened was unusual. Caleb was therefore encouraged to check this out again and record his next 10 college grades.

Case Study Active experiments: Laura's social anxiety

Laura (14) felt anxious in social situations, which she avoided. If she did participate, she engaged in many 'safety behaviours' designed to reduce her anxiety. Laura rarely spoke and, if she did, spoke in a very quiet voice. She was very self-focused, constantly monitoring what she said, fearing that she was boring and that people would laugh at her.

What thought or belief do you want to test?

▶ Laura agreed to test her thought that her 'safety behaviours helped her to feel less anxious'. She believed they did and rated her belief on a 1–100 scale as 85.

What experiment could you undertake to test this?

▶ Laura agreed to an experiment at the clinic where she engaged in a brief conversation with an unfamiliar member of staff. In one conversation, she would engage in her safety behaviours, and in the other she would explore what happened when she spoke more, in a louder voice, and focused on the conversation, not how she was performing. The conversations would be videotaped.

What do you think will happen?

▶ Laura thought that she would feel much more anxious if she didn't use her safety behaviours.

What happened?

▶ Laura looked at the videotapes and was surprised to see that she communicated better when she dropped her safety behaviours. She rated how anxious she felt in both situations and felt more anxious (rated 80) when she engaged in her safety behaviours that when she didn't (rated 50).

What have you found out?

▶ Laura was surprised to discover that her safety behaviours made her feel more anxious.

Has this changed your thought or belief?

▶ Laura's belief that her safety behaviours helped her to feel less anxious reduced to a rating of 50. Further work helped Laura to externally focus on the conversation and to reduce her critical self-focused internal evaluation.

Case Study Information gathering experiments: Adam's formulation

Adam (nine) was referred because of anxiety and panic attacks at school. These occurred at lunchtime and resulted in Adam refusing to eat or drink throughout the school day.

During the assessment it emerged that Adam was very concerned about his appearance. He wore designer clothes, had highlights in his hair, and took a great deal of care over his appearance. He commented that when he sat at the table at lunchtime, he often thought the other children stared at him. When asked why they were looking at him, Adam commented that they probably thought 'I looked ugly' or that there was 'something wrong with me'. Adam reported several anxiety symptoms at lunchtime, particularly a dry throat, racing heart, shortness of breath, and sweating. When Adam noticed these, he felt unable to eat his lunch and wanted to leave the dining hall. The formulation in Figure 6.4 was developed to explain what was happening.

Adam did not think this was right and produced an alternative formulation (Figure 6.5). He described how he liked to play football before eating his dinner. He ran around a lot chasing the ball and so felt hot, sweaty, and short of breath as he sat down to eat his dinner. He also had a dry throat and didn't want to eat his dinner, asking instead to go outside to cool down.

Adam's explanation made a great deal of sense. Whilst he did not make any reference to his cognitions, he did manage to integrate what was happening with his feelings and subsequent behaviour.

We discussed whether we could undertake an experiment to check out which of these provided the best explanation. Adam agreed to monitor

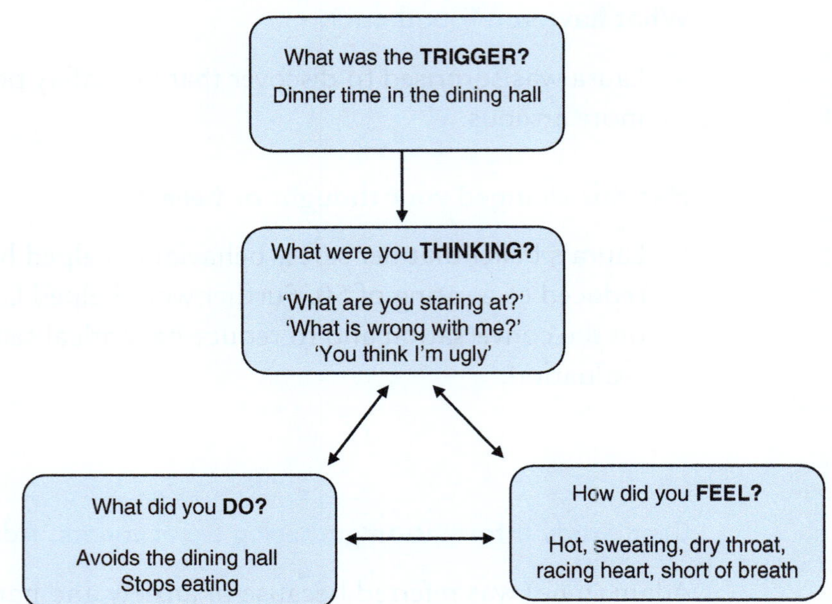

Figure 6.4   Adam's dining hall formulation.

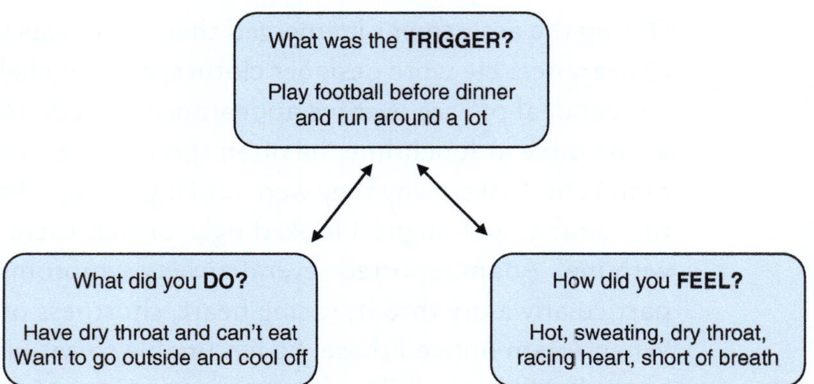

Figure 6.5   Adam's football formulation.

what happened on the next three wet playtimes. The children were not allowed outside when it rained and so Adam could not run around and play football. If Adam's explanation was right, then if he was unable to play football, he would not feel hot and would be able to eat his lunch. If he was still unable to eat his lunch, then there must be another explanation. The experiment showed that even though Adam had not played football he still did not eat his lunch. This led Adam to consider an alternative explanation.

CHAPTER SEVEN

E: Emotions

Demonstrates use of a variety of emotional techniques to facilitate therapeutic change

Work in the emotional domain aims to increase awareness of core emotions and to develop skills in emotional management. Emotional literacy is developed by understanding the body signals associated with each core emotion (happy, sad, anxious/stress, angry). Some body signals may be specific to particular emotions (e.g. tearful, swearing), whilst others (e.g. feeling hot) may be shared. Psycho-education helps the young person to discover that emotions do not randomly occur but are triggered by situations and events, what they think and what they do. This can empower the young person to take control of their emotions and to actively manage how they feel. Rather than living with their unpleasant feelings, young people are encouraged to use a range of strategies to help them feel better.

Develops emotional literacy by facilitating the identification of a range of emotions

Young people are often unaware of the different emotions they experience or may lump them together under general headings like feeling 'rubbish', 'stressed', 'OK', or 'mad'. Understanding different emotions is helpful and informs what the young person can do to help themselves feel better.

A Clinician's Guide to CBT for Children to Young Adults: A Companion to Think Good, Feel Good and Thinking Good, Feeling Better, Second Edition. Paul Stallard.
© 2021 John Wiley & Sons Ltd. Published 2021 by John Wiley & Sons Ltd.
Companion website: www.wiley.com/go/cliniciansguide2e

► Relaxation can help when a young person is feeling anxious or angry, but is less helpful if they are feeling sad.

► Behavioural activation can help when a young person is feeling sad, but may be less helpful if they are feeling anxious.

Emotional literacy is the ability to understand and express feelings. Whilst this is often taught in schools, it is useful to check the breadth of emotional vocabulary the young person has developed. This can be assessed in different ways.

► A series of photographs or flashcards of different facial expressions can be used to 'name the emotion'.

► A series of situations can be presented, and the young person asked to describe how they would feel. For example, if they were:

  ► given some money or a special treat;

  ► told off by a teacher;

  ► not invited to a party;

  ► accused of something they had not done.

► Video clips of people in different situations can be shown and the young person asked how they might feel if they were in those situations.

► A 'feelings word search' (TGFG p158) can be used as an activity to name and find different feelings and to identify which the young person relates to.

► Colour 'my feelings' (TGFG p160) can be used with younger children to show the type and amount of the feelings they experience. The child is asked to assign a colour to each of their feelings and to then colour in an outline of a person to show the amount of each different feeling inside them. As they select a colour for each feeling, the child is asked to name the feeling it relates to.

Once the emotional labels have been generated, it is useful to clarify how the young person is using them. For example, a young person may use a label like 'wound up' or 'stressed' to describe feeling both anxious and angry. Clarification of meaning can also be extended to parents, who may misinterpret how the young person is feeling. For example, parents may perceive that a young person is angry when in fact that are feeling frightened and unable to cope.

In terms of the degree of emotional literacy, it is usually important that young people are able to identify and label the basic core emotions of happy, sad, angry, and anxious.

Helps to distinguish between different emotions and identifies key body signals

Body signals

Once there is a shared understanding of core emotional labels, the young person can be helped to identify their specific body signals. Worksheets can be used to prompt the young person to consider a range of possible signals and to identify which apply to them when they feel:

- down (TGFB p147), e.g. tired, comfort eat, cry, can't concentrate, difficulty sleeping;

- anxious (TGFB p148), e.g. racing heart, dry mouth, feel hot, butterflies in tummy;

- angry (TGFB p 149), e.g. raised voice, clench fists, grind teeth, red in the face.

The exercise can help the young person identify which body signals they particularly notice, and which are their strongest.

An alternative approach with younger children is to help them attend to three different ways that emotions are conveyed, that is, facial expression, body posture, and behaviour. Worksheets can be used for each of the core emotions of feeling sad (TGFG p161), angry (TGFG p162), anxious (TGFG p163), and happy (TGFG p164), where the young person draws or writes what happens. Once the emotions are defined, the young person can be asked to rate how much of the time they notice each feeling.

If undertaking emotional recognition in groups, these activities can be scaled up. For example, a young person can lie down and be drawn around to create a life-sized body shape. The group can then draw on body signals relating to each emotion. Alternatively, this can be made into a game with younger children, where each child who notices a particular signal can be asked to stand up or move to a certain part of the room. Group activities like this help children to consider a number of possible body signals and to identify those that are most common and those that are shared by different emotions.

Feeling diaries

A key task is to help the young person understand that emotions are not random events but are triggered by specific situations, events, and thoughts.

With younger children, worksheets can be used to link different feelings with places (TGFG p159) or to identify the important places, people, and activities in the child's life that are associated with pleasant and unpleasant feelings (TGFG p157). Young people can be encouraged to keep a feeling diary (TGFB p151). Whenever they notice a strong feeling, they are encouraged to briefly write down the day and time, how they felt, what they were doing, and what they were thinking. The completed diary can be reviewed, and common patterns explored to identify possible triggers for their emotions.

Case Study William feels sad

William noticed that he regularly had strong feelings of sadness. William thought these feelings were random and couldn't identify any particular pattern. He kept a feeling diary for one week and made entries as shown in Table 7.1.

The diary helped William to discover a pattern that his sad feelings were more likely to be triggered when he was on his own. Typically, they started soon after he woke, when he was in his bedroom. William recalled various unhelpful thoughts tumbling around his head, particularly about his schoolwork, worrying that he couldn't understand his maths and that he would fail his exams. The diary helped William discover that his feelings were not random but were associated with first thing in the morning and his worries about schoolwork.

Table 7.1 William's diary.

Day and time	How did you feel?	What were you doing?	What were you thinking?
Monday morning	Tearful, tired, wanted to cut myself.	Just woken up, lying in bed.	'I can't get up and go to school.'
Tuesday morning	Tearful. Want to cut myself.	Just woken up, in bed.	'What's the point? I'm going to fail my exams anyway.'
Wednesday morning	Tearful and stressed.	Woke early (5.30), lying in bed.	'I haven't finished my work. I don't know what to do.'
Friday morning	Tearful and sad.	Lying in bed.	'I don't understand my maths work. I don't know what to do.'

Emotional logs

Emotional monitoring can help young people notice that feelings and their intensity change throughout the day (TGFB p152). At agreed predefined times, the young person is asked to rate the strength of the dominant feeling they have experienced during that time block. The exercise can demonstrate that feelings change and help to identify particular times associated with stronger and weaker feelings. This is then explored to identify what the young person was doing. For example:

▶ Feelings of sadness may be stronger at tea and bedtime. Exploration may reveal that the young person usually takes themselves off to their room on their own and spends time worrying about the next day.

▶ Feelings of anxiety may be stronger at lunchtime. Exploration may reveal that the young person is in a large dining room and often sits on their own, worrying what to say if anyone approaches them.

▶ Feelings of anger may be stronger on a Tuesday morning or Wednesday afternoon. This may be related to a particular lesson where the young person feels picked on by the teacher.

Case Study Isabella feels down

Isabella was feeling down and reported feeling really depressed 'all the time'. She couldn't identify any variation in her mood and so kept a mood log for a week. Isabella rated how down she felt on a 1–10 scale (1 really down, 10 really happy) at set times each day (Table 7.2).

The diary showed that Isabella was feeling very down in her mood and that she never experienced any positive feelings greater than 4. However, the diary also showed that these feelings were stronger in the morning when she woke and started to worry about her day. They were also stronger after school before tea when Isabella isolated herself in her bedroom and ruminated about how bad her day had been. Understanding this led Isabella to experiment with activity rescheduling to see if this helped to improve her mood.

▶ Could she do something else when she woke in the morning instead of lying in bed listening to her worries? She enjoyed music, so could she listen to the radio?

▶ Could she sit downstairs after school with her mother and sister instead of isolating herself?

Table 7.2 Isabella's mood diary.

Day	Woke up	Mid-morning	Lunch	After school	Team time	Bed
Monday	1	3	2	2	4	2
Tuesday	1	4		2		2
Wednesday	1		2	1	4	2
Thursday	1		4	1	4	1
Friday	1	3	3	2	2	
Saturday	2	4	4		3	1

Develops emotional management skills such as relaxation, guided imagery, controlled breathing, calming activities

Emotional management involves developing a toolbox of skills the young person can use to manage and tolerate their unpleasant emotions. The concept of a toolbox highlights the need for different skills that can be used at different times and in different places.

► Physical activity and self-soothing may prove difficult to undertake whilst at school but can be used at home.

► Diaphragmatic breathing can be readily used in many situations.

The process starts by identifying the techniques the young person is currently using to manage their emotions. They may already have some effective methods which could be enhanced. For example, a young person may count to three, a technique that could be developed into diaphragmatic breathing. They may also identify ways of managing unpleasant emotions such as gaming, self-harm, or, with older adolescents, drinking alcohol, smoking, or drug misuse, which need to be questioned. The potential risks, benefits, and limitations of these methods should be explored, and the young person encouraged to experiment with some alternative methods to manage their distress.

Progressive muscle relaxation

For young people presenting with arousal problems such as anxiety, anger, or physiological problems such as headaches, relaxation training can be a helpful way of reducing the unpleasant physiological symptoms they experience. Relaxation training induces a physiological state (relaxation) that is incompatible with the stress response and is a core component of many CBT programmes for young people (King et al. 2005).

Progressive muscle relaxation involves systematically tensing and releasing muscles in each of the major muscle groups until all tension in the body has been eliminated. The process helps to increase awareness of tension and to identify those parts of the body most affected.

Progressive muscle relaxation should initially be taught and practised together. This provides an opportunity to ensure that the young person is able to engage in the exercises and to address any problems they might encounter. After relaxation, the young person can be encouraged to reflect on the process (e.g. where they noticed most tension, any exercises they found difficult) and to rate their tension before and after to identify any change (TGFG p166). All new skills require practice, and in order to gain maximum benefit, the young person should be encouraged to practise relaxation at home (TGFB p161). The young person should be encouraged to do this when they notice that they are tense or when preparing for something that will be stressful. Alternatively, a good way of building this into their everyday routine is to practise relaxation as part of their night-time routine before they go to bed each night.

Relaxation should be introduced to the young person as a skill that is widely used by many athletes, celebrities, musicians, and television and film stars. As with all new skills, they need to practise, and initially the young person may not notice any significant benefits. To avoid disappointment, the young person should be prepared for this possibility, with the focus of the initial sessions being on learning how to do it rather than experiencing significant emotional change.

When at home, the young person should find a quiet, comfortable place that is free from distractions. They should turn their phone off and choose a time when they will not be interrupted for 10 minutes. They can sit in chair or lie on a bed or the floor, whichever they find most comfortable and convenient. They can choose to shut their eyes or keep them open as they focus on the process of systematically tensing and relaxing each major muscle group in turn.

Each muscle group should be tensed enough so that the young person notices the tension, but not tensed so hard that they might hurt themselves. After tensing for five seconds, the muscle is relaxed and the tension is released. As they do this, the young person is encouraged to focus on the difference between tension and relaxation and the feeling of calm as they release the tension. Each muscle group should be tensed twice before moving to the next. After tensing all muscle groups, the young person can be encouraged to take a few minutes to enjoy the feeling of relaxation.

There are various commercially available relaxation guides that provide instructions for relaxation. It is a matter of personal taste which to choose. One approach (TGFB p 154) guides the young person from their feet to the top of their head through the following muscle groups:

▶ feet and toes

▶ legs

▶ thighs

▶ stomach

▶ arms and hands

▶ back

▶ neck and shoulders

▶ face

A quicker form of relaxation (TGFB p155) can combine muscle groups to tense and relax as follows:

▶ arm and hands

▶ legs and feet

▶ stomach

▶ shoulders and neck

▶ face

For younger children, relaxation exercises can be made into a game (TGFG p177) such as 'Simon Says', where the child follows the instructions they are given.

▶ Back, arm, and leg muscles are tensed as the child is asked to march like a soldier.

▶ Leg muscles are tensed by running on the spot.

▶ Arms and stomach muscles are tensed by stretching up to the sky and pretending to be a tall tree with branches waving in the wind.

▶ Face muscles are tensed by making a scary face.

▶ All major muscles are then tensed by rolling up tightly into a ball.

Finally, the tension is released as the child is asked to become a big heavy elephant moving as slowly as possible before they lie on the ground to become a sleepy lion who has to stay as still as they can.

Calming imagery

Relaxing imagery is a helpful way to control anxious or unpleasant feelings. The process starts by asking the young person to imagine and describe their restful, calming, or happy place (TGFB p163; TGFG p178). The calming place can be either a real or an imaginary place, but somewhere the young person associates with pleasant feelings. To develop the image, the young person is asked to describe it, draw it, or bring a photograph of it. The aim is to create a vivid, powerful, multi-sensory image by helping the young person to attend to each of their senses in turn.

- What do you see? – Describe the scene, the colours, shapes, and size of the core features in the scene.

- What do you feel? – Can you, for example, imagine feeling the hot sand on your feet, the cold water on your face, or the icy snow on your hands?

- What can you smell? – Imagine the smell of the salty water, hamburgers cooking on a BBQ, or the scent of the pine forest.

- What can you hear? – Imagine the sounds of seagulls screeching, waves crashing on the beach, trees rustling in the wind.

- What can you taste? – Imagine salty water from the sea on your lips or the sweet taste of ice cream melting in your mouth.

The image is developed in detail and practised until the young person can generate their relaxing, calming, multi-sensory image. Once the image has been achieved, the young person is encouraged to imagine their calming place when they notice themselves feeling anxious or stressed to counter any unpleasant feelings.

Case Study Aisha's calming image

Aisha had severe asthma. When she had an asthma attack, she became very anxious, which affected her breathing and made her attack worse. Aisha created a calming image, which involved a café her mother's friend ran in a little seaside town.

- Aisha was firstly helped to describe the image.

  - 'The cafe is in a little courtyard behind the shops. There are three tables outside where people can sit. As you walk into the café, there are five more tables and then a counter where you could buy all sorts of drinks and cakes.'

► Aisha was given a number of prompts that helped her **visualise** the inside of the café in detail.

  ► 'Is there anything on the tables?' – 'Yes, on each table is a red and white checked tablecloth. There is a white sugar bowl and a red flower in a vase.'

  ► 'Are there any windows or curtains?' – 'Yes, the whole of the front of the café is glass so you can look out. At each window are red and white checked curtains.'

► Aisha was helped to attend to touch and to notice what **she felt**.

  ► 'What do the seats feel like?' – 'They are wooden seats, no cushions, they feel hard to sit on.'

► Aisha was prompted to **listen** for any sounds.

  ► 'There is a stream outside and you can hear the water rushing past. Inside, people are talking and there is music playing in the background.'

► Aisha was prompted to identify any **smells**.

  ► 'The whole place smells of freshly ground coffee.'

► Aisha was prompted to identify any **tastes**.

  ► 'Can you buy any cakes?' – 'You can buy homemade scones, fruit-cake, carrot cake, and a wonderful chocolate fudge cake.'

  ► 'What is your favourite?' – 'The chocolate cake.'

  ► 'And what does it taste like?' – 'It has sweet, soft chocolate fudge on top. It is soft and sticky and tastes wonderful.'

Diaphragmatic (controlled) breathing

Shallow breathing and shortness of breath are common symptoms of the anxiety response. Abdominal or belly breathing is a method of countering this by deeply breathing using the diaphragm, the large muscle at the base of the lungs. This helps to slow down breathing, reduce heart rate, and helps the body to relax.

It is a simple and quick method which can be used in many different situations when the young person needs to release their tension and regain control. Young people can be asked to imagine a large balloon in their belly which they have to slowly fill and empty. They are asked to place one hand on their stomach and to slowly breathe in through their nose to fill the balloon. They will notice the hand on their stomach rise as the balloon fills. Once it is full, they are asked to slowly breathe out through their mouth and to notice the balloon empty and their stomach fall. This is repeated three or four times as the young person regains control of their breathing and begins to relax.

Controlled breathing is another method used to slow down rapid shallow breathing and to regain control. When the young person notices their breathing becoming fast and shallow, they are instructed to try 4-5-6 breathing (TGFB p 156; TGFG p 171). The young person breathes in through their nose to the count of 4, holds their breath to the count of 5, and then slowly breathes out through their mouth to the count of 6. This is repeated three or four times until the young person has regained control of their breathing.

For young children, controlled breathing can be practised by asking them to imagine blowing out candles on a birthday cake one by one. The child needs to breathe in through their nose. As they hold their breath, they need to select one candle and to carefully take aim. They then breathe out slowly through their mouth to extinguish the candle. The process is then repeated.

Change the feeling

The idea of changing the feeling encourages the young person to actively do something to feel better. Often, people notice symptoms of strong unpleasant feelings like anxiety or depression but do little to regain control and change them. Rather than allowing the feelings to be in control, the young person is encouraged to actively change the feeling and to make themselves feel better.

- If feeling tense, do something to relax. For example, a long bath, listen to music, read a book, draw, or paint.

- If feeling unhappy, do something to cheer yourself up. For example, watch an episode of your favourite box set, paint your nails, make a drink of hot chocolate, or play with your pet.

- If feeling angry, do something to calm down. For example, hit a cushion or punch bag, pop bubble wrap, go for a walk, play an instrument.

A worksheet (TGFB p164) can be used to help the young person identify activities that are associated with pleasant feelings. This can remind the young person what they can do when they feel strong unpleasant feelings in order to change that feeling.

Develops emotional management skills such as physical activity, letting feelings go, emotional metaphors, and imagery

Physical activity

For some young people, physical activity offers a natural way of systematically tensing their muscles and then releasing that tension. Obviously, this can only be undertaken in certain situations, but there may be opportunities to build physical activity into their daily routine.

- A young person enjoyed cycling and found it helped him to relax. When he came back from school feeling tense, he experimented to see if a short, brisk cycle ride helped him to unwind.

- A young person discovered that she always felt more relaxed after she had taken her dog for a walk. When she noticed herself feeling tense, she took her dog for a quick walk.

Physical activity does not necessarily mean sport. There are other physical things, such as doing a dance routine, going for a walk, cleaning the bedroom, washing the car, or walking to the shops, that could be tried (TGFB p162: TGFG p179). The young person needs to identify the physical activities that work for them.

Let the feeling go

Strong emotions can be frightening for young children. A way of helping them to let go of their unpleasant feelings is to show them how to externalise them and put them somewhere safe, like a feeling 'strong room' (TGFG p175). The child is encouraged to make a 'safe' or 'strong room' out of a box and to decorate it how they wish. Whenever they are troubled by strong emotions, they are encouraged to externalise the feeing by drawing a picture or naming the feeling on a piece of paper. The feeling is separated from the child and the paper is then placed in the strong room, where it can be kept safe. The strong room can be periodically opened, and the unpleasant feelings reviewed with someone the child can trust.

Emotional metaphors

Metaphors provide a useful way of helping young people to understand their emotional build-up. For young people with anger issues, the anger volcano (TGFG p176) is a familiar way to discuss their anger outbursts. The metaphor can help the young person to plot the stages their volcano goes through before they blow their top. They are helped to attend to their thoughts, emotions, behaviours, and experiences at different stages of their anger build-up, as in the following examples.

▶ Calm and relaxed: *Speak in a normal voice and volume, feel calm.*

▶ Irritated and annoyed: *Aware that people are winding me up. Feel hot.*

▶ Getting angry: *Grit teeth, clench fists, start to threaten. Think to myself 'I am going to hit you.'*

▶ Very angry but still in control: *Start to swear, go red in the face, not listening. Thinking to myself 'I am going to end this and have the last word.'*

▶ Start to lose control: *Become detached from what is going on, everything seems to happen in slow motion.*

▶ Blow your top: *Physically lash out, hit, kick, throw things.*

Once the signals in the anger build-up have been identified, the young person is encouraged to respond to symptoms at a lower level to initiate emotional strategies to prevent the volcano from blowing.

Emotive imagery

Emotive imagery provides a way of changing the nature of an anxiety- or anger-creating image to one that is more neutral. Emotive imagery was described by Lazarus & Abramovitz (1962) as 'those classes of imagery, which are assumed to arouse feelings of self-assertion, pride, affection, mirth and similar anxiety-inhibiting responses'. The young person is helped to develop adaptive emotional imagery that allows them to confront and overcome their problems. The image provides the young person with a method of countering any unpleasant emotions by changing the emotional content of problematic situations.

For example, emotive imagery can be used to change anxiety to laughter. This concept may be familiar to young people who have read the stories by J.K. Rowling about the boy wizard Harry Potter. In the third book, Harry is taught to overcome his biggest fears (e.g. Boggarts) with laughter. The frightening image is therefore changed to one that is humorous. Emotive imagery can transform a frightening image of a spider to one where the spider is wearing a ballet dancing tutu, big boots, and a silly hat.

Case Study Anthony's humorous image

Anthony (15) was often in trouble at school and was now in danger of being excluded. He was rude, would argue with the teachers, and, when he was corrected, became angry, throwing his bag and books around the classroom, kicking over desks, and walking out of the class. All of the major incidents occurred with one teacher. Anthony didn't like this teacher, who he felt unfairly picked on him. He entered these lessons expecting an argument and so was determined to have the first and last word. Anthony recognised that this wasn't helpful and was interested in exploring whether imagery could help him to remain calm.

During the assessment, Anthony mentioned that he had recently seen this teacher in a school pantomime dressed as an elf. He clearly found this image funny and was able to describe how his teacher was dressed in detail. We decided to experiment to see whether Anthony could use this image as a way of remaining calm so that he replaced his anger with humour. Anthony practised initiating the image and rehearsed how he could use it to keep calm. Anthony then conjured up the image as he walked into the classroom with this teacher or when he felt himself becoming angry. The humorous image provided a useful way of helping Anthony to remain calm. It was difficult for Anthony to become wound up or take what he perceived to be his teacher's critical comments seriously when he looked so ridiculous.

Develops emotional management skills such as self-soothing, mind games, and mindfulness

Self-soothing

An alternative approach to changing or reducing feelings is to learn to tolerate them. This encourages young people to look after and be kind to themselves by developing ways of self-soothing. This can be facilitated by focusing on each sense to identify those experiences that are soothing and pleasant.

▶ Smell – favourite perfume, soap, ground coffee, or scented candle.

▶ Touch – a smooth stone, soft toy, silky fabric, or warm bath.

▶ Taste – strong mint, tangy apple, or soft marshmallow.

▶ Sight – inspiring quotes, photographs of pleasant memories, or watching a fish tank.

▶ Sound – uplifting music, birds singing, or sounds of waves.

These can be collected into a soothing toolbox (TGFB p165), providing quick access to a range of materials that can be used whenever needed.

Mind games

This is distraction, a method of purposefully focusing attention away from unhelpful thoughts and unpleasant feelings. Focusing on unpleasant thoughts and feelings tends to make them worse. Instead, the young person directs attention from an internal focus (e.g. unpleasant thoughts and body signals) to an external focus (e.g. what is going on around them).

This can provide a short-term way of coping when a young person is feeling overwhelmed by their emotions or has an urge to act impulsively with unhelpful behaviours like self-harm. Mind games encourage the young person to stand back from their emotions and to focus their attention on something external. This can be anything that helps to maintain attention, such as:

▶ counting backwards from 175 in sevens;

▶ spelling their name or those of their friends backwards;

▶ naming an animal for each letter of the alphabet.

Mindfulness

An alternative approach to actively managing and changing unpleasant emotions is mindfulness. This is a method for focusing attention in a curious, non-judgemental way on what is happening here and now. When feeling emotionally overwhelmed, the young person is encouraged to notice but to stand back from their emotions as they learn to tolerate rather than change them.

The process of mindfulness can be developed through the steps summarised by the FOCUS acronym. This involves learning to focus (F) attention on the here and now as the young person learns to observe (O) what is happening in a curious (C) way. The young person is encouraged to use (U) all their senses as they suspend (S) judgement and observe how they feel in an open way.

The process helps the young person to notice feelings in a non-judgemental way. Feelings are not labelled as positive (e.g. happy, calm, or brave) or negative (e.g. angry, sad, or frightened), right or wrong. Instead, the young person simply notices how they are feeling with acceptance and curiosity. They learn to understand and accept their emotions rather than worrying about experiencing them or actively attempting to change them.

A helpful exercise is to 'let feelings float away' (TGFG p64). This involves the young person imagining that they are looking through a zoom lens on a camera as they actively focus their attention on their emotions.

▶ **Observe how you feel.** The young person is asked to direct their attention towards their emotions and to notice how they are feeling. They are encouraged to observe their body signals and to identify where in their body they notice each emotion.

▶ **Name the emotion.** The young person is encouraged to label the emotion but to detach themselves from it. Instead of 'I feel sad' or 'I feel angry', they are encouraged to note that 'this is sadness' or 'this is anger'.

▶ **Accept how you feel.** Rather than attempting to push this feeling away or to deny that it is happening, the young person is encouraged to step back and to accept how they feel. They learn to be aware of how they feel and to embrace their feelings with compassion and understanding.

▶ **Let feelings pass.** The young person can be helped to notice that their feelings come and go by imagining clouds floating in the sky or waves crashing on the beach. They can imagine writing the name of each feeling on a cloud or wave and watching as they float by or as each wave crashes on the beach. As one disappears, another cloud or wave takes its place.

▶ **Be curious.** The young person is encouraged to be curious and to explore what might be causing them to feel as they do. Rather than attempting to control how they feel, the young person embraces and accepts the feelings as passing emotions.

Talk with someone

Sometimes it can be useful to talk with someone else about how you are feeling (TGFB p166). Often, unhelpful thoughts and strong unpleasant emotions become stuck and keep rolling around in our minds and bodies. Talking with someone provides a way of redirecting attention away from these powerful feelings and can help the young person feel better.

▶ Who could the young person talk with and who makes them feel good? Encourage them to make a list of their 'feel good' people.

▶ What does the young person want to tell them? They may want to tell them how they are feeling or may prefer to talk about something else.

▶ What does the young person want them to do? Do they want them to change the feeling, to sort out their problems, or to listen and acknowledge how they are feeling?

▶ How will they contact them? Social media, text, email, call?

▶ When will they do this? Rather than putting this off, it can be helpful to set a date and time and talk as soon as possible.

F: Formulations

Develops a coherent understanding of relationships between events, cognitions, emotions, physiological responses, and behaviour

A formulation is a shared understanding of the onset and/or maintenance of the young person's presenting problems described within a cognitive behavioural framework. It is a prerequisite for any individual intervention. The formulation is developed collaboratively and evolves over time, with the emerging formulation being discussed, tested, and revised until a mutually agreed working model is agreed. The formulation is therefore dynamic and provides the explicit shared working hypothesis that directs and informs the specific content of the intervention.

Provides a coherent and understandable rationale for the use of CBT

Formulations are a useful alternative to static diagnostic classifications and provide a functional, coherent, and testable way of bringing together important variables that explain the onset of the young person's difficulties and/or current maintaining factors. The formulation is at the heart of good clinical practice and serves important functions.

For the young person, the formulation is the vehicle by which they understand and make sense of their difficulties. Individual symptoms, thoughts, behaviours, and experiences that often feel unconnected are brought together in an understandable way. The development of this shared understanding during the early stage of the intervention models the active, open, and collaborative process that will continue throughout therapy. The construction of the formulation also clearly acknowledges the importance of the information the young person and their carer possess and introduces the concepts of self-discovery and self-efficacy.

Clinically, the formulation is used to assess the onset and development of the young person's problems against theoretical explanatory models and provides the mechanism by which theory and practice are bound together (Butler 1998; Tarrier & Calam 2002). It provides the empirical model that directs and informs the content of the intervention and ensures that the intervention remains focused and effective. The formulation lies at the very heart of CBT and 'guides the practitioner in planning and delivering the right intervention, in the right way at the right point towards the collaboratively agreed goals for therapy' (Kuyken & Beck 2007).

The specific detail contained in the formulation will differ depending upon its purpose. For clinicians, different levels or types of cognitions may be important to specify and compare with theoretical models. This level of sophistication and analysis may not necessarily be required by young people or their parents/carers. They need enough information to be helpful without becoming overburdened by too much detail.

The formulation is developed in partnership. The young person provides the content and specific detail whilst the clinician provides the theoretical framework and structure which helps to organise this information. The process is descriptive, in which the young person describes in their own words their feelings and the meanings they attribute to events. This information is organised to highlight and explore the relationships between the core systems of the CBT model, that is, what was happening, what was the young person thinking, how did they feel, and what did they do? (TGFG p75). Formulations therefore educate the young person and their parents/carers about the cognitive model and provide the rationale for the intervention.

▶ The formulation may highlight that a young person engages in unhelpful ways of thinking resulting in them not doing things because they think they will be unsuccessful. The intervention might focus on challenging these thoughts to develop more balanced and helpful ways of thinking.

▶ The formulation might highlight that a young person experiences strong feelings of anxiety resulting in them avoiding situations. The intervention might focus on helping the young person to develop ways to manage and tolerate these feelings and to face the situations they are avoiding.

▶ The formulation might highlight that the young person spends a lot of time at home on their own. The intervention might focus on encouraging the young person to become busier so that they have less time to listen to their upsetting thoughts.

Once developed, the formulation should be diagrammatically summarised (Kuyken et al. 2008). This provides a powerful, permanent visual representation that can be referred to during each session and revised accordingly. The young person and their carers can take a copy home, which will allow them to reflect upon the accuracy of the formulation and to discuss and share it with others who did not attend the appointment. In addition, formulations can be empowering and facilitate the development of self-efficacy. By providing a coherent explanation of the current situation, the parent/carer and young person can begin to consider potential ways in which these unhelpful patterns can be changed.

The process of developing a formulation involves the elicitation and identification of relevant information which is then arranged according to a theoretical or explanatory model to understand the origins, development, and /or maintenance of the presenting problem (Tarrier & Calam 2002). A formulation therefore depends upon the careful identification and selection of key information. This process has the potential to become overly inclusive and complex as attempts are made to assimilate the wealth of information gathered during an assessment into a single formulation, resulting in everyone becoming overwhelmed and confused. This tendency should be avoided. As a guiding principle, formulations need to be simple so that they are readily understandable and do not exceed the cognitive capacity of the young person. The aim is therefore to provide the minimum amount of information necessary to helpfully summarise the problems and to provide the rationale for the intervention (Charlesworth & Reichelt 2004).

Provides a collaborative understanding of events which links thoughts, emotions, and behaviour (maintenance formulations)

Mini-formulations (two- or three-system models)

The simplest formulations focus on the associations between two (e.g. What was happening and how did you feel?) or three (e.g. What was happening, how did you feel, and what were you thinking?) of the core systems of the CBT model. These are particularly useful during the early stages of CBT when the young person and their parents/carers are new to the cognitive model. Their simplicity is helpful for young children, who may have a limited cognitive capacity and may initially find the abstract relationship between all the elements of the CBT cycle difficult to understand. Focusing upon each relationship in turn (i.e. cognitions and associated emotional reaction; emotional reaction and associated behavioural response) provides a simple, understandable, staged way of developing the model. Mini-formulations can then be joined together to develop a fuller formulation involving all core elements of the CBT model.

Case Study Rhiannon is unhappy and scared

A mini-formulation was used to help Rhiannon (8) understand how her worries about the other children at school resulted in her feeling frightened and playing on her own. The first step was to help Rhiannon describe what happened in the school playground during playtimes. This was summarised in the diagram in Figure 8.1.

Next, Rhiannon identified how she felt when she was in the school playground (Figure 8.2).

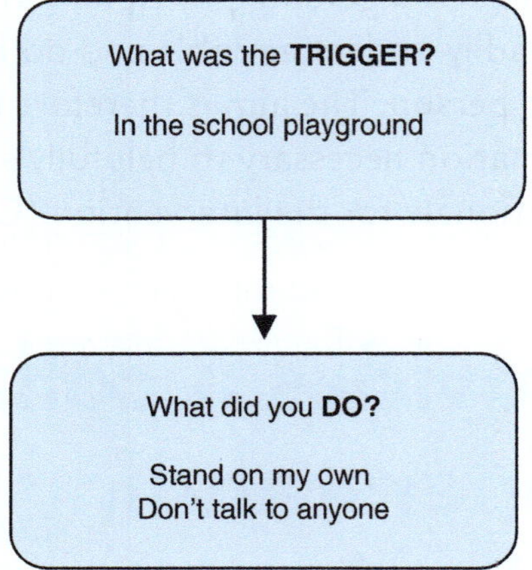

Figure 8.1   Rhiannon's situation and behaviour link.

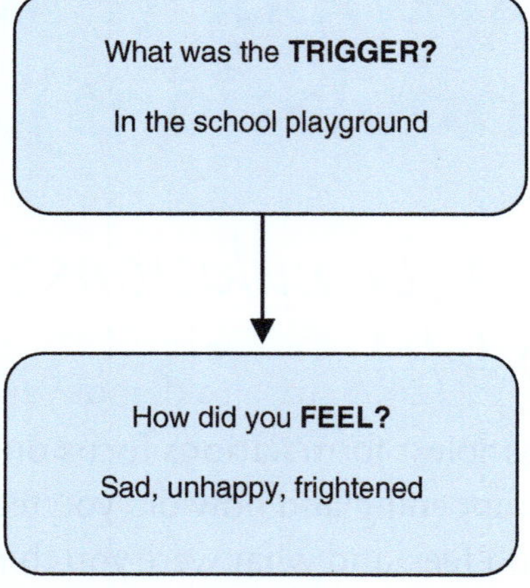

Figure 8.2   Rhiannon's situation and feelings link.

Rhiannon was helped to identify the thoughts that tumbled through her head when she felt sad and frightened in the playground (Figure 8.3).

These diagrams were then combined to provide a simple mini-formulation that highlighted the link between what Rhiannon thought, how she felt, and what she did in the school playground (Figure 8.4).

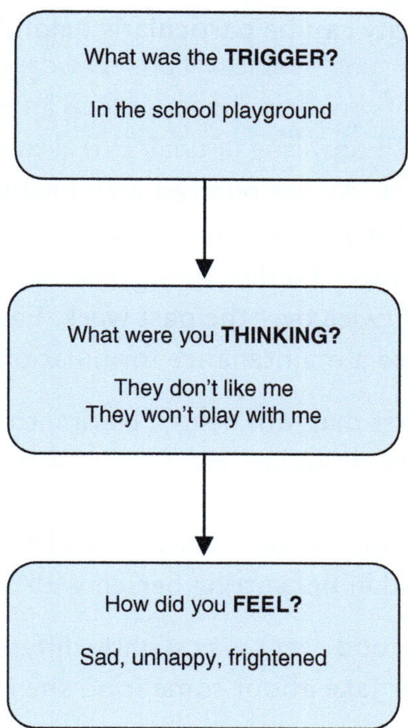

Figure 8.3 Rhiannon's thoughts and feelings link.

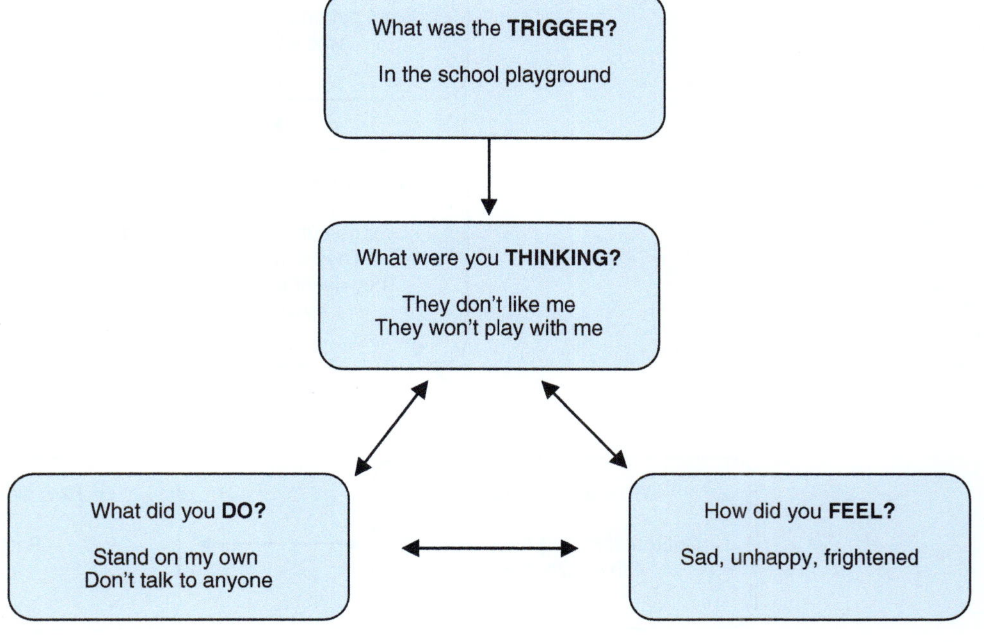

Figure 8.4 Rhiannon's mini-formulation.

Maintenance formulations

Maintenance formulations bring together the core elements of the CBT model: triggering event/situations, thoughts, feelings, and behaviour (TGFG p76). In many situations, young people are interested in understanding what is happening here and now. Simple maintenance formulations highlight the important relationships between thoughts, feelings, and behaviour, and their simplicity can be particularly helpful for younger children.

Case Study Naomi cuts herself

Naomi (14) was referred with problems of depression and self-harming. The self-harming involved Naomi cutting her arms and the top of her legs with a razor blade. During assessment, Naomi reported that she had cut herself twice over the past week. Each of these events was tracked to produce a maintenance formulation using the Negative Trap template.

This first diagram helped Naomi to recognise the importance of her negative thoughts. Her family went out together leaving Naomi at home on her own. Naomi found herself thinking that her parents 'didn't like her' and never took her out. These thoughts made Naomi sad and tearful and resulted in her cutting herself with a razor blade (Figure 8.5).

The second event was slightly different. Naomi had an argument with her brother Jake about some food she had eaten from the fridge. Jake was

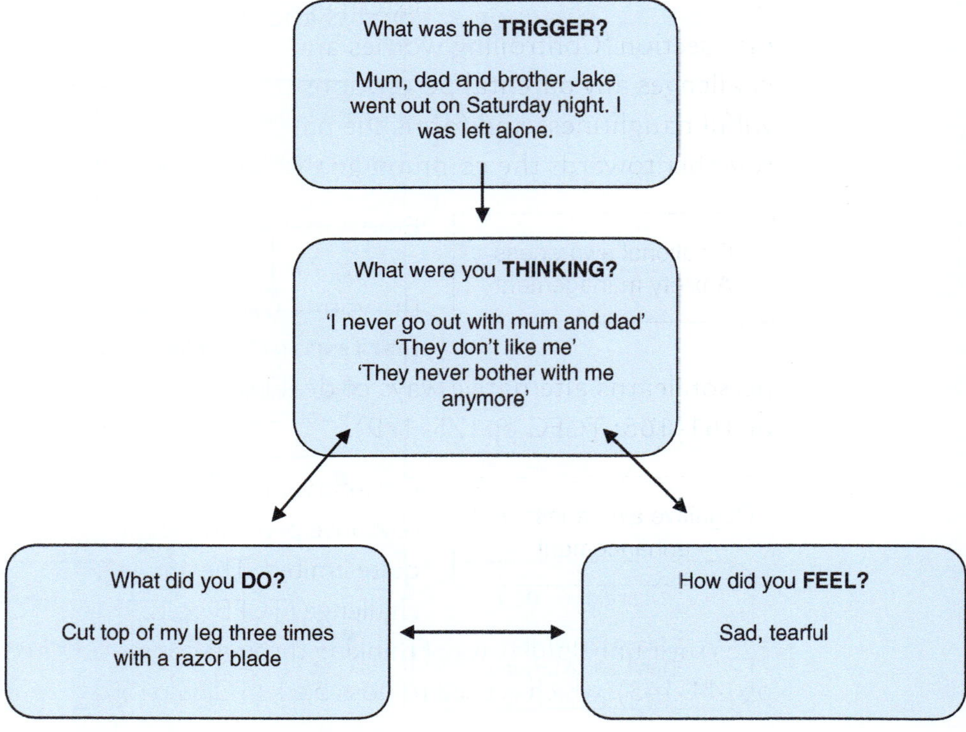

Figure 8.5   Naomi is at home on her own.

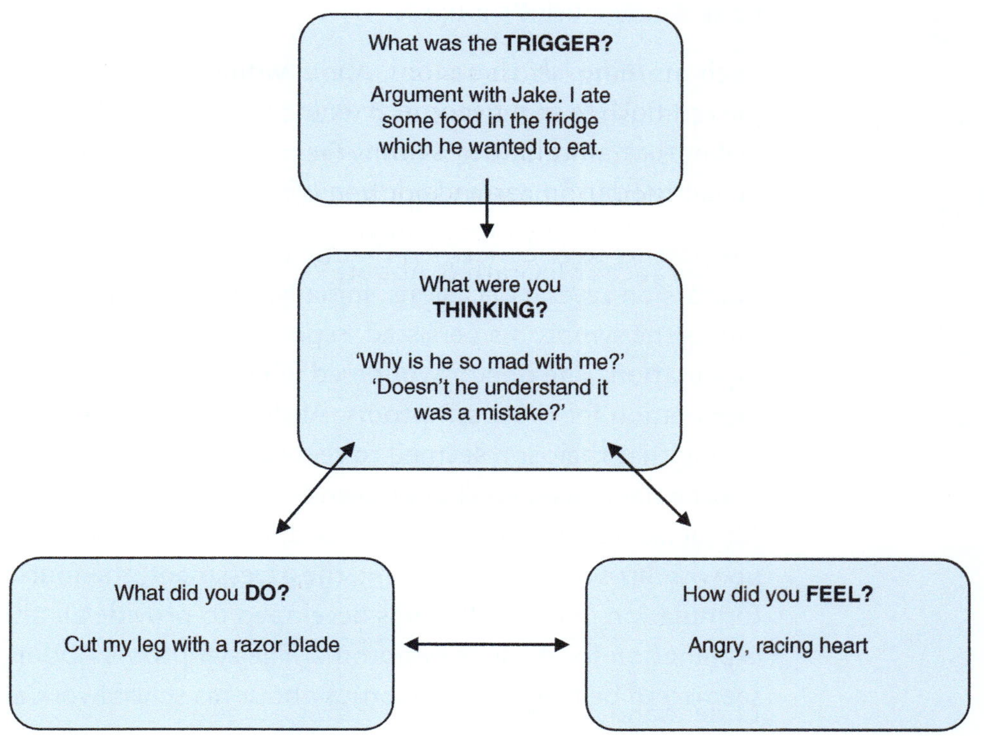

Figure 8.6   Naomi argues with her brother.

saving this food and was angry when he found that Naomi had eaten it. Whilst this was a mistake, Naomi found herself thinking that her brother 'hated her'. The argument and these thoughts made Naomi angry and resulted in her cutting herself (Figure 8.6).

Both these situations involved Naomi thinking that people (her parents and brother) didn't like her. The feelings these thoughts created were very strong but different (sad and anxious). This helped Naomi to understand how she found it difficult to tolerate and cope with any strong unpleasant feelings. The way she coped was to cut herself, with the physical pain taking away the emotional pain.

Four-system formulations

Combining emotions and physiological responses as feelings helps to keep the core model simple. However, in some situations, it can be helpful to differentiate between feelings (moods) and somatic symptoms (bodily changes). The formulation therefore starts with the trigger and adds a fourth system (symptoms) to the three systems previously identified (thoughts, feelings, and what you do). All systems interact with each other, giving rise to the name the 'hot cross bun' formulation (Greenberger & Padesky 1995). This can be particularly useful with young people if physiological symptoms are being perceived as signs of physical illness.

Case Study Abdul's anxiety

Each morning before school, Abdul would complain of feeling unwell. He looked flushed in his face and would complain of feeling hot, sweating, feeling sick, and having a funny feeling in his stomach. Because he seemed unwell, Abdul's parents kept him off school.

His parents were concerned that he was often ill and had taken him to the doctors on several occasions. Initially, the doctor put this down to a virus, but as the symptoms persisted, repeated tests could not find any medical explanation. The doctor wondered whether there might be a psychological explanation for these symptoms. Abdul's parents also wondered about this, noting that their son seemed to recover quickly if he stayed off school and that he never seemed ill at weekends or during school holidays. Although Abdul liked school and worked hard, he had been finding it difficult to keep up with his schoolwork. During the assessment, the four-systems formulation in Figure 8.7 was developed to provide an alternative explanation for Abdul's symptoms. The symptoms Abdul complained about seemed to be triggered by worries about his schoolwork and are common

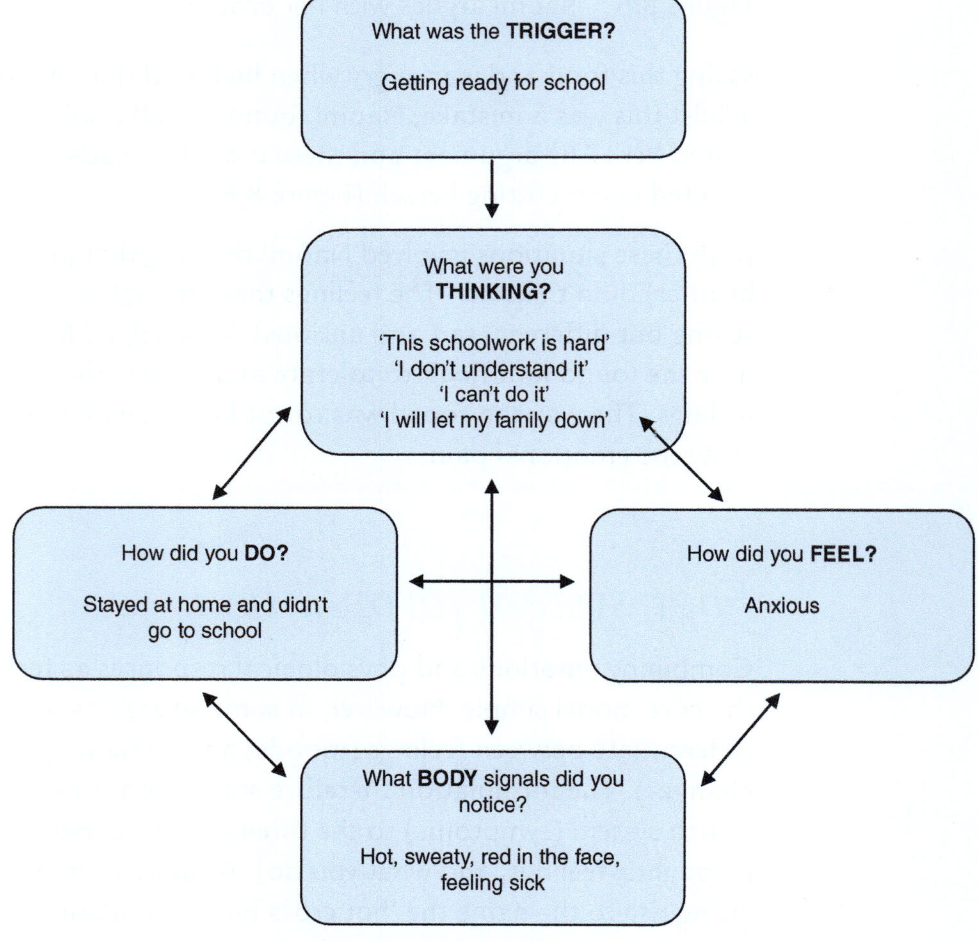

Figure 8.7   Abdul gets ready for school.

anxiety symptoms. This helped to understand why they only occurred on school days and how staying off school made his worries about coping with his work worse. The more he stayed off school, the further behind he fell with his work and the more worried he became that he was not coping.

Remember the strengths

Problem formulations provide a useful summary of the current difficulties. However, this problem focus ignores the strengths and skills the young person possesses that can help them to overcome their difficulties and build future resilience (Padesky & Mooney 2012). These skills and strengths may be unrelated to the young person's problems but focusing on them will provide examples of how they have been successfully used.

The Find your Strengths worksheet (TGFB p 52) explores several areas in the young person's life where strengths may be found. These can include:

- what the young person does (e.g. music, art, acting, gaming, or looking after animals);

- activities the young person likes (e.g. walking, jogging, dance, keep fit, or swimming);

- what the young person does at school/work (e.g. favourite lessons/ activities or well organised);

- any achievements (e.g. learned something new, or did something special like setting up their own website or blog);

- personal attributes (e.g. kind, try hard, clever, good listener, or funny);

- interpersonal qualities (e.g. popular, trusted, kind, or loyal).

Once these strengths have been identified, the young person can be encouraged to consider how these, or the process by which they acquired them, can be applied to other parts of their life.

- A young person may have important acting parts in a play. This may help to discover how they manage their nerves when performing or learning their lines. Could these skills be applied to other anxiety-provoking situations or learning situations (e.g. preparing for exams)?

- A young person may enjoy running. Could this be used as a mood-lifting activity, where they go for a run when they notice their mood dropping?

- A young person may struggle with their maths work at school but nonetheless keep trying to get it right. How can this determination be used to overcome their problems socialising with their peers?

► A young person may be particularly good at gaming. How did they acquire these skills, and can this process of perseverance and practice be applied to other situations where they need to learn new skills?

► How can a personal attribute like a good sense of humour be used when a young person is beating themselves up over something trivial? Can it help them to be more compassionate to themselves and to keep events in perspective?

► How can a young person use their interpersonal attributes, such as helping friends deal with their problems? Can this help them learn to speak more kindly to themselves and to challenge their self-critical and negative thoughts?

Including a box on personal strengths in the formulation can be a helpful way of highlighting strengths that the young person may be able to draw upon to overcome their difficulties. In the earlier examples:

► Rhiannon was a very good footballer and by taking her ball to school she was soon playing with the other children.

► Naomi had artistic skills that provided her with a way of letting out her feelings by drawing how she felt rather than cutting herself.

► Abdul had determination to do well with his schoolwork, which helped him to take his symptoms with him and return to school irrespective of how he felt.

The process of identifying and using personal strengths often requires active direction and encouragement (Padesky & Mooney 2012). Young people in particular may find it hard to identify their strengths and skills and to think how they can be applied to other parts of their life. The approach needs to be proactive, positive, and persistent as the young person is helped to identify their strengths and to consider how these might help with their problems.

Provides an understanding of important past events and relationships (onset formulations)

Young people and carers may be interested in understanding how they became caught in their Negative Traps and how their unhelpful patterns developed. Onset formulations provide a developmental explanation of how past experiences have shaped important cognitions and behaviours (see Figure 8.8). The onset formulation highlights how significant events and experiences result

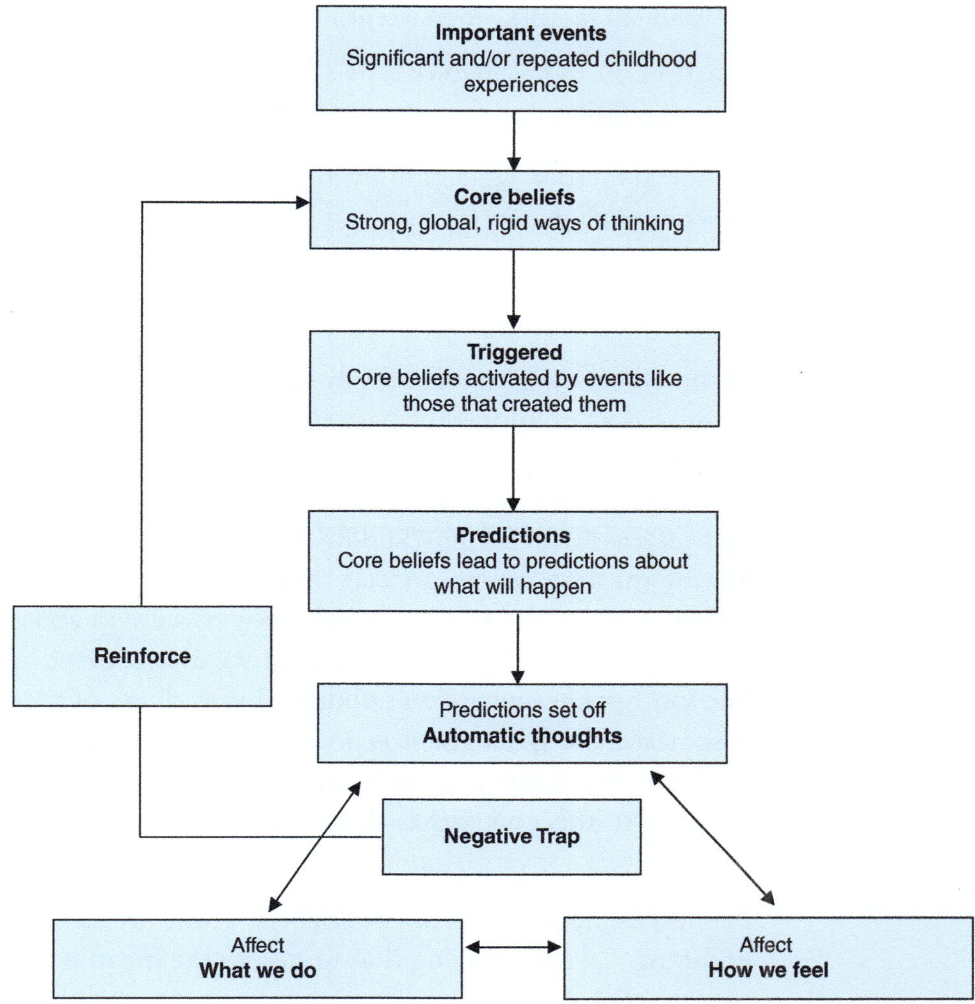

Figure 8.8 Onset formulation.

in the development of important beliefs/schemas/assumptions that determine how the young person perceives themselves, their performance, and their future. In developing onset formulations, it is important to consider potentially significant family factors and relationships, important or traumatic events, school experiences, and relationships with peers.

The key elements of the cognitive model proposed by Beck provide a helpful way of structuring an onset formulation and disentangling the different levels of cognitive processes (TGFB p100; TGFG p74).

Important events and experiences are central to the development of strong, rigid, and enduring ways of thinking called maladaptive core beliefs or dysfunctional schemas. Potentially important negative experiences could include:

▶ family factors – death, illness, poor or violent parental relationships, parental separation, poor parental mental/physical health;

▶ relationship issues – separation from parents, poor or ambivalent attachment, rejection, failed relationships, multiple carers;

▶ medical factors – persistent health problems, disability, chronic illness, repeated or prolonged hospitalisation;

▶ educational issues – school failure, learning problems, bullying;

▶ social factors – rejection from friends/peers, isolation, delinquent/criminal behaviour;

▶ trauma – abuse, single or multiple traumatic events, discrimination.

Some events may not objectively appear particularly significant and could be dismissed as unimportant or irrelevant by a third party. It is therefore important to assess the meaning the young person ascribes to these events so that their potential significance can be determined. For example, a girl of 16 was referred with a longstanding history of OCD related to germs and health. During the assessment, a range of possibly important events emerged, although most appeared comparatively trivial. However, further questioning clearly revealed the personal significance of one event in which the girl fell and cut her knee whilst on holiday. The vividness of the memory and her associated thoughts – 'this is not going to stop bleeding', 'no one will know I am hurt', 'I am going to die' – clearly highlighted the importance she had ascribed to this comparatively minor everyday event.

The model proposed by Beck identifies different levels of cognitions, with the deepest being schemas or core beliefs. These are strong, global, fixed, and enduring ways of thinking that underpin the meanings and interpretations that we make about ourselves, what happens, and the future. These cognitive filters provide a framework for quickly making sense of our world and select the information we attend to and how it is interpreted. We are more likely to attend to information that is consistent with our mental filter and are likely to interpret anything that is inconsistent as an exception or will attempt to make it fit by minimising its importance. Core beliefs and schemas can be functional and enabling, but some are overly rigid, negative, and dysfunctional. For example, a young person with mild learning problems or overly critical and demanding parents may develop a cognitive schema that they are a 'failure' who always gets things wrong.

We develop several schemas that are triggered by events reminiscent of those that produced them. The young person's belief that they are a failure may be triggered by school exams. Once activated, attention-, memory-, and interpretation-processing biases filter and select information that supports the schema. Attention biases result in attention being focused upon information that confirms the schema (poor school marks) whilst neutral or contradictory information (good marks) is overlooked. Memory biases result in the recall of information that is consistent with the schema (poor performance in a past exam), whilst interpretation biases (rubbishing positive performance) serve to minimise any inconsistent information.

This information would help to predict what will happen in an upcoming examination and will fuel a string of automatic thoughts or self-talk. These are the most accessible level of cognitions and represent the stream of thoughts that race through our minds providing a continuous commentary about events. The content of these is related to our beliefs/schemas. Functional beliefs produce more empowering and enabling self-talk, whilst dysfunctional and unhelpful beliefs produce more negative and disempowering automatic thoughts. Often these will be biased and self-critical and generate unpleasant emotional states, for example, anxiety, anger, unhappiness, and maladaptive behaviours such as social withdrawal or avoidance. The unpleasant feelings and maladaptive behaviours associated with these dysfunctional cognitions and processing biases serve to reinforce and maintain them as the individual becomes trapped in a self-perpetuating negative cycle.

Case Study Mary's anxiety

Mary (15) was urgently referred with acute anxiety. Mary lived in an isolated cottage in the countryside with her mother. Her parents separated when she was five years old. Her mother had a series of violent relationships, and although Mary was not abused by any of her mother's partners, she witnessed violence between them. Approximately seven months ago, one of her mother's ex-partners followed her home from school trying to find out where her mother was. The police were informed.

Her current problems started about three weeks ago and coincided with two nights where the electricity supply to their house was switched off. Her mother described Mary as going 'hysterical'. She was pacing, complaining of a racing heart, hyperventilating, short of breath, and worrying that she would pass out. Since this time, Mary has continued to be acutely anxious. She will check that the windows and the doors are shut and bolted several times each night to 'make sure they are safe'. She will check under her bed and in wardrobes for intruders. There was an incident three years ago when their house was burgled. Mary was the first home and hadn't noticed that this had happened until her mother returned. Her mother recalled that Mary was very anxious after this and kept asking her, 'What would have happened if the burglar was still in the house?'

On the day of our appointment, Mary had not slept for several nights. She described how she now stays awake at night to watch out for anyone breaking into their house. She reported how 'she could hear things' and wondered if 'someone is here'. When asked what she thought might happen, Mary reported that 'someone will hurt me'.

The onset formulation (Figure 8.9) helped Mary and her mother to understand how the past experiences of her mother's violent relationship, the house burglary, and the intimidating incident with her mother's ex-partner made Mary feel vulnerable and unsafe. This led Mary to develop a belief that 'people will hurt me'. This belief was activated by the power cut and her house being thrown into darkness. Mary described how she thought someone had cut the power cables to the house and was going to break in and hurt them. Her belief about being hurt was operationalised through her predictions that 'if I lock the doors and stay awake, I will be safe'. However, each night when it became dark, Mary lay awake and noticed many noises thinking 'Is someone here? They will hurt me. I can hear something.' These thoughts made Mary panic and resulted in her going around the house checking that doors and windows were locked and searching under her bed for intruders. In turn, her preoccupation with keeping safe tended to strengthen her belief that people will hurt her.

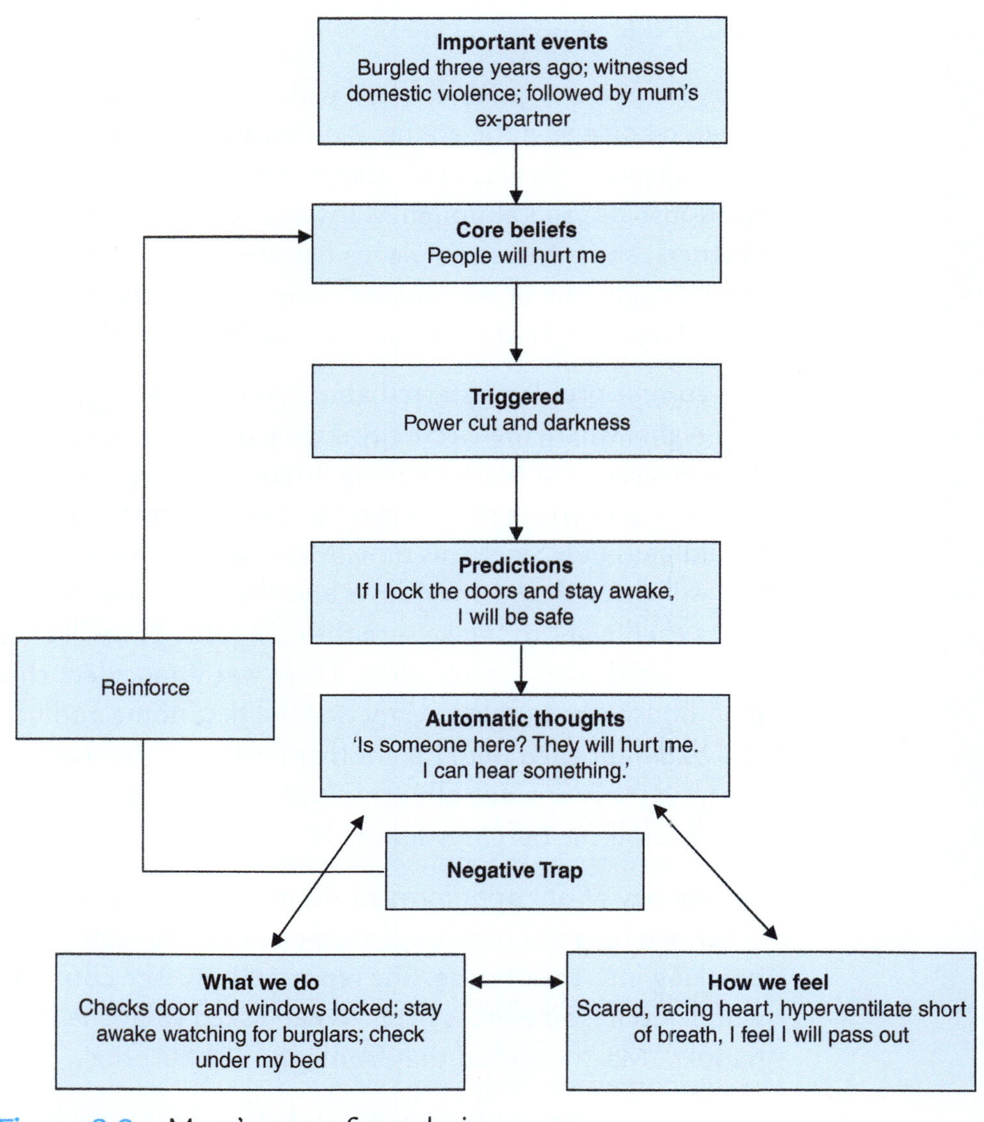

Figure 8.9 Mary's onset formulation.

Includes, as appropriate, the role of parent/carers in the onset or maintenance of the child/young person's problems

There are times when it is helpful to develop a more complex formulation in which the role of carers or other significant parties in the onset or maintenance of the young person's problems can be identified.

Case Study Sally's anxiety

Sally (eight), an only child, lived with her mother and father. Her father worked away during the week and was only at home at weekends. The family was very close, had few family friends and little contact with relatives, and so spent most of the time together on their own. The relationship between Sally and her mother was especially close, and Sally's mother would spend considerable time helping her daughter with her homework and listening to her worries and would regularly take up any of her daughter's issues with the school.

Sally had always been anxious. She was reluctant to separate from her mother at playgroup and did not play with the other children or talk with staff. Her mother recalls how she would have to stay with her daughter for the first four months of playgroup. The same happened when she started school, resulting in her mother helping in the class to reassure Sally that she was nearby.

Academically, Sally was clever, but she often set herself very high standards and became upset if her performance fell short of these. This had become a problem recently since she had a new teacher. Sally didn't like her teacher, reporting that she became cross and shouted if children got things wrong or misbehaved. Her teacher had spoken with her mother about how Sally was not completing work in class. She always appeared to be correcting and changing her work and never handed anything in. Sally said that she felt anxious, fearing that she would make errors and be told off.

The situation had continued to be difficult, resulting in Sally being referred with excessive worrying and anxiety. Her mother did not like to see her daughter so upset, so she introduced 'worry time' to show her daughter that she cared by making time each night to listen to her worries. Similarly,

Mary refused to do her homework on her own and insisted that her mother help. Her mother therefore made time to help Mary with her schoolwork. However, no matter how she helped, Mary constantly worried, 'What if I get it wrong. I can't do this. What if my teacher is cross and shouts?' As the evening progressed Mary would become more anxious and would panic, cry hysterically, and complain of feeling ill and wanting to stay at home or sleep with her mother. There had been a few days recently where Mary had stayed at home and not attended school.

The formulation (Figure 8.10) highlighted important factors (always anxious, only child) and experiences (family socially isolated, no friends, mum and Sally spend lots of time together) that resulted in Sally and her mother developing a very special relationship. Sally came to rely on her mother when she felt anxious (starting at playgroup and school) and developed a belief that 'I cannot cope without mum'. This belief was

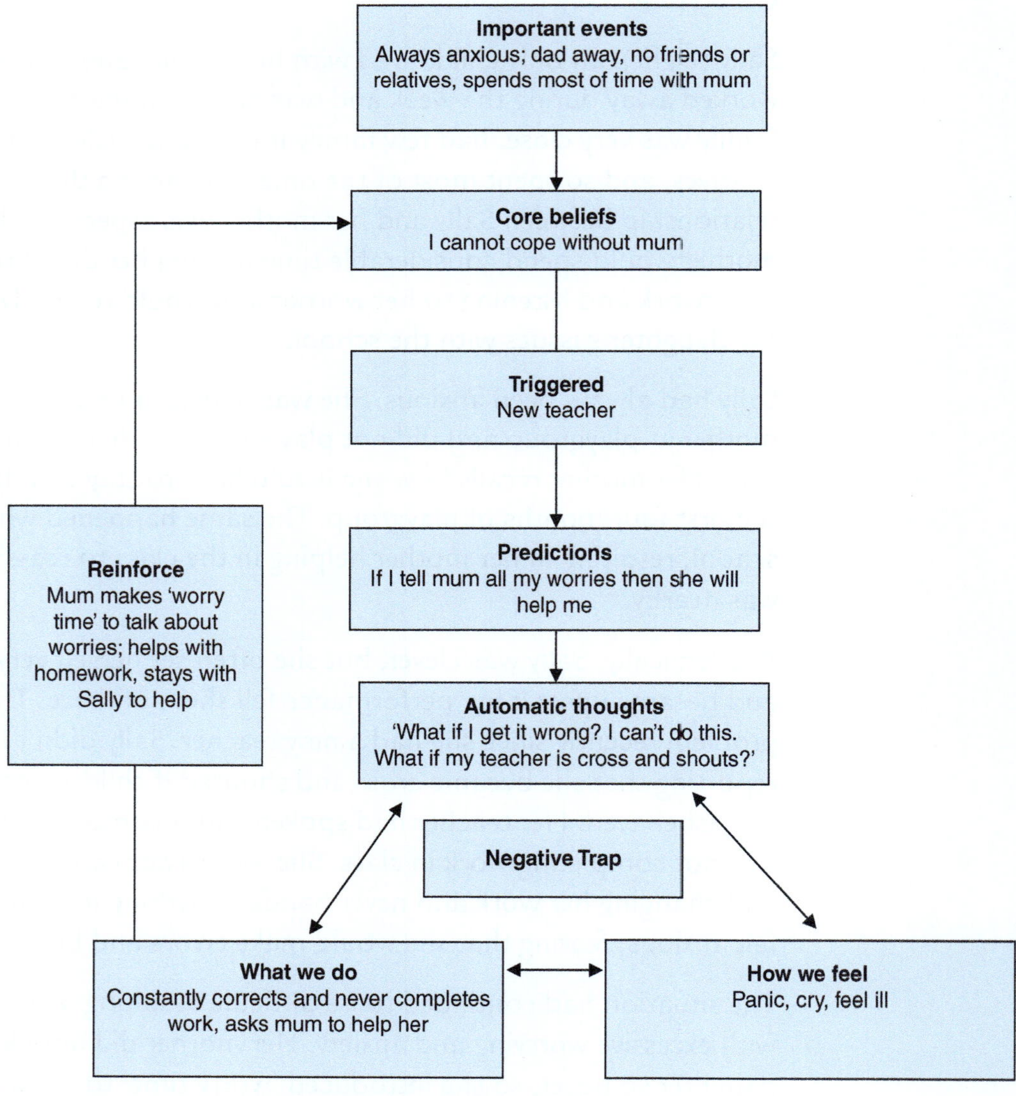

Figure 8.10   Sally's onset formulation.

triggered by her new teacher, who she didn't like and who she thought was cross and shouted at people. Sally thought that she could prevent this from happening if she told her mother all her worries and asked her to help with her schoolwork. When her teacher set work, Sally worried, 'What if I get it wrong. I can't do this. What if my teacher is cross and shouts?' These thoughts made Sally anxious and she would cry and complain of feeling ill and would constantly correct her work and never finish anything. She would then take it home and ask her mother to help her with it. Sally's mother didn't like to see her daughter upset and so made special 'worry time' each night to talk through her worries and made time to help her with her schoolwork. This didn't help. Sally spent more and more time talking about her worries and, as she spoke, became increasingly anxious. The more time Sally spent focusing on her worries, the more anxious she became.

Activities and goals/targets are clearly linked to the formulation

Individualised formulations provide explanations within a CBT framework which guide and inform the intervention. The young person and their parents/carers are encouraged to reflect on the formulation and what might need to change for them to break out of their current unhelpful cycle. With Sally, the formulation suggested many ways in which her problems could be addressed.

▶ Is the teacher the problem? Sally's anxieties and worries about her teacher may be justified. If the teacher is constantly shouting and criticising the children, then Sally's response may be appropriate, and the intervention should focus on how the teacher's behaviour could be addressed.

Sally's mother had already looked in to this. She had spoken with the teacher, observed her with the children, and talked with other parents, but no one else had noted any such difficulties. Parents were reporting that although the teacher was strict, children liked her and were being rewarded with stickers for their work. Sally had also returned home with many stickers for good behaviour.

▶ Is 'worry time' helpful? It was understandable why Sally's mother had given her daughter the chance to talk about and resolve her worries. However, the more time she spent reassuring her daughter about her worries, the more worries Sally discovered and the more anxious she became. This resulted in Sally spending most of her time talking about how she couldn't cope rather than how she could cope. Worry time wasn't helping Sally to deal with her worries. It was having the opposite effect of making them worse by reinforcing her belief that she cannot cope without her mother.

Sally needed to know that there was space for her to discuss her worries, but this needed to be limited and considerably shorter. Sally was encouraged to write her worries down throughout the day (TGFG p148), and for 15 minutes each night she would review these with her mother. A number of her worries had passed (e.g. 'Who will sit next to me in the dinner hall?') and the remaining worries were sorted into those that Sally could do something about (e.g. 'Have I got my PE kit?') and those that she couldn't (e.g. 'Will my teacher be in a good mood?'). Sally and her mother then took some of the worries that could be solved and planned how Sally could deal with them. For her PE kit, Sally wrote on the calendar when she had PE, wrote a list of what she needed to take, and put her packed bag by the front door ready for the next day. Those that she couldn't do anything about were noted, but the time was spent problem solving and developing coping skills (TGFB p131).

▶ Do we need to check Sally's belief: 'I can't cope without mum'? Sally was not completing her schoolwork and was constantly asking her mother to help her, which had the effect of strengthening her belief that she was unable to cope. This belief could be challenged by shifting the focus to coping. Sally's mother agreed that the time they spent together each evening would focus on when Sally had coped or been successful. Sally was encouraged to talk about her day, but this time to highlight her successes, the positive things that happened, the situations she coped with, and the nice things that may have been said. These were written down and, as the list grew, provided a way of challenging Sally's belief that she couldn't cope (TGFG p143).

▶ Do we need to help Sally manage her anxiety? Sally did not have any ways of controlling her anxious feelings. Her anxiety escalated until she experienced a distressing anxiety attack, leaving her exhausted. Developing emotional management skills to prevent this build-up and to manage this anxiety could help Sally recognise that there may be things she can do to cope with her feelings. Sally and her mother spent time together practising a range of relaxation skills such as controlled breathing (TGFG 171) and calming imagery (TGFB p163; TGFG p178).

▶ Do we need to check whether Sally's behaviour is helpful? Sally is constantly correcting her work but is not finishing it at school. Sally and her mother agreed to talk with her teacher and to try an experiment for one week to see what happened if she did things differently. Sally set up an experiment to check this out (TGFB p185; TGFG p141) and agreed with her teacher that she would hand her work in at the end of each lesson. Her teacher understood that Sally was worried about this and so reassured her that she would not be critical and wanted to help Sally. At the end of the week, Sally and her mother met with the teacher and compared her work from the time she was taking it home to finish to what she had achieved at school. There were no differences in her marks, and indeed, her teacher thought that her work was tidier without so much correcting. Sally's mother also thought this was better. When she was helping Sally at home, her daughter would become upset, and this hadn't happened over the past week.

▶ Do we need to think about Sally's parents? The family were socially quite isolated, with Sally's mother spending all her time during the week with Sally. Although her father worked away during the week, we discussed ways in which he could become more involved in helping Sally. He was able to Skype home and used this time reviewing with Sally her list of how she had coped. He also spent time at the weekend reviewing Sally's progress and tried to spend more time with the family each Sunday afternoon.

Sally's mother also thought about herself. She had enjoyed helping at the local nursery and so offered to volunteer two mornings each week. This gave Sally's mother a new focus and provided her with social contact with other adults.

Common problems

Difficulty identifying thoughts or feelings

It is sometimes difficult to identify the young person's cognitions or feelings. The young person may talk in a descriptive, matter-of-fact way in which events are objectively and factually described. However, attempts to directly elicit thoughts or feelings may be unsuccessful.

Direct questions can be helpful, particularly for those adolescents who are often ready to volunteer their ideas. Embedding questions in specific events or situations often makes them clearer, understandable, and easier to answer. A young person may find it easier to answer, 'What was going through your head as you walked up to Mike in the playground?' rather than, 'What do you think when you meet people?'

Carefully listening to apparently factual descriptive accounts often reveals a wealth of thoughts and assumptions. At other times, the use of indirect or non-verbal approaches can be helpful as younger children often feel more relaxed and able to volunteer their thoughts when engaged in an activity. Useful methods to consider are:

▶ the use of thought bubbles;

▶ wondering what a third party/best friend might think in a similar situation;

- the use of puppets to act out a situation;
- drawing a picture about the difficult situation;
- telling a story.

If the appropriate means of communication are found, young people can volunteer some of their thoughts or feelings.

Is it important to distinguish between different levels of cognitions?

Greenberger & Padesky (1995) highlight the importance of being aware of different levels of cognitions, noting that they require different methods of assessment and interventions. Automatic thoughts are the most accessible and are often amenable to assessment through thought diaries or become apparent when talking through difficult situations. These can be modified by the method, commonly used with young people, of replacing negative and dysfunctional automatic thoughts with positive self-talk (TGFG p144). The young person is therefore encouraged to practise alternative, more helpful thoughts that can be used in difficult situations.

Predictions are rarely directly verbalised but can be identified through behavioural experiments in which the young person is asked to predict (i.e. operationalise their cognitions) what will happen. Behavioural experiments also provide a useful way of challenging and testing predictions and can lead to cognitive restructuring. However, whilst behavioural experiments may provide information that challenges the young person's core beliefs, this alone will not be enough to change them. By definition, core beliefs are the deepest and most enduring cognitions and are typically resistant to new or conflicting information. If working with core beliefs, the therapeutic aim is to develop an alternative belief rather than attempting to disprove the existing belief. This process can be facilitated by using ratings, so that subtle changes in the strength of existing beliefs can be highlighted.

I can't seem to put this together in a formulation

The key is to identify important information and to organise this in a cognitive framework that helps the young person to understand their problems. It is easy to become overwhelmed by the amount of information collected during the assessment and to struggle to incorporate this into a simple, understandable, or coherent formulation. This difficulty often arises for two main reasons.

Firstly, the relevant information to develop the formulation may not have been identified. This may be due to inexperience, assessment questions not being sufficiently specific or detailed, or the collection of enormous amounts of information that may not be directly relevant to the current problems. It is therefore helpful to carefully consider the structure of the interview to ensure that relevant areas included in the onset formulation are assessed. If the information gathered is not sufficiently detailed, then paying greater attention to the type and content of the questions may help to elicit clearer and more specific information. If these difficulties persist, then clinical supervision will be particularly important to develop clinical practice.

The second common reason is that a clear formulation framework to select and organise the information has not been used. The mini-formulation provides the simplest structure and helps focus upon identifying a triggering event and tracking through each of the accompanying key elements of the CBT cycle, that is, thoughts, feelings, and behaviour. If necessary, feelings can be further subdivided into the emotional reaction and physiological/somatic changes. These can then be combined to develop a maintenance formulation.

I'm not sure if the formulation is right

It is important to ensure that the formulation is accurate and is consistent with a cognitive explanatory model. There are, however, times when this preoccupation with getting it 'correct' is counterproductive and can result in the emerging formulation not being shared. The opportunity to educate the young person and their family about the cognitive model is delayed. The process moves from an open collaborative model to one that becomes closed and secretive. The failure to freely share information implicitly shifts the process of CBT away from shared empiricism towards that of an 'expert-led model'.

Formulations are not static and therefore can never be totally 'correct'. They are dynamic, constantly updated and revised during the intervention as new information emerges or behavioural experiments confirm or disprove aspects of the model. However, at any one time, the formulation is the shared understanding, the working hypothesis. Adopting a collaborative, dynamic approach ensures that the formulation is developed and shared early during the intervention.

I can't seem to find all the information to complete the formulation

In developing a formulation, there will inevitably be times when it is difficult to identify specific information. Core beliefs are the deepest cognitions and often the least accessible. Assumptions can prove difficult to access, and young people may not have the language to adequately describe their emotions. At these times, information can still be organised within the CBT framework but with missing information being highlighted. This is often useful to do visually so that the incomplete boxes are clearly visible. At other times, it might be helpful to simply acknowledge that 'we don't know what to put in this box yet' and to leave a question mark. The missing section of the formulation is therefore highlighted and can be returned to during subsequent sessions to explore whether new information has emerged that will allow the missing section to be completed.

CHAPTER NINE

G: General skills

Is well prepared and conducts treatment sessions in a calm and organised way

Meetings need to be organised and well managed to ensure that CBT remains focused and is efficiently provided. Sessions should be planned and prepared so that any worksheets, formulations, outcome measures, and audio or video clips are available. Any disruptive behaviour needs to be actively managed so that it does not interfere with the delivery of the intervention. Sessions need a clear agenda and a predictable structure. Routine outcome and goal ratings should be completed, home assignments and learning reviewed, the session topic introduced, skills practised, and home assignments agreed. Sufficient time for each topic is required to ensure that the agenda is completed during the allocated time. Sessions need to be suitably paced to match developmental and learning abilities. They need to be responsive to the young person, with the agenda being flexibly adjusted to respond to any issues that may emerge. Finally, progress should be regularly reviewed, and sufficient time allowed to prepare for endings and the development of a relapse-prevention plan.

Prepares and brings the necessary materials and equipment to the meeting

Sessions need to be well prepared so that all required resources are available. Failing to have the necessary resources will inevitably result in the session being less coherent, efficient, and effective.

A Clinician's Guide to CBT for Children to Young Adults: A Companion to Think Good, Feel Good and Thinking Good, Feeling Better, Second Edition. Paul Stallard.
© 2021 John Wiley & Sons Ltd. Published 2021 by John Wiley & Sons Ltd.
Companion website: www.wiley.com/go/cliniciansguide2e

- ▶ Core materials for any CBT session include paper, pens, worksheets, and a laptop/tablet to play videos with an Internet connection.

- ▶ Routine assessments and goal ratings need to be available to monitor change and provide a quick way of gauging how much progress the young person feels they are making. Past and current rating scales need to be available for comparison.

- ▶ A visual summary of the current formulation should always be present. During the assessment stage, this will be evolving as new information is being collected and assimilated. Once a working formulation has been established, the formulation will inform and direct the intervention.

- ▶ Previous home assignments and completed materials should be present for reference and used to link previous sessions and the concepts covered.

- ▶ Materials to facilitate the planned focus of the session need to be available. For example, worksheets to identify different types of thoughts (TGFG p89, p90), diaries (TGFB p109: TGFG p87), or handouts for developing new skills such as mindfulness (TGFB p79; TGFG p62) or self-kindness (TGFB p65, p67). If video clips or audio instructions are to be used, then reliable technology must be accessible.

- ▶ If undertaking implementation tasks such as exposure, access to the feared stimuli is necessary and the session may need additional time to ensure that exposure has been successful and anxiety has reduced.

To make CBT more engaging and motivating, materials can be personalised according to the young person's interests. For example, if a young person likes sport, worksheets can be created around a sporting theme. If they like music, a young person can be encouraged to identify songs that make them feel good or a particular song that expresses how they feel. Diaries can easily be personalised with the addition of the young person's name and some relevant images. Personalisation is motivating and makes young people feel special and valued.

Manages the young person's behaviour during sessions

Disruptive behaviour needs to be appropriately managed to ensure that it does not negatively interfere with the intervention. A contract with the young person is a helpful way of clarifying expectations. This may involve basic requirements about arriving on time and switching off their mobile phone or expectations about participating in skill-development sessions and completing home assignments. To signal the importance of the contract, it should be signed by the young person and the clinician, with a copy being available at each session to refer to if required.

Disruptive behaviour may arise due to anxiety, as can occur with young people with autism spectrum disorder (ASD). If this is the case, the session can be structured to make it predictable. For example, the basic session agenda can be written on a board so that it is immediately visible to the young person as they enter the room.

For young people who find it difficult to maintain their focus, sessions can be shorter and different materials used to stimulate and maintain their attention. A session could, for example, involve drawing on a whiteboard, completing a worksheet or quiz, engaging in a role play, and watching a video. For those who find it hard to sit still, consider making sessions more active, for example, go for a walk or break up passive activities with more active ones. For example, a young person who is socially anxious could be guided around the clinic or hospital building to practise greeting people.

If disruptive behaviour becomes a regular problem, consider the use of contingency management, where a formal reward or tick chart can be established. It may be possible to provide a small reward, which could be linked to the young person's problems and the skills they are acquiring. For example:

▶ A young person who becomes anxious in group situations could be rewarded with a drink from the local coffee shop;

▶ A young person who is anxious eating in public could be taken to a coffee shop and rewarded with a piece of cake.

On other occasions, contingency management can occur within sessions, for example, 'Once we have completed our agenda, you can go on YouTube and you can show me those videos you like.'

Another form of behaviour that needs to be managed is procrastination. This often occurs as a way of putting off or avoiding challenging tasks. Once noted, this should be discussed with the young person, their anxiety acknowledged, and a plan with clear deadlines agreed. Wherever possible, seize the moment in a clinical session to move from discussion to action.

▶ 'Let's go and do this now.'

▶ 'Let us find out what happens.'

Finally, some young people will be very talkative and this may result in the agenda not being covered. The young person needs to be given time to talk, but limits need to be placed around this. If it becomes an issue, it can be directly raised with the young person and problem solving used to explore how this can be dealt with.

> ▶ 'I am aware that there seems too much to talk about and that in our last couple of meetings we haven't managed to get through all of our agenda. It is important that we cover everything, and I wondered what we can do about this?'

Ensures that sessions have an agenda and clear goals and are appropriately structured

Sessions need to remain focused and have a clear agenda and structure. This should be made explicit during the first session, where a clear rationale for agenda setting should be provided.

> ▶ 'At the start of each session we will agree an agenda. This will set out what we will talk about and will help us to remain focused on helping you to achieve your goals.'

The agenda should be developed collaboratively with prioritisation ensuring that the most important issues are addressed. The agenda will include a balance of task-focused activities, that is, those helping the young person to secure their treatment goals, and those items that maintain and strengthen the relationship. These may focus on the young person's interests or on specific issues that the young person would like to discuss.

> ▶ 'What would you like to put on the agenda today?'

> ▶ 'Has anything important happened this week that we need to think about?'

The agenda should be written down, items prioritised, and time agreed.

> ▶ 'What is the most important thing to cover today?'

> ▶ 'Which of these things do you think will help you most?'

> ▶ 'We have 45 minutes, so how much time do you think we should spend on this?'

Although the process is collaborative, the clinician is responsible for ensuring that the agenda is feasible within the time available. The agenda therefore needs to be manageable and not become too large and overwhelming.

In terms of content, the agenda needs to be relevant to the stage of the intervention and clearly relate to the problem formulation and the young person's goals. The agenda will usually include a general update, completion of outcome measures, home assignment review, the session content, home assignment, and session summary and feedback.

General update

At the beginning of the session, it is useful to obtain a brief update about any significant events that have occurred since the last meeting that might contribute to the young person's problems or potentially interfere with their progress.

▶ 'Has anything important happened since we last met that it would be helpful for me to know about?'

This provides an opportunity for the young person to share any particular concerns or problems.

▶ 'Mum and dad have been having lots of arguments and they are both very angry at the moment.'

It also provides opportunities to celebrate anything positive or discuss important unplanned events that have occurred.

▶ 'You know I don't like going out much. Well, on Monday, my friend invited me round to their house, and I went.'

Outcome measures update

Routine outcome measures and goal ratings should be completed at the start of each session. These provide an immediate opportunity to review progress, and the intervention can then be adjusted and paced accordingly.

Completing these brief measures does not take long and experience suggests that young people like to complete them. It can often be easier for a young person to complete a symptom or goal scale rather than trying to verbally explain how they are feeling or what happened. Young people are also interested in finding out how their problems are changing over time. If positive change is occurring, reviewing previous assessments can be empowering and motivating. If there is lack of change or progress is limited, then an exploration of possible reasons would be indicated and, if appropriate, a new plan agreed.

Home assignment review

The task agreed in the previous meeting should be reviewed. If completed, success needs to be celebrated and the young person encouraged to reflect on what they have learned or discovered.

▶ 'Well done, Caz, you have managed to find three hot situations. What have you found out? Have you noticed any patterns or themes?'

If the task was not completed, potential barriers need to be explored and a plan agreed as to how these might be addressed.

▶ 'We all forget to do things, Jack, so don't worry about that. I wonder if we could look at how you can be reminded to do this next time.'

Session topic

Most of the session will focus on the main topic. This will be guided by the formulation and will ensure that the intervention remains focused on developing the skills to achieve the young person's goals. The session may focus on psycho-education, skill development, or the practice of new skills from the cognitive, emotional, or behavioural domain. In addition, time can be allocated during each session to briefly practise helpful skills such as mindfulness, relaxation, or gratitude.

Home assignment

The relevance of the topic to the young person's difficulties will be emphasised and a home assignment agreed. Depending on the stage of the intervention, this might involve collecting assessment data through some form of monitoring, practising skills, or undertaking implementation tasks such as discovery experiments or behavioural activation.

Home assignments are important and provide the bridge between clinical sessions and the young person's everyday life. They also provide continuity between sessions, where the home assignment agreed at the end of one session is reviewed at the start of the next, with this linking to the content of the session. Home assignments bring the young person's daily experience into the meeting and facilitate the application of clinical discussions and skills into daily life.

Session summary and feedback

Finally, feedback from the young person should be sought about how they found the session. Questions can be rated on a 10-point scale ranging from 'not at all' (0) to 'totally' (10) and can assess core dimensions, including:

▶ feeling heard: 'Did you feel listened to?'

▶ contribution: 'Were you able to say everything you wanted to say?'

▶ understanding: 'Did you understand what was talked about?'

▶ involvement: 'How involved were you in planning the home assignment?'

Young people may be reticent about providing feedback. They may worry about upsetting or criticising the clinician, feel unsure about what will happen if they say something critical, or be concerned that they will be told off or get into trouble if they say the 'wrong' thing. It is therefore important for young people to be provided with a clear explanation of why they are being asked to provide feedback and how this can be helpful.

▶ 'I want to check how you have found our session today. I want to make sure that you have felt involved and listened to and that you have had a chance to share your ideas and say what you wanted to say. Please be honest so that we can make these meetings as helpful as we can.'

It is not unusual for young people to rate sessions highly. However, it is not so much the rating itself but any change that is important. If a young person gave the last session a rating of 7 for feeling heard but gave this session a 6, then this needs to be explored.

▶ 'Looks as if I haven't been listening to you as well as I did last time we met. Do you have any ideas about what would help you feel that you had been heard?'

Similarly, if a rating has increased, this should be briefly discussed.

▶ 'You have rated your involvement in the session today higher than last time. What do you think has happened today to make you feel more involved?'

Ensures good timekeeping so that all tasks are completed

As part of agenda setting, items should be prioritised and notional time allocated. Time will need to be monitored and the agenda adjusted accordingly to ensure that all items are provided with sufficient attention. The clinician should take responsibility for timekeeping, but decisions to reprioritise agenda items or to reallocate time should be taken collaboratively with the young person.

In order to ensure that sessions are conducted in an efficient way, they need to be actively managed. Lengthy discussions which may prevent the agenda being covered need to be sensitively handled and concluded using summaries and paraphrasing.

▶ 'It seems, Maria, that there are lots of things that make you anxious. You told me about situations where there are lots of people – going to new or unfamiliar places and social situations. This is really helpful, and I wonder if we can now move on to look at the sort of thoughts that race through your head in these situations.'

Whilst the agenda should form the structure for the session, this needs to be flexibly managed. There is no point in racing through an agenda simply to complete it. Once again, this can be agreed with the young person.

> 'You had a lot you wanted to talk about today and that has helped me catch up with what has been happening. We need to make sure that we have enough time to discuss the things on our agenda, and I don't think we have enough time to cover everything. I wonder what we should do?'

The young person can be involved in finding a solution, which might involve starting with any unfinished items next meeting.

Ensures that the session is appropriately paced, flexible, and responsive to the needs of the young person

Agenda setting involves prioritisation and time allocation, and this will inform the pace of the session. The pace needs to reflect the young person's developmental capacity and allow enough time for learning and processing of information. The clinician therefore needs to judge the length of the agenda and to maintain an overview of the session to ensure that the pace is appropriate. The pace should be consistent so that the later agenda items are not rushed. However, the session will need constantly monitoring and the pace should be adjusted and responsive to the young person's responses.

> For those young people who find it hard to sustain their concentration, sessions can be made shorter.

> If the young person appears disinterested, then consider how different materials can be used to maintain their interest.

> If the young person appears overwhelmed, adjust the amount of information that is being provided into smaller, more focused chunks.

> If the young person appears bored, then check whether the session is appropriately paced. If too slow, the young person might become bored. If too fast, the young person might not understand and lose interest.

Session pace is also determined by content and how much information/focus is required before key messages are understood and assimilated.

- How much does the young person already know? If the young person already has a good understanding of key parts of the CBT model, then less time needs to be spent in these areas.

- Is information provided at a sufficient level? Some young people will assimilate ideas quickly, whilst others will require the material to be presented a few times before it is understood.

- Has the information been provided in sufficient depth? Children, for example, might need to identify different types of thinking traps, whilst adolescents might want more information about how they developed.

A well-paced session should therefore have enough agenda items to be covered in the allocated time for the young person to understand, integrate, and apply to their personal situation.

The pace should be neither too fast nor too slow. Unnecessary repetition is not efficient and runs the risk of the young person feeling patronised and bored. Similarly, sufficient time is required for the young person to understand, apply, and adapt new information to their own individual situation. This can be assessed by asking the young person to summarise what they have heard and how it can be applied to their problems.

- 'Tina, could you summarise for me in your own words what we have been talking about?'

- 'How do you think this can help you to deal with your problems?'

To maintain momentum, talkative young people need to be sensitively managed and steered back from extended peripheral discussions to the agenda. Whilst the agenda helps to maintain a clear focus, it is important not to be completely driven by this structure. If, for example, a young person volunteers information about self-harm or suicidal thoughts, this needs to be assessed in order to ensure their safety.

If a decision is made to deviate from the agenda, this needs to be made explicit and the reason for this clarified.

- 'It seems that you are really worried, Katie, by this change in your mum's behaviour. Although we hadn't planned to talk about this, you seem very upset by this. I wonder whether we should leave our agenda and explore what you can do to help mum and yourself to feel better?'

Responsive

It is important to remain flexible and responsive to the young person's emotional responses, important events that occur outside of sessions, or spontaneous and unplanned therapeutic opportunities.

A young person may attend in an emotional state or become emotional during a session. This should not be ignored but needs to be acknowledged and sensitively explored. Without appropriate exploration and discussion, it is probable that this highly aroused emotional state will prevent the young person from attending to the planned sessional content.

Similarly, the intervention needs to be considered within the wider context of the young person's everyday life. There are many events which may impact on them and their ability to prioritise the intervention. These could include:

▶ family issues, e.g. arguments with parents or siblings;

▶ friendship issues, e.g. relationships ending or bullying;

▶ educational issues, e.g. exams or academic pressures;

▶ community issues, e.g. violence or drug pressure;

▶ health issues, e.g. family or personal health.

Whilst the agenda provides opportunities for brief updates, there will be times when this will need to be flexible and responsive to immediate issues and allow a longer exploration of these events.

Case Study Gary is worried about germs

Gary (16) had many worries about germs. Upon arrival for his clinical session, he appeared very anxious and revealed that he had stood on a used condom that was lying outside on the pavement. He was convinced that he was now infected with HIV.

The planned focus of the session was on psycho-education about the CBT model. However, given this opportunity, we discussed whether we should instead find out more about this situation which had made Gary so anxious. Rather than sitting in the room and talking about this, Gary was invited to show the clinician what had made him so anxious. They went outside, where Gary pointed to something white on the floor. This 'hot situation' was used to identify Gary's catastrophic thoughts as he was encouraged to look at this and describe the thoughts tumbling through his head. The situation was used to highlight how Gary is sensitive about germs and is actively looking for situations where he might be contaminated. In this situation, the white item on the floor that Gary had identified as a condom was in fact a wet tissue.

Prepares for endings and relapse prevention

CBT is a time-limited intervention and, from the first session, the young person should have an indication of the intervention duration and/or when progress will be reviewed. The young person should therefore be clear that this is not an open, ongoing process. This focus on the end of the intervention is reinforced throughout meetings as regular reviews of progress and routine outcome measures and goal-based ratings quantify change and determine progress. However, symptom change and goal acquisition are not the only outcomes upon which to base decisions about ending. The ultimate aim is for the young person and/or their parents to become their own therapist, so increased awareness and self-efficacy are also important. Positive reasons for ending an intervention include:

▶ initial problems being resolved;

▶ symptoms reducing to a manageable level;

▶ the development of effective coping skills to deal with future problems;

▶ increased self-awareness to understand common traps and pitfalls;

▶ the development of self-efficacy.

Enough time should be allowed to prepare the young person for ending. This should be explicitly highlighted as a positive development, particularly in the latter sessions whilst the young person is consolidating their skills. This consolidation phase will typically be accompanied by a longer period between appointments, allowing the young person more opportunities to deal with any issues that might arise on their own.

Whilst many young people will be pleased by the ending of the intervention, some will be worried. They may doubt their self-efficacy and ability to cope or fear the ending as being abandoned or another experience of rejection from someone they value. It is important to recognise this and to discuss the ending of the intervention in an empowering and thoughtful way. The young person's fears need to be recognised and normalised. Their strengths and skills need to be highlighted and included as part of a relapse-prevention plan. Similarly, when and how future help could be sought should be made explicit.

Relapse prevention

The final sessions focus on relapse prevention. These encourage the young person to reflect on those aspects of the intervention that have been most helpful, prepare them for possible setbacks, and help them to develop a contingency plan in case problems do re-emerge. Areas to cover may include some or all of the following.

What helped?

This should briefly summarise those elements of the intervention that have been most important for the young person (TGFB p214). These might include:

- important messages, e.g. 'the less you do, the more time you have to think';
- useful ideas or skills, e.g. 'doing something to look after myself when I am down';
- techniques to feel better, e.g. soothing toolbox or what helps to cope with their unhelpful thoughts, e.g. 'treating myself like I would treat my friend'.

Build helpful skills into daily life

Find ways in which helpful skills can become part of everyday life. Encourage the young person to think about the different parts of their daily life and how they can build in helpful activities.

- As they brush their teeth in the morning, can they practise speaking kindly to themselves?
- As they eat their dinner, can they eat three mouthfuls mindfully?
- As they prepare for bed, can they practise their relaxation skills?

Remember to practise

Skills will become more effective the more they are used and practised. Encourage the young person to make time each week to review their use of helpful skills. Reinforce attempts at practice, explore barriers that stopped the skills being used, and plan whether any skills may be particularly helpful over the coming weeks.

Prepare for setbacks

It is important to normalise the likelihood of setbacks so that the young person is prepared for this possibility. There will be future challenges, problems will re-emerge, and there will be times when new skills do not seem to work. However, these need to be reframed as temporary setbacks rather than a sign that the previous problems have returned and that their new skills no longer work.

Know your warning signs

Being aware of personal warning signs can help to detect potential problems early and prevent them escalating (TGFB p215). Encourage the young person to identify and monitor their unhelpful ways of thinking, body signals associated with unpleasant feelings, and ways of behaving that might indicate that things are slipping.

Watch out for difficult times

Becoming aware of triggers can help to predict difficult events (TGFB p216). Transitions, going somewhere new, exams, new social situations, and disagreements may all be events that could trigger a return to unhelpful patterns. Becoming better at spotting these can help the young person prepare to cope and to practise the skills they have found helpful.

Be kind to yourself

Useful skills for life are acceptance, compassion, and gratitude. Encourage the young person to accept that things will go wrong and people will be unkind. Rather than them expecting everyone to be against them or blaming themselves for things that go wrong, encourage them to develop compassion, both for themselves and for others. Encourage them to show gratitude by seeking out positive events and experiences and showing appreciation. Often, these are small everyday events that evoke a positive emotion, such as being given a lift to meet friends or that favourite top being washed ready for a night out. These are often overlooked.

Stay positive

Things will go wrong, and setbacks will occur. However, rather than being overwhelmed by these, encourage young people to stay positive, to focus on their strengths, and to remind themselves what they have achieved.

Know when to seek help

Sometimes the young person may become trapped in their old unhelpful ways. When this happens, agree a clear written plan about who they will talk with and their contact details. Seeking help is a sign of strength, so the sooner this happens, the quicker they will be able to do something to make themselves feel better.

Watch out for strong unhelpful ways of thinking

During relapse-prevention planning, it is important to highlight what the young person has achieved and how they are responsible for this success. This is particularly important since many of their unhelpful thinking patterns involve external, global, and stable attributions.

▶ Depressed young people may attribute success to external factors rather than internal changes in how they are coping.

▶ Anxious young people may present with global attributions by which they underestimate what they can achieve and worry whether they will cope with future challenges.

▶ Angry young people may attribute their explosive tendencies as a stable trait which they will not be able to change.

These attributions need to be clearly challenged during the response prevention stage.

▶ Global attributions, for example, not being able to cope, can be challenged by highlighting successes that put limits around them: 'Whilst you do still worry about social situations, let us review what you have been able to achieve. You have been out with friends to eat, been to a party, are part of the sports team, travel with them to away games, and sit with three friends at lunch time at school.'

▶ External attributions about the reasons for change need to be challenged and internal attributions highlighted. This can be done by reviewing the skills the young person has learned and how these are related to changes in symptoms and the achievement of their goals.

▶ Stable attributions can be challenged by identifying and highlighting those occasions when the behaviour did not occur. For example, when the young person was provoked and did not lose their temper.

H: Home assignments

Uses home assignments to gather and transfer knowledge and skills between clinical meetings and everyday life

Home assignments are the bridge between clinical sessions and the young person's everyday life. Their purpose is related to the phase of the intervention, for example, psycho-education, monitoring, practice, skill development, or experimenting with new ways of behaving or responding to situations. Home assignments should be collaboratively agreed, developmentally appropriate, and tailored to the needs and interests of the young person. They should have a clear purpose, be linked to the problem formulation, and provide a logical development of the work undertaken during clinical sessions. Assignments should be manageable, well defined, and safe, with the outcome being reviewed and learning discussed.

Negotiates home assignment tasks

Home assignments provide opportunities to gather information or to test new skills in the environments in which they occur and will be used. They are essential in transferring session content to daily life and in bringing experiences from the home environment to clinical sessions. They extend the curious, objective scientific practitioner role that underpins CBT to encourage the young person to discover what happens and what works.

Home assignments should be tailored to the young person's unique experiences and circumstances. Assignments should therefore be introduced

A Clinician's Guide to CBT for Children to Young Adults: A Companion to Think Good, Feel Good and Thinking Good, Feeling Better, Second Edition. Paul Stallard.
© 2021 John Wiley & Sons Ltd. Published 2021 by John Wiley & Sons Ltd.
Companion website: www.wiley.com/go/cliniciansguide2e

during the initial sessions as a core part of CBT, and it should be made clear that an assignment will be undertaken after every session.

> ▶ 'We will need to find out what is happening and which of the ideas we discuss are helpful and which are not. To do this, you will need to do some work outside of our meetings. This might be completing a diary, practising a new skill, or trying a new way of behaving to see what happens.'

With young people, it is important not to call assignments 'homework', since this has several negative connotations. Homework is usually set by someone else, often young people do not want to do it, and typically homework is assessed and marked. In CBT, assignments are collaboratively agreed, have a clear purpose, and are not assessed. Homework has therefore been defined as Show That I Can (STIC) tasks (Kendall 1990), practice or between-session tasks (Fuggle et al. 2012), action plans (Beck et al. 2016), or home assignments (Stallard 2019a, 2019b).

The primary purpose of home assignments is discovery. During the early stages of the intervention, home assignments will be psycho-educational, designed to increase the young person's understanding about common psychological problems. For example, a young person with low self-esteem might undertake an assignment involving an Internet search to identify famous people with high or low self-esteem and to describe how they behave (TGFB p54). Similarly, a young person with depression might be encouraged to find out the common symptoms of depression. An assignment might also be agreed on to educate the young person in the CBT model.

> ▶ 'I've talked about this way of helping called CBT. I wonder if you could search the Internet and find out more about what that means for how we will work together.'

Monitoring assignments contribute to the assessment and help to develop and inform the formulation.

> ▶ 'I can't live with you 24/7 to see what happens when you become anxious. I wonder if you could keep a brief diary to record how often this happens over the coming week?'

Depending on need, monitoring assignments could identify situations that trigger unpleasant feelings (TGFB p151), establish common thoughts (TGFG p88), or cause strong body signals (TGFB p152).

As the intervention progresses, home assignments will focus on the development and practice of new skills. The focus will be informed by the formulation but could include practising relaxation (TGFB p161), finding kindness (TGFB p67; TGFG p48), or mindfulness (TGFG p61).

> 'You have done really well with our mindfulness today. Like any new skill, mindfulness will become more helpful the more you practise. I wonder if we could agree times when you could practise this at home?'

During the implementation stage, home assignments will typically focus on the adoption and implementation of new skills in daily life.

> 'We need to find out whether these skills we have been practising during our meetings work for you when you need them at school. Would it be possible to agree a time when you will use them?'

Assignments could involve becoming more active (TGFB p206), dealing with problems in different ways (TGFG p215), or undertaking experiments to check out predictions (TGFB p185).

Finally, the process involved in setting home assignments provides an important framework that can be used during relapse prevention. It provides a simple structure that can be applied to gather information, test assumptions and beliefs, or evaluate new ways of responding. The young person therefore has the tools to become their own self-helper, which they can continue to use after sessions have finished.

Once the home assignment has been agreed, it is helpful to check that the young person fully agrees with and understands the assignment.

> 'Is the task clear or are there things we need to clarify?'

> 'Can you remind me what we hope to discover from this assignment?'

> 'Do you have all the support and help you need to complete this assignment?'

The aim is for the assignment to be completed successfully in order to promote self-empowerment, rather than reinforcing beliefs about failure. It is therefore important to have an open and honest discussion about the assignment and what the young person is realistically able to undertake. A young person may feel ambivalent or unable to undertake an assignment. The reasons for this need exploration, for example, fear of failure, lack of motivation, disorganised. Ultimately, if a young person does not feel able to undertake an assignment, this should be acknowledged. Home assignments are not essential during the initial assessment stage since helpful information can still be obtained by reviewing events during clinical meetings. They are more important during the latter stages of the intervention when the young person needs to implement their new skills in their daily life. By this stage, the young person's difficulties in completing assignments can be addressed, and they will hopefully be more motivated and prepared to try.

Finally, sufficient time within the session should be allocated to assignment setting. This usually occurs towards the end of the session and so there may be a tendency to rush this process and squeeze it in to whatever little time is available. This should be avoided. During agenda setting, home assignments should be prioritised and sufficient time allocated for this activity.

Ensures assignments are meaningful and clearly related to the formulation and clinical session

Home assignments are an extension of the clinical session and as such need to clearly relate to the session content, the problem formulation, and the young person's goals. Home assignments are not a random selection of uncoordinated tasks but need to be relevant and meaningful and to enhance the intervention. There is no point in establishing an assignment just to have an assignment. Similarly, an assignment should not reiterate what is already known or what has already been established. Multiple assignments demonstrating, for example, that someone becomes anxious in social situations are unnecessary and tedious.

Home assignments should link the end of one session to the start of another and by so doing create a sense of momentum for the intervention. They should clearly relate to the formulation and can be used to test, develop, and explore relationships between the core elements of the cognitive model, that is, thoughts, feelings, and behaviour.

▶ 'When you feel sad, you don't want to be with people and take yourself off to your room on your own. When you are on your own, your sad feelings become worse and you become more troubled by your unhelpful thoughts. Do you think it would be helpful to explore what would happen if you did something else when you felt sad?'

The formulation can also be used to identify what skills might be helpful to develop and practise during home assignments.

▶ 'You keep going over your unhelpful thoughts in your mind and constantly beat yourself up. Would it be helpful to check out whether it is possible not to listen to these thoughts and to just let them come and go?'

The assignment should therefore be relevant, meaningful, and clearly defined so that the young person fully understands what it will help them to discover.

Ensures assignments are consistent with the young person's developmental level, interests, and abilities

Assignments need to reflect the developmental level of the young person. Younger children may be more motivated to engage in assignments by encouraging them to become a detective. Their job is to find clues to find out what happens. In *Think Good, Feel Good*, the Thought Tracker helps with assignments about thoughts, the Feeling Finder with emotional assignments, and Go Getter with behavioural tasks.

Developmentally, assignments need to be consistent with the young person's cognitive, reading, and writing ability. If a young person finds writing difficult, then an alternative way of completing a monitoring assignment should be agreed. The diary below (Figure 10.1) uses emojis as a simple visual way of demonstrating the child's strongest feelings during a specified period.

Technology can be used with young people to support and undertake assignments. Young people can be encouraged to create their own diaries (TGFB p108, p109) on their tablet or computer. The exercise where young people are encouraged to 'download their head' (TGFB p110) to find their thoughts can be undertaken using a smartphone. The young person can download their head directly onto their phone rather than writing on paper.

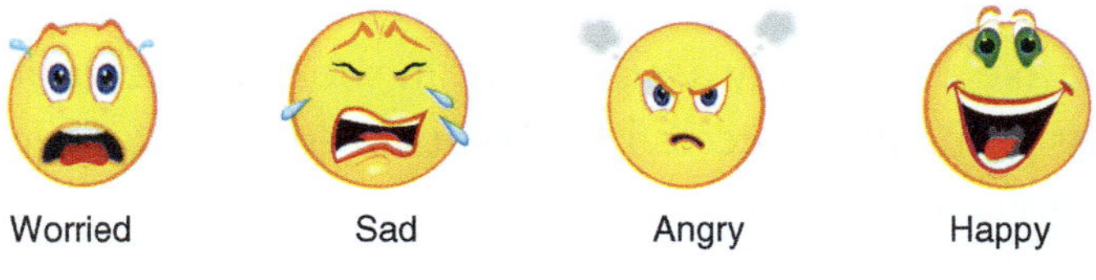

Day	Morning	Afternoon	Evening
Monday	Worried	Angry	Angry
Tuesday	Worried	Happy	Happy
Wednesday	Worried	Happy	Happy

Figure 10.1   Emotional faces diary.

Similarly, they may prefer to download their head into an email. Smartphones can be used to undertake Internet searches. Apps can be downloaded to provide instructions for practice assignments or to develop skills such as mindfulness or relaxation.

Cameras on smartphones can be used to take pictures of difficult situations which can then be used to plan discovery assignments. If a young person prefers not to write, smartphones can be used to create photo libraries. For example, a young person can take photographs for an assignment in which they are looking for the positives (TGFB p53; TGFG p143) or finding their strengths (TGFB p52). Short videos can be made of young people undertaking practice or discovery assignments. These videos provide useful opportunities to review the everyday application of skills and to inform how they can be enhanced. Alarms and prompts can be set on smartphones to remind a young person to undertake an assignment. Similarly, the young person's kinder inner voice (TGFB p66) can be saved on their phone as a screen saver or as an easily accessible prompt which they can access when they are beating themselves up.

Assignments can be made into fun, engaging games and practical exercises. Parents of children with separation anxiety can create treasure hunts to encourage their child to leave their side and independently find the hidden treasure. A mindfulness assignment may involve making a clutter jar (TGFG p62) in which a jar is filled with glitter and water and shaken to represent the thoughts swirling around in their head. They are encouraged to focus on the jar and to notice how the water clears as the glittery thoughts no longer swirl around and clutter up the jar.

With younger children, it will be important to involve their parents in any home assignments. Their involvement may range from awareness that their child is monitoring or practising a skill through to supporting their child to undertake a discovery assignment. In the latter case, in order to ensure that the assignment is successful, parents need to be fully involved in planning and agreeing the task.

It is important to be clear about the role of parents and that of the young person in undertaking the assignment. Parents will usually have a supporting and facilitating rather than a leading role. This needs to be explicit, and the young person needs to be aware that although they are responsible for completing the task, they can request support and help from their parents if required. The clinician therefore needs to be sensitive to the possibility of parents taking a more proactive and dominant role in securing the completion of the assignment. This takes away responsibility from the young person and can reduce their motivation, ownership, and involvement in future home assignments.

If a young person fails to complete an assignment, this will be reviewed during the next meeting and, unless previously agreed, does not need any active intervention from parents. This will avoid any negative or critical parent–child interactions that may result in home assignments being perceived as negative or unhelpful. However, positive engagement in home assignments does need parental recognition and reinforcement. Parents have a key job in recognising, acknowledging, and highlighting the importance of what the young person has achieved. The way in which this is done can be agreed as part of the assignment planning.

Assignments are realistic, achievable, and safe

Fully involving the young person in determining the assignment will increase their ownership of it and the likelihood that it will be competed. The task needs to be realistic, with the nature and extent of the assignment being openly discussed and agreed. This provides opportunities to discuss any concerns the young person may have about the assignment demands and the practicalities of how it will be undertaken, and to clarify exactly what is involved.

In terms of assignment demands, the frequency and/or length of time that is realistic should be clarified.

- Can the young person complete a dairy of all events for one week or perhaps capture two examples?

- Can the young person practise their new skills every day or perhaps twice during the course of the week?

- Can the young person experiment with their new skills each morning as they walk to school or on those days they find most difficult?

Potential practical issues that may interfere with assignment completion need to be discussed and a plan agreed.

- Whilst at school, can the young person record a mark somewhere on their phone every time they spot a negative thought?

- Do they have a secure place where they can keep their diary private so that their siblings cannot read it?

- Can practice assignments be scheduled on those nights when the young person does not have any other regular commitments?

It is important that the assignment and expectations are clear and that potential motivational issues are addressed. Avoidance is common with anxiety, and young people may repeatedly put things off. Similarly, young people with low mood may find it hard to initiate an assignment. If the assignment does not clearly specify when it will be undertaken, there is a danger that it will be put off or not completed. Rather than a vague or general assignment, for example, 'practise relaxation a couple of times', it can be useful to make the instructions very specific, for example, 'practise relaxation on Monday and Thursday night before bed'. Avoid imprecisely defined assignments that are ambiguous and open to interpretation. Agree with the young person exactly what the task involves.

Like discovery experiments, assignments should be carefully planned to mitigate against potential problems, as in the following examples.

▶ Is a parent able to support their child's exposure on a Saturday morning or does that interfere with other events such as shopping or visiting relatives, suggesting a different day would be better?

▶ If the assignment involves phoning a friend to ask them to the cinema, what would the young person do if they were unavailable?

▶ If the young person is staying the weekend away from home, how will they be able to practise their relaxation or mindfulness exercises?

To ensure the assignment is achievable, the task needs to be small. A smaller but successfully completed assignment is preferable to an idealistic task that is too large and runs the risk of not being completed. If a task is too large, a smaller, more modest, but nonetheless informative assignment should be considered. The process used in the fear ladder (TGFB p195) can help to identify some of the smaller steps that might result in more achievable assignments.

Assignments should be safe and should not expose the young person to any physical danger. If a young person is being bullied, for example, an alternative option for resolving this could involve being assertive and standing up to the bullies. Before agreeing this as a discovery assignment, the positive and negative consequences need to be carefully considered (TGFG p213). If this option might increase the risk that the young person will be exposed to greater physical bullying in response to their increased assertiveness, an assignment such as this is not appropriate.

Finally, some assignments may sound simple but may be very challenging. For example, a depressed young person may be so familiar with their negative and critical thoughts that they find it very difficult to identify anything positive that might happen. In these situations, it can be useful to start the assignment in the meeting with the young person.

▶ 'Let us think about what has happened today and see if we can find one positive thing to start the diary.'

This provides an opportunity to model how this can be approached, as the young person is guided through their day to identify some of the positives that have happened. Clearly, attending the meeting is a positive event which shows that the young person is keen to help themselves and to change what is currently happening. Similarly, it is all too easy to dismiss everyday events like getting to school on time as unimportant, although if the young person did not get to school on time they would be in trouble.

Starting the assignment in the meeting provides opportunities to model and define the task and to resolve any problems, thereby increasing the likelihood of successful completion.

Refers to goals when planning assignments and to rating scales when reviewing progress

Once goals have been identified, prioritised, and agreed, they can be translated into home assignments.

Case Study Harry wants to get fitter

Harry (14) had been feeling low in his mood and had stopped doing many of the things he used to enjoy. He would seldom go out, would spend a lot of time in his bedroom on his own, and, although he used to enjoy sport, had not done anything physical for several months. He had put on weight, felt physically unfit, and was feeling very unhappy.

During the assessment, Harry identified that he would like to get fit. This was turned into a SMART goal – specific, measurable, achievable, relevant, and timely.

▶ Specific: 'If you were fitter, what would you do?' – 'I would be able to run again, something I used to enjoy.'

▶ Measurable: 'How would you know if you had achieved it?' – 'I would use my Fitbit to measure how far I was able to run.'

▶ Achievable: 'Is this something you could realistically achieve?' – 'I used to regularly run five kilometres, so I could run one kilometre.'

▶ Relevant: 'How will this make a difference to you?' – 'If I can start running again, it will get me out of the house and I will become fitter and start to feel happier.'

▶ Timely: 'Can you do this within the next two weeks?' – 'Yes, I haven't got any plans at the weekend so can go for a one-kilometre run on Saturday.'

Once the goal was agreed, it was translated into an assignment, with the skills that would help Harry to be successful being explored.

- ▶ Harry realised that whilst he felt enthusiastic, this feeling did not last and he often felt unmotivated. What could Harry do to maintain his motivation?
  - ▶ Would it be helpful if his parents were involved to remind and support him to run on Saturday?
  - ▶ Could Harry set himself a caring message as a screen shot on his phone to empower him to attempt his challenge?
- ▶ Harry recognised that he would feel very self-conscious going for a run. He had put on weight and was worried that other people would laugh and stare at him.
  - ▶ Could Harry choose a time and route where there might be fewer people around?
  - ▶ Would relaxation exercises like Change the Feeling (TGFB p164) help him to feel more relaxed before he went out on his run?
  - ▶ Could Harry be more compassionate to himself? Instead of criticising himself, could Harry practise talking to himself with a kinder voice (TGFB p66)? 'I am feeling anxious, but everyone feels like that if they haven't done something for a while. I am trying to help myself feel better.'
- ▶ Harry was feeling down, and he found it hard to recognise or acknowledge anything positive he did.
  - ▶ How would Harry celebrate and reward himself after his run (TGFG p200)?
  - ▶ Could Harry keep a diary of his successes so that he remembers what he has achieved (TGFB p53)?
- ▶ Rating scales were used to assess Harry's mood each week. His goals were systematically increased until he achieved his goal of running five kilometres twice per week.

Case Study Fatima's unhelpful thoughts

Fatima was experiencing many unhelpful thoughts, which were making her feel sad. These thoughts were very self-critical (e.g. 'I can never get things right'), devaluing (e.g. 'I am not important, so can't bother people with my problems'), unkind (e.g. 'I am stupid'), and uncaring ('I might as well not be here, no one would notice'). Fatima wanted to feel better in her mood but did not know how to develop this into a goal until she understood more about how she could deal with her critical thoughts. Understanding her choices helped Fatima to clarify her goals and the activities that would help her to secure them.

- ▶ One approach would be to directly challenge her unhelpful thoughts. This is based on the premise that Fatima's thinking is biased and selective and that she is failing to notice or acknowledge the more positive things that happen. This would involve identifying her common unhelpful thoughts (TGFB p108; TGFG p89), exploring whether she had fallen into a thinking trap (TGFB p117; TGFG p103), challenging her thoughts (TGFB p129; TGFG p117), or undertaking an experiment to check them out (TGFB p185).

- ▶ A second approach would be for Fatima to change her relationship with her thoughts. This is based on the assumption that her problems are not because she is having these unhelpful thoughts, but because she believes that these are true. This would involve Fatima changing the relationship with her thoughts and discovering that she is not her thoughts. She would develop mindfulness (TGFB p77). Instead of trying to stop or change her thoughts, she would learn to decouple herself from her thoughts and to stand back and observe them (TGFB p78; TGFG p63). Instead of thinking 'I am stupid', she would notice that she is having a thought that she is stupid.

- ▶ Another approach would be for Fatima to develop more self-compassion. Her current way of thinking is very critical, uncaring, and unkind, which has a negative effect on her mood. She would develop more self-compassion and kindness by learning to speak kindly to herself (TGFB p64, p66; TGFG p44), accepting who she is (TGFG p45), caring for herself (TGFB p65; TGFG p46), and acknowledging her strengths (TGFB p52).

Agreeing the approach helped Fatima to clarify her goals. The goals were used to inform the intervention and home assignments, with her progress being reviewed during each session.

Assignments are reviewed and reflection encouraged

If an assignment has been agreed, it is essential that it is reviewed during the following session. If it is overlooked or forgotten, it sends a message to the young person that assignments are not important and do not need to be undertaken. The assignment review highlights their importance and provides a chance to acknowledge what the young person has achieved and an opportunity to promote self-efficacy, reflection, and discovery.

If the assignment has been completed, the young person should be praised and encouraged to reflect on what they have discovered.

- 'It is great that you did that Internet search we agreed last meeting. Tell me what you have found out.'

- 'Well done, this monitoring chart looks really good. Have you noticed any patterns?'

- 'You've done really well practising these skills. Which of these do you think will be most helpful?'

- 'Fantastic that you have completed this task. What have you discovered by doing things differently?'

It is important to promote self-discovery since this reflective process needs to continue once meetings have finished.

There will be times when assignments are not completed or have been undertaken in a less than ideal way, for example, diaries being completed retrospectively on the day of the meeting rather than as they occurred. The reasons for this should be reviewed in an open, curious, non-judgemental way and the young person should not be criticised. Instead, the focus should be on the barriers that prevented the young person from undertaking the assignment. Understanding the barriers can inform the design and successful completion of subsequent assignments. There are a variety of barriers that can be explored.

- **Levels of distress are too high.** The young person may be too anxious and frightened, too depressed and lacking in motivation, or feeling too angry and hopeless to be able to complete the assignment. When distress is high, assignments need to be smaller so that they feel more achievable.

- **Assignment is too complex.** Although the young person may have agreed to the assignment, it may prove too complicated or demanding or exceed their cognitive abilities. In these cases, future assignments need to be simpler and tailored more carefully to the young person's developmental abilities.

- **Assignment is unclear.** The young person may be confused or unclear about the assignment. This indicates that future assignments should be more specific, and a written summary provided for the young person to take away. Starting the task in session demonstrates what is required.

- **Forgot.** The young person may be chaotic or disorganised and may have forgotten to undertake the assignment. Building reminders, such as writing on a calendar or telephone prompts, into future assignments may be helpful.

- ▶ **Fear of failure.** The young person may be anxious about the task or a perfectionist fearing that they will not do it correctly. Tasks should be more clearly specified, and their rationale defined, stressing that there are no right or wrong answers or ways of approaching this.

- ▶ **Not engaged.** The failure to undertake an assignment might indicate a lack of engagement or motivation. This should be reassessed and, if necessary, brief motivational interviewing undertaken before continuing with the intervention.

Once the reasons for non-completion have been established, the assignment should be undertaken in the meeting.

- ▶ If the home assignment was one of monitoring, the young person can be asked to verbally review incidents.

- ▶ If the home assignment was to practise skills, the skills can be practised there and then.

- ▶ If assignment was one of implementing new skills, it may be possible to engage in a role play.

Completion during the session highlights the importance of the assignment and signals that the assignment will not be forgotten or avoided.

Finally, discovery assignments are undertaken in an open and curious way, and the outcome may confirm the unhelpful core belief or assumption that is being checked. This possibility needs to be considered at the planning stage so that the information obtained is helpful whatever the outcome.

CHAPTER ELEVEN

Putting it together

The CORE philosophy, the PRECISE process, and the ABC of specific techniques need to be brought together to form a flexible intervention tailored and adapted to the young person's needs. This individualised approach is grounded in a clear case formulation which informs the selection, timing, and pacing of specific CBT techniques.

There is growing evidence from randomised controlled trials using manualised programmes to highlight the combinations of techniques and strategies that have been found helpful in the treatment of childhood problems. These trials have typically involved standardised treatment packages, so the specific contribution of each element is largely unknown. Similarly, the relevance and importance of each specific component for individual children will vary. In terms of age, most trials have been undertaken with young people aged 7–16 years, so comparatively less is known about younger children. Several studies have been conducted in research clinics with young people recruited via media adverts, thereby raising the question of whether these programmes are as effective with the young people with multiple problems referred to clinical settings within mental health services. These caveats having been acknowledged, the following core components are presented as typically having been included in standardised CBT programmes for the treatment of anxiety disorders, obsessive-compulsive disorder, depression, and post-traumatic stress disorder.

A Clinician's Guide to CBT for Children to Young Adults: A Companion to Think Good, Feel Good and Thinking Good, Feeling Better, Second Edition. Paul Stallard.
© 2021 John Wiley & Sons Ltd. Published 2021 by John Wiley & Sons Ltd.
Companion website: www.wiley.com/go/cliniciansguide2e

Anxiety

Effectiveness

There is growing evidence from systematic reviews of randomised controlled trials that CBT for the treatment of childhood anxiety is effective (James et al. 2015; Reynolds et al. 2012; Wang et al. 2017; Zhou et al. 2019). Many of the studies that have evaluated manualised CBT interventions are based upon variants of the original generic 16-session *Coping Cat* programme that was developed by Phillip Kendall (1990). The first eight sessions of the programme are concerned with education and skill acquisition, with the remaining eight focusing upon exposure-based practice. The programme includes psycho-education, emotional awareness and management, cognitive restructuring, hierarchy development, and exposure. This is consistent with a large review of treatment components of established interventions for childhood anxiety where 88% used exposure, 62% cognitive techniques, and 54% relaxation training (Higa-McMillian et al. 2016). Many anxiety programmes are trans-diagnostic, that is, they can be used with children with a variety of anxiety disorders. Whilst some research suggests that specific disorders (e.g. social anxiety) may not respond so well to trans-diagnostic interventions (Hudson et al. 2015), other reviews have found that these approaches are effective (Ewing et al. 2015).

New, anxiety disorder-specific programmes are being developed and have shown encouraging results, for example, the single-session exposure intervention for children with specific phobias (Öst & Ollendick 2017) and the cognitive intervention for children with social anxiety (Leigh & Clark 2018). Similarly, there is emerging evidence that the new, "third wave" CBT interventions such as acceptance and commitment therapy (Hancock et al. 2018) and mindfulness (Borquist et al. 2019) are also effective.

Rationale informing the intervention

The underlying model for anxiety-focused CBT is based upon the premise that anxiety is a conditioned response (Compton et al. 2004). When an individual confronts an anxiety-arousing situation, there is an increase in unpleasant feelings (e.g. increased heart rate, shortness of breath, sweating) and cognitions (e.g. I won't be able to cope). These unpleasant feelings and thoughts are minimised by removing or escaping from the threatening situations. This brings immediate emotional relief and results in the young person learning to reduce their anxious feelings by avoiding anxiety-provoking situations. The young person never learns to beat their anxiety and to face and cope with such situations.

In addition, parents may have a role in the development and maintenance of the young person's anxiety. The young person's bias towards appraisals of threat and their avoidant behaviour may be encouraged, reinforced, and modelled by their parents (Barrett, Rapee, et al. 1996). Parents of anxious children may also be more protective and over-involved. This conveys a sense of continual danger to the young person, with their parents' over-involvement limiting their chances of developing appropriate coping mechanisms or acquiring problem-solving skills.

Core components of CBT interventions for anxiety disorders

Psycho-education

As with all programmes, the intervention starts with psycho-education. This covers the cognitive model (TGFB p89), the theoretical rationale underlying the use of CBT, and an understanding of the fear response and the avoidance trap (see section 'Beating anxiety' in Chapter 12, Resources).

Emotional awareness / Anxiety management

The intervention then typically shifts into the emotional domain. Emotional awareness is increased as the young person learns to identify the specific physiological anxiety cues (TGFB p148; TGFG p163) their body uses to signal feelings of anxiety. To counter these unpleasant feelings, the young person learns relaxation skills (TGFB pp161–166; TGFG pp177–179) and is encouraged to practise these when they become aware of their anxious feelings.

Cognitive awareness and enhancement

Important cognitions associated with these anxious feelings are then identified (TGFB pp101, 108–109; TGFG pp87, 156). These beliefs, assumptions, and automatic thoughts are often referred to as 'self-talk'. Young people are helped to identify their anxiety-generating cognitions or thinking traps (TGFB p117; TGFG p103) and to replace these with anxiety-reducing cognitions or positive self-talk (TGFB p130; TGFG p144). Alternatively, mindfulness (TGFB pp77–80; TGFG pp59–64) can help the young person to develop a less critical and more compassionate relationship with their thoughts and a greater acceptance of anxiety-provoking situations and events that they are unable to control.

Self-reinforcement / Exposure and practice

The emotional and cognitive elements promote self-awareness and evaluation, and young people are encouraged to develop self-reinforcement (TGFG p200) and to praise their own attempts at using coping self-talk (TGFG p145) and relaxation strategies. Once these positive coping skills have been mastered, the young person embarks upon a process of exposure. Feared situations or events are identified and arranged in a hierarchy of fearfulness (TGFB pp194–195; TGFG pp196). Starting with the least fearful, the young person systematically faces (exposure) each situation. They are encouraged to use their new emotional and cognitive strategies as they confront their fears (TGFB p196; TGFG p198) and learn to overcome their anxieties.

Relapse prevention

Finally, the young person is encouraged to consolidate their new skills and to identify what has been particularly helpful (TGFB p214). They are helped to identify warning signs (TGFB p215) and potential difficult events (e.g. changing school) and to develop a coping plan to deal with any issues that might arise (TGFB p216).

Parents

Programmes have augmented child-focused sessions with parent sessions designed to address parental factors that might be maintaining the young person's anxiety (Barrett, Dadds, et al. 1996). Programmes typically teach contingency management techniques (praise courageous behaviour and ignore anxiety-talk) and help parents to identify and confront their own anxious behaviour and develop problem-solving and communication skills.

With younger children, interventions can be delivered via parents trained and supported in the use of CBT (Creswell et al. 2017; Kennedy et al. 2009). Parents are helped to manage their child's avoidant coping, to reduce parental overprotection, and to encourage child independence. Core treatment components include psycho-education about childhood anxiety, identification and testing of anxious thoughts, graded exposure, and problem solving.

Little research has investigated the specific contributions of individual treatment components, although contingency management, cognitive restructuring, and particularly exposure appear important (Manassis et al. 2014; Peris et al. 2015).

Important cognitions

Young people with anxiety disorders tend to have more expectations that negative events will occur, make more negative evaluations about their performance, are biased towards possible threat-related cues, and perceive themselves as being unable to cope with any frightening events that do arise. Barrett, Rapee, et al. (1996) found clinically anxious children were more likely to interpret ambiguous situations as threatening and were more likely to select avoidant ways of coping with these situations. The tendency for anxious children to be biased towards possible threat was also found by Bögels and Zigterman (2000). In addition, the authors found that anxious children rated themselves as less competent at dealing with threatening situations. The nature of the association between these cognitions and the presence of anxiety, that is, causal or a consequence, is unclear.

With generalised anxiety disorders, cognitions tend to focus upon worries about future or past events. These could be about what was said ('I hope Nina didn't think I was talking about her when I said that people get on my nerves'), how one behaved ('They will all think I'm stupid for missing that goal'), or what might happen ('My teacher will be really cross with me tomorrow'). The cognitive focus in separation anxiety centres around cognitions about being separated from others and, in particular, whether the child will cope ('I don't think I can go to the shops without mum') or whether their parents will be safe ('I bet something bad will happen to mum if I don't stay to look after her'). Phobias tend to involve cognitions specific to the feared object ('That dog will bite me'), whereas social phobia is characterised by cognitions associated with negative social evaluation ('They will laugh at these clothes; I know they don't like me'). Panic disorder typically involves catastrophic interpretations ('My heart is racing; I am going to have a heart attack and die') of internal physiological symptoms such as palpitations.

Depression

Effectiveness

There are a growing number of well-conducted randomised controlled trials that have evaluated CBT for the treatment of depression. Systematic reviews which combine these results have shown that CBT is an effective intervention for mild to moderate adolescent depression (Pennant et al. 2015; Zhou et al. 2015) and has been identified as a psychological treatment of choice in the United Kingdom and the United States (Birmaher et al. 2007; NICE 2019). Unfortunately, there have been few studies undertaken with children under the age of 12, so it is less clear how effective these programmes are with this younger age group (Forti-Buratti et al. 2016).

One of the most frequently evaluated standardised programmes for the treatment of depression in young people is the *Coping with Depression Course* developed by Lewinsohn (1990) and colleagues. The programme adopts a psycho-educational approach in which the young person develops a toolbox of skills to help them cope. Skills include restructuring negative cognitions to increase cognitions associated with positive mood, behavioural activation to increase pleasant events ('activity scheduling'), and the development of social, problem-solving, or conflict resolution skills. Cognitively informed programmes have been heavily informed by the work of Beck (1976). They typically involve 12–16 sessions and include components focusing on emotional recognition, self-monitoring, self-reinforcement, activity scheduling, challenging negative thinking and cognitive restructuring, social problem solving, and communication skills (Goodyer et al. 2007). In terms of treatment components, positive effects have been reported for behavioural activation (getting busy), challenging thoughts, and learning problem-solving and social skills (Kennard et al. 2009; Oud et al. 2019).

Finally, there is growing evidence that the new wave of CBT interventions, such as mindfulness (Dunning et al. 2019), compassion-based therapy (Marsh et al. 2018), and acceptance and commitment therapy (Twohig & Levin 2017), can also be effective interventions for depression.

Rationale informing the intervention

The theoretical rationale underlying CBT programmes for children with depression is based upon two main models. The first, based on social learning theory, assumes that depression is a product of low levels of positive reinforcement arising from cognitive distortions and interpersonal and problem-solving skill deficits. These deficits lead to repeated failure, increased unpleasant emotional affect, negative cognitions about performance resulting in avoidance, fewer opportunities to engage in potentially reinforcing activities, and the development of depressive symptoms (Seligman et al. 2004).

The second is the distortion model and is based upon the cognitive model developed by Beck (1976). Important negative and distorted cognitive processes are viewed as the primary cause of negative affect. The young person therefore develops a negative and biased cognitive framework of themselves, their performance, and their future characterised by cognitions related to low self-esteem, blame, helplessness, and hopelessness. Events are selected and distorted to fit within this framework, leading to reduced affect, behavioural avoidance, and lack of motivation, which serves to reinforce the young person's negative cognitions.

In addition, the role of the family has been identified as important. For example, everyday conflicts between the young person and their parents often serve to reinforce negative cognitions and beliefs about personal failure and inadequacy. Similarly, the young person's social withdrawal and isolation may be the focus of arguments as parents struggle to understand what is happening and how they can help.

Core components of CBT interventions for depression

CBT programmes for depression address important emotional and behavioural skill deficits that may lead to repeated failed experiences and the cognitive processes that lead to a biased and distorted perception of events.

Psycho-education

The theoretical model, process, and goals of CBT are firstly explained (TGFB p89). Many depressed young people have become socially disengaged and inactive, resulting in them spending considerable time listening to their negative thoughts and ruminating about their perceived failings. The intervention therefore aims to promote a sense of mastery and acceptance rather than dwelling upon and rehearsing negative cognitions (see section 'Fighting back depression' in Chapter 12, Resources).

Activity monitoring Behavioural activation

Activity monitoring (TGFB p204; TGFG p192) and scheduling and behavioural activation (TGFB p205; TGFG p195) are comparatively undemanding first steps and provide a useful overview of the young person's daily routine. This can lead to affective monitoring (TGFB p152; TGFG p161) whereby the young person rates the strength of their depressed mood throughout each day to identify particularly difficult times. The young person's daily activity level is then increased and previously enjoyable activities that they had stopped are reintroduced, particularly at those times of very low mood (TGFB p206). Increased activity often results in an improvement of mood so that the young person is better able to engage in cognitive work.

Cognitive awareness and enhancement

This involves becoming more aware of common negative thoughts, beliefs, assumptions, and cognitive traps (TGFB pp108, 109, 117, 120; TGFG pp91–93, 104). These may be actively evaluated and challenged (TGFB pp129–130; TGFG pp116–117) as the young person is helped to develop an alternative, balanced, and more helpful cognitive framework. Alternatively, the young person may prefer to develop a different relationship with their thoughts through mindfulness (TGFB pp77–80; TGFG pp59–64) and the development of self-compassion (TGFB pp64–67; TGFG pp44–48) instead of self-criticism.

Skill development

Potential deficits in social and problem-solving skills (TGFG pp211–216) are identified and solutions generated, rehearsed, and evaluated. This occurs within a positive and supportive relationship where the young person is encouraged to identify their strengths and to acknowledge and celebrate their successes. Skills to manage symptoms of depression, such as how to improve sleep (TGFB p55), are developed.

Relapse prevention

Finally, the young person consolidates their new skills and identifies what has been particularly helpful (TGFB p214). They are encouraged to identify how helpful skills can be incorporated into daily life, recognise their early warning signs, and develop a coping plan (TGFB p215), which includes when and how to seek help if required.

Parents

Caregivers are involved in different ways in CBT interventions for the treatment and prevention of depression (Dardas et al. 2018). Several programmes focus solely on the young person, although there is emerging evidence that parental involvement might result in enhanced outcomes (Oud et al. 2019). Where they are involved, programmes typically focus on psycho-education about depression and the CBT model, problem solving, conflict resolution and communication skills, and how to support and reinforce the young person's attempts at change. In addition, programmes allow the parent's own mental health needs to be identified and appropriate signposting and support to be arranged. However, as emphasised by Dardas et al. (2018), it appears important to involve parents in joint sessions with the young person rather than seeing them separately.

Important cognitions

Young people with depression are more likely to attend to the negative features (particularly sadness-related) of an event (Platt et al. 2017). They have negative views and expectations of themselves (Kendall et al. 1990), their performance, and their future and attribute positive events to external rather than internal causes (Curry & Craighead 1990). They tend to have more negative attributions about events, are more likely to report guilt and worthlessness, and are more likely to generalise failure in one domain (e.g. schoolwork) to other areas (e.g. sport) (Kaslow et al. 1988; Seligman et al. 2004; Shirk et al. 2003).

The cognitive style of young people with depression tends to be characterised by global, internal, and stable attributions (Seligman et al. 1979). Global attributions generalise specific negative events to other areas, for example, 'I did really badly in that exam; I'm going to leave school without any qualifications.' Internal attributions personalise negative events rather than attributing them to external circumstances, for example, 'I am stupid for not understanding that work.' Stable attributions fuel hopelessness that negative events and beliefs are unchanging over time, for example, 'I will never have any friends; people just hate me.'

The aim of CBT is to challenge these attributions and to develop more balanced thinking styles which are specific, external, and unstable. Specific attributions counter generalisations by putting limits around global statements. Instead of 'I'm never going to get any qualifications,' a specific attribution might be 'I am not very good at maths, but I usually do OK in my other subjects.' Internal attributions are countered by recognising the external context within which events occur. Instead of 'I am stupid,' an external attribution might be 'Everyone said how hard that work was today.' Finally, stable attributions are countered by looking for times when these events have not happened. Instead of 'People hate me,' an unstable attribution might be 'There are a couple of people who hang out with me.'

Finally, mindfulness and compassion-based approaches do not directly attempt to challenge or change cognitions. Instead they encourage the young person to change their relationship with their negative and critical ways of thinking by focusing on the here and now in an open, curious, non-judgemental way. Thoughts are therefore seen as passing mental activity rather than evidence of reality that the young person needs to engage with. The aim therefore is to help the young person change their relationship with their thoughts, rather than to directly challenge or change their content. Paying attention to the present moment helps to reduce negative rehearsal and rumination, whilst developing self-compassion counters negative, self-critical thoughts.

Obsessive-compulsive disorder (OCD)

Effectiveness

Systematic reviews for the treatment of OCD have concluded that CBT is an evidence-based intervention and the psychological treatment of choice for adolescent OCD (Franklin et al. 2015; Freeman et al. 2018; Geller et al. 2012; NICE 2005; Öst et al. 2016). There is also evidence that family-based CBT is effective for the treatment of OCD in young children aged five to eight (Freeman et al. 2014).

The earliest manualised CBT programme, *How I Ran OCD Off My Land* (March & Mulle 1998), is both acceptable and effective (Watson & Rees 2008) and has informed subsequent programmes (Barrett et al. 2004; POTS 2004). The programme consists of approximately 12 sessions and involves psycho-education about OCD and CBT, mapping OCD obsessions and rituals, contingency management, and systematic exposure and response prevention. Parents are typically involved in most sessions to support the young person and to encourage exposure and practice at home. Some interventions have a more extensive focus on family factors and aim to reduce feelings of guilt and blame, improve problem-solving and family communication skills, and increase treatment compliance and disengagement from the young person's OCD (Barrett et al. 2004; Piacentini et al. 2011).

Rationale informing the intervention

CBT for the treatment of OCD involves either exposure and response prevention, cognitive therapy, or a combination of both. Exposure and response prevention are the foundations of many programmes. Exposure ensures that the young person systematically confronts feared situations (e.g. touching items associated with germs) and continues in their presence until the associated anxiety decreases. During this time, engagement in the previously learned rituals or compulsive behaviours (e.g. hand washing) that the young person has used to reduce their anxiety are prevented. The young person therefore learns that anxiety levels can be reduced without engaging in compulsive behaviours. A third element involves the removal of parental attention, which would reinforce the young person's rituals thereby extinguishing their occurrence.

Whilst behavioural interventions have proven effective, recent interest has turned towards assessing the applicability to children of the cognitive model of OCD developed from work with adults (Salkovskis 1985, 1989). The model emphasises that it is not the obsessional intrusive thoughts themselves that cause distress but rather the way the individual appraises these. Important appraisals involving blame or an inflated responsibility for harm to oneself or others produce intolerable discomfort, which is reduced by engaging in neutralising behaviours such as compulsions, avoidance, and reassurance seeking to prevent these events occurring. The model suggests that overestimation of both harm probability and severity is central to the development and maintenance of OCD. In addition, other important cognitive processes associated with the maintenance of OCD include thought-action fusion (I think it, therefore it will happen), self-doubt (leading to indecisiveness), and a perceived lack of cognitive control (which leads to increased intrusive thoughts) (O'Kearney 1998).

In terms of family characteristics, parents and siblings have been found to accommodate and become involved in their child's OCD, which in turn serves to maintain their symptoms (Barrett et al. 2004). Family accommodation can include engaging in the young person's rituals, assisting with avoidance by modifying daily routines, or the provision of excessive reassurance (McGrath & Abbott 2019).

Core components of CBT interventions for OCD

Psycho-education

The CBT model and process are explained (TGFB p89). Intrusive thoughts are normalised, the function of rituals explained, and OCD externalised as separate from the young person (see section 'Controlling worries and habits' in Chapter 12, Resources). This challenges any parental perceptions that the young person's OCD is due to wilful naughtiness and forms the parent/young person team working together towards the common goal of beating OCD.

Emotional awareness Anxiety management

Emotional awareness (TGFG pp160, 163) and anxiety management typically follow. This provides the young person with an understanding of the fear response. Once this is understood, the young person learns alternative ways of dealing with their anxious feelings (TGFB pp161–165; TGFG pp175–179).

Cognitive awareness and enhancement

For interventions primarily based on exposure and response prevention, the cognitive component is quite limited. The young person is encouraged to challenge (TGFB pp129, 140; TGFG pp116, 117, 125) their unhelpful ways of thinking through coping and positive self-talk (TGFG pp144–145), which is used to boss back (TGFG p150) their obsessional thoughts.

Interventions based on cognitive models have a more extensive focus on the young person's attributions and assumptions that are driving their OCD. The aim is to increase awareness of these cognitions and to highlight and evaluate common thought traps, for example, cognitions about responsibility and increased probability for bad things happening (TGFB p187) and unhelpful cognitive strategies such as thought suppression.

Exposure, response prevention, rewards

Once armed with a range of emotional and cognitive strategies, the young person maps their obsessional thoughts and compulsive behaviours and the degree of distress associated with each, and a hierarchy is developed (TGFB p195; TGFG p197). Starting with the least fearful step, the young person confronts and overcomes each step of their fear hierarchy without engaging in any compulsive behaviours (TGFB p196; TGFG p199). A series of rewards (TGFG p200) acknowledge and praise the young person's success and increase their motivation to attempt the next step.

Relapse prevention

The programme ends by focusing on relapse prevention. Early signs of relapse are identified and a coping plan to address this is detailed.

Potentially difficult future situations and events over the coming year are identified and a coping plan agreed (TGFB pp214–216).

Parents

The role of parents in the original programme developed by March and Mulle (1998) was limited and was mainly concerned with psycho-education. Subsequent programmes have developed a more extensive role for parents (Freeman et al. 2008; Piacentini et al. 2011). This involves developing problem-solving skills and reducing family accommodation and unhelpful patterns of communication, as well as helping parents to become effective coaches during exposure and response prevention (Barrett et al. 2004; Peris et al. 2017).

Important cognitions

The cognitive model of OCD (Salkovskis 1985,1989) has provided a useful framework for assessing potentially important cognitions and processes in young people. The model suggests that obsessional thoughts are interpreted in a maladaptive way, particularly appraisals of inflated responsibility (for harm), exaggerated estimates that unwanted events will occur (thought-action fusion), and a need to control these thoughts. Young people with OCD have been found to have significantly higher appraisals of responsibility, harm severity, and thought-action fusion and less cognitive control than a group of non-referred children. (Barrett & Healy 2003). Similarly, Libby et al. (2004) found that young people with OCD had higher scores on measures of inflated responsibility and thought-action fusion and that inflated responsibility predicted OCD symptom severity.

Post-traumatic stress disorder (PTSD)

Effectiveness

Randomised controlled trials and systematic reviews have demonstrated that trauma-focused CBT (TF-CBT) is effective in the treatment of PTSD in young people (Mavranezouli et al. 2020; Morina et al. 2016; Smith et al. 2019). There is also evidence that modified CBT is effective for younger children aged three to seven (Dalgleish et al. 2015: Scheeringa et al. 2011). These positive findings have resulted in TF-CBT being recommended in the United Kingdom and the United States as the first-line treatment for persistent PTSD in children and young people (Cohen et al. 2010; NICE 2018).

The most widely evaluated programmes are those of TF-CBT developed by Cohen et al. (2004) and cognitive therapy for PTSD (CT-PTSD) developed by Smith et al. (2007). Both programmes involve approximately 12 sessions and include: psycho-education about PTSD; development of a shared treatment rationale; behavioural activation; relaxation training; imaginal exposure to the trauma memory (imaginal reliving); cognitive restructuring and memory updating; and planned exposure to trauma triggers and reminders. The programmes differ in the emphasis they place on cognitive work.

Parents are typically fully involved in the intervention in either co-joint or parallel sessions. Interventions involve psycho-education; behaviour management and parenting skills; relaxation; affective expression and management; cognitive coping and processing; trauma narrative; and enhancing future safety and development (Cohen et al. 2006).

Rationale informing the intervention

CBT models are largely based on learning theory and assume that stimuli associated with the trauma become conditioned with emotional reactions. Distress is moderated by avoidance, which in turn serves to reinforce intrusive traumatic images and cognitions. Interventions therefore use exposure (imaginal and in vivo) to facilitate emotional processing of traumatic memories.

Cognitive models focus more on the way that traumatic events are appraised and processed. Symptoms of PTSD are reduced by modifying negative and unhelpful trauma appraisals. The model assumes that the traumatic event is not cognitively processed and is poorly integrated into memory. The traumatic event is negatively viewed as catastrophic or devastating, and the young person misinterprets their symptoms (e.g. 'I am going mad'), which creates a sense of current threat. The use of avoidant behaviours and cognitive strategies such as rumination or thought suppression prevent the trauma being processed and serve to reinforce their sense of current threat.

Core components of CBT interventions for PTSD

TF-CBT targets the cardinal features of PTSD in the cognitive (trauma re-experiencing), emotional (increased arousal), and behavioural (avoidance) domains.

Psycho-education

TF-CBT starts with psycho-education about traumatic reactions (see section 'Coping with trauma' in Chapter 12, Resources) and the CBT model (TGFB p89). This helps the young person understand common reactions to traumatic events and begins the process of normalising their reactions and challenging their beliefs about their symptoms ('I must be going mad'). The possibility of achieving positive change is reinforced, and the young person is encouraged to resume everyday or pleasant activities that they had stopped (TGFB pp205–206).

Manage emotional arousal

Arousal management skills are learned, and the young person is taught to rate their feelings (TGFG p166), skills that will be helpful during the next stage of exposure. This might involve learning relaxation techniques (TGFB pp161–165; TGFG pp177–179), anger management skills (TGFG p176), or how to improve sleep.

Cognitive awareness and enhancement

The young person is helped to process their trauma by developing a narrative in which the event is reconstructed from beginning to end (TGFG p77). Important cognitions are elicited (TGFB pp109, 120, 187; TGFG p88) and discussed (e.g. responsibility, blame, shame) (TGFB p187), and dysfunctional cognitive processes that prevent processing of the trauma (thought suppression, avoidance) are discouraged. Repeated imaginal exposure to those parts of the trauma that are most distressing is undertaken until the associated distress reduces.

Exposure and reclaiming life

This is followed by in vivo graduated exposure (TGFB pp195, 196; TGFG pp149, 196,198) to feared situations/places associated with the trauma, and behavioural experiments (TGFB pp185–186; TGFG p141). This helps the young person to confront and cope with any events or trauma reminders that are being avoided. In addition, any specific symptoms which impair everyday functioning, such as poor sleep (TGFB p55) or lack of activity (TGFB p56), are addressed.

Relapse prevention

The programme ends by identifying potentially difficult future situations and events and agreeing a coping plan (TGFB pp214–216). Finally, the issue of future safety and how and when further help should be sought is discussed.

Parents

Most programmes involve a parent component where parents are involved with their young person, either together or in parallel sessions. Parents are helped to develop effective behavioural skills to manage any behavioural problems that might arise, such as increased irritability, angry outbursts, or poor night-time routine. A range of supportive behavioural skills might be developed, including contingency management, selective attention, positive reinforcement, communication, and problem-solving skills. Parents are helped to understand trauma reactions and, by listening to the young person's trauma narrative, understand how they are appraising the event and the attributions they have made. Through this, parents are encouraged to identify and challenge their own maladaptive cognitions about what happened (e.g. should have kept them safe or protected them). They are encouraged to support the young person during exposure tasks and learn to be less protective towards or over-involved with them.

Important cognitions

A number of potentially important cognitions have been identified as contributing to the onset and maintenance of PTSD. These include attributions about the event (e.g. as life-ruining) or symptoms (e.g. 'I am going mad'). Attributions about perceived responsibility for the trauma happening (e.g. 'I am to blame for this'), shame about how they behaved ('I didn't try to stop this'), and guilt about what they should or should not have done ('I ran away instead of trying to help') need to be elicited and challenged. Finally, the use of dysfunctional cognitive coping strategies such as thought suppression, rumination, and avoidance are discouraged.

When it doesn't go right

Whilst these intervention plans summarise the key components of evidence-based manualised CBT programmes, there is no guarantee that they will be effective. As with all interventions, they will not work in all situations for everyone. It is therefore inevitable that some young people will not make progress despite careful adherence and implementation of the intervention plan. The question therefore arises as to what has happened.

Chorpita (2007) discusses this issue in his modular approach to CBT and identifies four core areas for consideration. He advises that attention should be paid to the young person's readiness to change, the focus of the intervention, the case formulation, and the way the intervention has been delivered. Exploration of these issues needs to go beyond simply describing what happened, to a deeper understanding of why this might have occurred.

▶ A young person might have failed twice to undertake home-based monitoring assignments.

　　▶ Is this an indication that the home assignment has been poorly explained or negotiated?

- ▶ Is the young person unmotivated and not fully engaged with the therapeutic process?

- ▶ Does the young person understand the value and relevance of the task?

▶ Behavioural activation, getting busy, may have been discussed with a young person but abandoned because they were unable to identify any activities.

- ▶ Should this be abandoned, and the clinician move on?

- ▶ Could the clinician have explained this in a different way with greater exploration of possible activities?

- ▶ Is the young person feeling overwhelmed by their depression and feeling hopeless about the possibility of change?

▶ A young person struggled with the cognitive element of an intervention to challenge unhelpful cognitions.

- ▶ Should this cognitive focus continue, or the intervention shift to the emotional or behavioural domains?

- ▶ Has the PRECISE process been well implemented, and the intervention pitched at the right level for the young person to access?

- ▶ Does the young person understand the rationale for CBT, or should a different approach such as mindfulness be explored?

There are many possible explanations for the issues that arise during the delivery of an intervention. Understanding these is important and will inform what needs to be done. For example:

▶ provide more psycho-education to facilitate greater understanding of the rationale for CBT, the importance of home assignments, and how realistically they can be undertaken;

▶ review the PRECISE process and the partnership and whether the intervention has been appropriately explained and pitched at the right level;

▶ confirm the formulation to see if it needs to be updated with any new information or the problem focus revised;

▶ reassesses the young person's engagement and commitment to change;

▶ put the CBT intervention on hold whilst engaging in a process of motivational interviewing to help the young person feel more hopeful about the possibility of change.

Is the young person motivated to change?

Once a problem has been identified, clinicians are keen to discuss and initiate an intervention. Identification of a problem does not necessarily imply that the young person is motivated to engage in a process of change. Motivation can be affected by feelings of hopelessness, doubts about self-efficacy, ambivalence about whether change is possible, and external and internal drivers to change, as well as timing.

▶ Hopelessness – Do you think it is possible to do something about your problems?

Young people may be overwhelmed by their problems. Their problems may have been present for a long time, so that it is hard to imagine how things could be different. Initial enthusiasm and hope may fade as the young person questions whether their problems can really be changed. Comments such as, 'I've tried everything, and nothing seems to help' or, 'What's the point? I won't feel any better' signal a sense of hopelessness.

In these situations, the young person needs an opportunity to verbalise their hopelessness whilst being helped to recognise how the current intervention is different. This might include highlighting the available support, the use of routine outcome measures and goal ratings to carefully monitor change, or perhaps examining how the aim of the intervention might be different from what has previously been tried, for example, learning to accept what is happening rather than actively trying to change thoughts and emotions. In these situations, the aim is to engage in a Socratic dialogue to help the young person to question their hopelessness and to notice how the intervention might be different, in order to empower them to embark on a process of change.

▶ Self-efficacy – Do you think you can beat your problems?

Whilst many young people would like things to be different, they often doubt their ability to bring about change. They may feel powerless and unable to recognise the skills and strengths they possess and how they can be used to help with the current problems. They may be concerned about failing and reluctant to engage in a process of change for fear of being unsuccessful. In these situations, the young person is doubting their ability to positively influence events to secure their desired outcome.

If this is the issue, the Socratic dialogue should focus on helping the young person discover and acknowledge their strengths and skills. The conversation needs to shift from what the young person cannot do and focus instead on what they have been able to successfully achieve. Once past situations have been identified, the young person can be encouraged to explore what helped them to be successful, that is, what skills, strengths, or support they utilised. This positive conversation focuses on evidence of success, thereby challenging beliefs about powerlessness, and helps to identify past strategies and strengths that may help with the current difficulties.

► Ambivalent about change – Are you ready to change?

Ambivalence about readiness to change is common and fluctuates over time. If the young person or their carer is ambivalent, a process of motivational interviewing may be considered. This should involve a limited number of sessions designed to help the young person explore and resolve their ambivalence. The aim is to develop a discrepancy between the current situation and what the young person would ideally like.

► 'I hear that you want to go to college next year, but at the moment you are not attending school. What needs to happen for you to be able to attend college?'

► 'You say that you want to have a better social life and to go out with people and have fun. For the last three months you have stayed at home and you haven't been out at all. If this continues, you won't achieve your goal, so what needs to change?'

Motivational interviewing is a focused and directive technique in which the young person's ambivalence is viewed as the central obstacle that needs to be resolved in order to initiate change. It is this discrepancy between the here and now and future aspirations that provides the motivation to embark on a process of change. The goal is to actively facilitate the young person's expression of ambivalence and is based on a number of core principles.

► Firstly, motivation is elicited from within, not imposed from without. The early stages of motivational interviewing are therefore concerned with helping the young person to identify their potential targets for change. Attempts to elicit motivation by external threats, 'You know that you will be excluded from school if you don't try to control your temper', or persuasion, 'I am sure this can be different so why don't you give it a try', should be avoided.

► Secondly, the aim of motivational interviewing is to help the young person articulate their concerns and express both sides of their ambivalence. They are helped to identify and weigh up the potential advantages or disadvantages of action or inaction so that they can make an informed choice about the path they would like to pursue. This process can be done verbally or as a visual exercise using the Scales of Change.

▶ Thirdly, direct persuasion is not effective and serves to increase resistance. If the young person has no ownership of a problem, they will have no commitment to or investment in change. With adolescents, direct attempts at persuasion can be counterproductive. Attempts at persuasion often result in increased verbal hostility as the young person counters persuasive arguments by adopting a more rigid position, which they feel obliged to defend and justify. The process becomes combative instead of collaborative.

▶ Fourthly, readiness to change will fluctuate over time. During motivational interviewing, the clinician needs to pay attention to signs of resistance and denial and to use these to alter the focus and pace of the interview. A young person may, for example, seem committed to securing change at the end of one session but appear resistant during the subsequent session. This may be due to a variety of intervening events that have served to increase their uncertainty. Alternatively, positive signals of agreement may have been misread as signs of self-motivation rather than as a passive acceptance aimed to please and end the session.

▶ Finally, motivational interviewing occurs within a positive and supportive relationship in which the young person is an active partner. Their ideas are welcomed and respected even if they conflict with those of others. Responsibility for determining and securing change resides with the young person, with the clinician attending to, and reinforcing, any positive signs, such as the young person attending appointments, talking about problems, or sharing their ambivalence and feelings.

Case Study Sam's costs of change

Sam (14) was keen to become friends with Surinder but was very reluctant to talk with her. The Scales of Change helped Sam communicate his ambivalence (Figure 11.1).

Although it looked as if there were more reasons for Sam to talk with Surinder, this changed when Sam was asked to rate the importance of each item. Sam was very worried about being shown up and ignored, and this far outweighed all the potential benefits. The costs of change were too great for Sam.

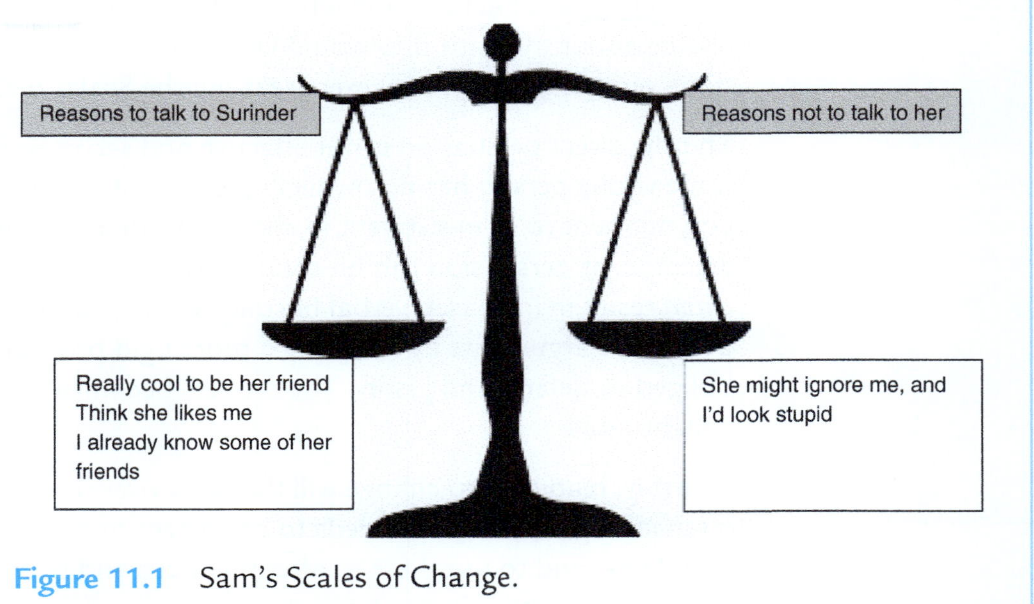

Figure 11.1   Sam's Scales of Change.

▶ Drivers to change – Is this something which is important to change?

Young people seldom refer themselves for help and are typically dependent on parents recognising and acknowledging their problems. Motivation to seek help is therefore heavily influenced by external drivers, particularly parent or school concerns. Often there is a crisis, a tipping point, which precipitates help-seeking. However, once the immediate crisis has passed, parents may question the need for an ongoing intervention, and motivation might reduce. Other factors that might affect parental motivation include concerns about being blamed for the problems, stigma associated with seeking psychological help, or their child being labelled. In these situations, parental ambivalence and negative beliefs associated with help-seeking need to be elicited and explored.

Similarly, the internal readiness and commitment of the young person will vary over time. The young person may find themselves returning to the contemplation stage as they rehearse their doubts, worries, and uncertainty about being able to bring about change. Internal readiness to change can be assessed by using questionnaires (TGFB p 88).

▶ Timing – Do you think this is the right time to try and change things?

Whilst the young person's psychological health is clearly important, this presents within a wider systemic context. For example, there may be other issues within the family, such as a house move, change of job, or physical or mental health issues, that the young person and their family may want/need to prioritise. Similarly, whilst there might be a commitment to change, the timing of the intervention may not be right. The young person may, for example, have school exams and may prefer to focus on these before addressing their specific problems.

In these situations, a hopeful and positive position needs to be adopted as the right time to focus on the young person's problems is clarified. The intervention should then be postponed and rescheduled for a future date.

Are the young person and their family engaged with the intervention?

The degree to which the young person and their parent/family are engaged with the intervention is important. They need to believe that CBT is a helpful way of addressing their problems, that the goals are meaningful and important, and that the intervention is focused on the right problem. In addition, they need to believe that the clinician can work with them to bring about change.

▶ Intervention – Do you think this way of working (CBT) will help you?

Although the young person may have been provided with an explanation of what CBT involves (TGFB p 89), it may feel very abstract until they have experienced it. They may have been provided with opportunities to ask questions but found it hard to verbalise their questions or concerns.

CBT does not suit everyone. Some people may doubt the basic premise of CBT and the focus on cognitions. There may be concerns about some methods, such as exposure, where the young person will learn to beat their anxiety by facing their anxiety-creating situations. Some may be reluctant to engage in an active process and may not be committed to undertaking home assignments or practice. Others may see the reason for their problems residing in others. For example, a young person with anger outbursts may understand the reason for these as their teacher unfairly picking on them. They will therefore have no engagement in changing what they do, instead seeing the teacher as the one who needs to change.

Further explanation of the rationale for CBT, the active process of collaboration and guided discovery, and the importance of home assignments may be helpful. The young person may find it reassuring to know that home assignments and exposure tasks will be jointly agreed and will be undertaken in a staged way to ensure that they will be successful. Similarly, whilst the young person may see the reason for their difficulties residing elsewhere, it could be helpful to explore how they could minimise any adverse effects on themselves.

▶ Problem focus – Do you think we are focusing on the most important problem?

The assessment will identify the extent and nature of the young person's problems and will clarify their goals. Where there are multiple problems, it is important to establish which will be the initial focus of the intervention, since the sequencing and use of specific CBT techniques will vary. For example:

▶ Interventions for depression typically start by changing behaviour, whereas those for anxiety focus on emotional awareness and management.

▶ Whilst relaxation training might be helpful for an anxious young person, these skills may be less helpful for one with depression.

▶ Exposure is an essential component of interventions for anxiety and PTSD, but not for depression.

The formulation is the process which brings together the young person's problems within the CBT framework. The formulation is developed collaboratively and provides a shared understanding of the problems. It makes sense of what may feel like a random selection of unrelated events, thoughts, emotions, and behaviours.

The formulation is dynamic and evolving and will be revisited and revised during each session to accommodate new information and to inform the intervention. The formulation is therefore a powerful way of bringing complex information together and guiding the intervention. It clarifies what work needs to be undertaken in which domain and provides a clear rationale to inform the selection and sequencing of specific techniques.

Given the central role of the formulation, it is important to regularly revisit this and to check that it is focused on the right problem. At other times, young people can be helped to prioritise multiple problems by asking about the impact they have on their life or the achieving of their goals.

▶ 'You have told me that you feel down in your mood, become anxious in social situations, and are not getting on with your mum and dad. If you could change one of these, which would make the biggest difference to your life?'

▶ 'You identified a goal of wanting to go out with your friends. Which of your problems, anxiety or low mood, is the biggest barrier that is stopping you from being able to do this?'

Problems may change, and the dynamic nature of the young person's psycho-social and systemic environment means that the intervention focus should be regularly reviewed and agreed.

Case Study Jade is anxious and depressed

During the assessment, Jade (15) presented with significant symptoms of anxiety and depression. She completed the Revised Child Anxiety Depression Scale, which confirmed that she had significant symptoms of both anxiety and depression. Jade identified what she wished to achieve: being able to go out with her friends.

To clarify the primary problem, a recent situation was tracked which was summarised in a maintenance formulation (Figure 11.2).

The trigger was a social situation where her friend Tracey asked if she wanted to go to the cinema. Jade hadn't been to the cinema for a long time and found herself thinking that she would not be able to cope. She recalled feeling anxious and scared at the prospect of going out but also sad that she was trapped at home on her own. She decided that she could not go and instead stayed in her bedroom all night crying.

The discussion as the formulation was developed clarified that the primary problem for Jade was one of anxiety. It was her anxiety that prevented her from going out, with her low mood being a consequence of being trapped at home on her own.

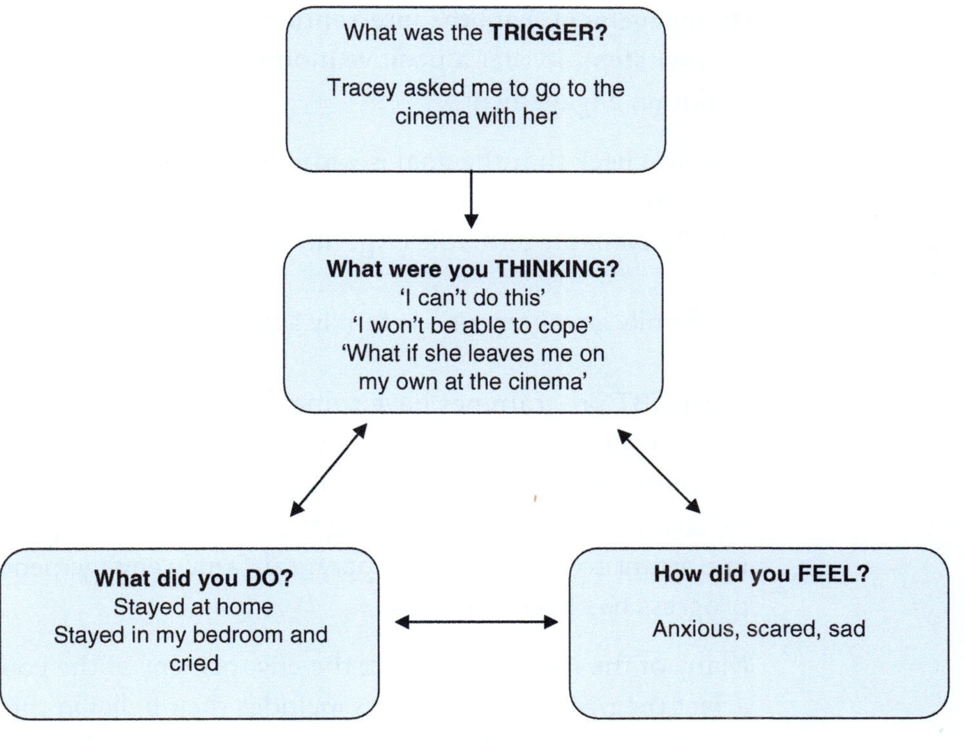

Figure 11.2   Jade is invited to the cinema.

► Meaningful goals – Are the goals meaningful and important?

Engagement will be influenced by the intervention goals and what the young person is working to achieve. It is therefore helpful to check that goals are relevant and meaningful to the young person.

A young person may have simply agreed with the goals suggested by others and have no real interest in securing their achievement. For example, parents may be keen for their child to be more sociable and to attend social activities or join clubs, whilst the young person may feel content with their current level of social activity and friendships. In addition, goals need to be personally meaningful. Whilst a goal of going to the supermarket may help someone who is anxious about facing a crowded situation, it may not be relevant or important for them. Perhaps going to the local music shop on a Saturday afternoon might be more meaningful and motivating. Similarly, goals should relate to the young person's values. If the young person values personal fitness, a more meaningful goal would be to go to the local gym, sports hall, running track, or swimming pool.

Whilst meaningful and important goals may have been identified, it is helpful to check that they are clear and achievable. A goal of 'feeling happier' does not clarify what the young person needs to do to improve their mood. Making sure that goals are SMART (specific, measurable, achievable, relevant, and timely) will help to clarify what the young person is working towards and when they will achieve it. In addition to being unclear, a goal of 'feeling happier' is too ambitious and will inevitably result in failure and disengagement from the intervention. Large goals need to be broken into smaller steps so that a positive momentum of success can be established to maintain engagement.

Finally, check that the goal is within the gift of the young person to achieve. For example, a goal of 'going to the cinema with my friend' requires a friend who is available and able (e.g. money, interest, transport) to attend.

► Family engagement – Is family support available?

Most CBT programmes have some degree of parental/family involvement. This ranges from providing practical support to help the young person attend appointments through to attending sessions to directly modify parent/family behaviours that are maintaining the young person's problems. It is therefore important to check that the parental/family engagement necessary to secure progress has been achieved.

Many of the issues that affect the engagement of the young person will also affect the parents/family. This includes their belief in the CBT model and process, understanding of the young person's problem, and agreement with the formulation, problem focus, and goals. Parents may have knowledge of, or themselves be engaged in a process of, CBT, and this experience will influence their perception of what is involved and how helpful this might be. Their recognition of the young person's problems and how they can support their child needs clarification. Do they understand that depression, for example, is different from normal adolescent moodiness, or that OCD routines are not deliberate or wilful? The formulation provides a personalised explanation of the young person's problems and informs the subsequent intervention. Do the parents/family understand the problem formulation and agree with the intervention focus and the goals that will be focused upon? The formulation may highlight parental behaviours that are maintaining the young person's problems, resulting in parents feeling criticised, blamed, or responsible for what has happened. It is therefore important to adopt an open, no-blame approach that uses the formulation to positively plan how the parent/family can help to secure change and move forward. Finally, parents may have different goals and priorities from those of the young person. These need to be heard, acknowledged, and parked to be returned to later.

Once the parents/family are engaged with the approach and goals, it is helpful to check their ability to support the intervention.

▶ Are parents able to tolerate their child's anxiety and distress in order to support exposure tasks? Is the family able to stop accommodating the young person's OCD?

▶ Can parents support and reinforce attempts by their depressed young person to get busy?

▶ Can a parent tolerate listening to their child's appraisals of their trauma?

Factors such as these may reduce engagement and limit progress, and, if identified, alternative solutions need to be explored.

▶ Is there another family member who can support exposure or reinforce attempts to change?

▶ Can the family be helped to become more confident to stop accommodating by practising with one small ritual?

This process may also highlight parental mental health needs that require specific intervention. For example, a parent may have been involved in the trauma with their child and require a referral to adult mental health services to help them process their experience.

Finally, it is important to be mindful about whether CBT is the most appropriate intervention and what it can realistically achieve. In some situations, responsibility for family dysfunction can be inappropriately assigned to the young person. Scapegoating in this way is inappropriate, and an alternative, family-focused intervention needs to be suggested. Similarly, the parents/family may refuse to engage with the intervention, believing that it is the young person, not them, who needs to change. Once again, this needs to be directly challenged, the parent/family support required clearly identified, and the more limited goals that the intervention would have without their involvement clarified.

▶ Clinician and young person fit – Do you feel that I am hearing what you have to say?

The PRECISE process ensures that CBT is suitably tailored towards the young person. However, sometimes the 'fit' between the clinician and the young person does not work and there isn't a strong, positive relationship. This can be very hard for a young person to verbalise. They may be worried about upsetting the clinician or about what might happen if they did voice their concerns.

The routine use of a session rating scale can identify this possibility. Scales can assess aspects of the therapeutic relationship, such as whether the young person felt listened to; whether they had opportunities to talk about the things they wanted to; whether they felt that this way of working was helpful for them; how satisfied they were with the session; and what could be done to make the meeting more helpful. Session ratings are often high, so it is useful to focus on any variations that might occur between sessions. This might highlight ways in which the young person's feedback can be accommodated so that they feel more engaged with the process. However, there may be times when an open and honest discussion leads to a conclusion that an alternative therapist may be required.

How has the intervention been delivered?

There will be times when a clear formulation has been developed and the appropriate problem agreed. The young person is motivated and ready to embark on a process of change, and the appropriate intervention has been provided. However, routine outcome measures and goal rating scales fail to show any progress. At times, this may be expected as the young person learns and develops the skills to address their problems. However, on other occasions, it is important to review how the intervention has been provided.

▶ Has the intervention been pitched at the right level?

An initial session of mindfulness may have been unsuccessfully undertaken resulting in a conclusion that the young person 'does not get it'. Should the clinician learn from this unsuccessful session and repeat the session in a different way, or should they move on?

▶ Has information been provided in enough depth?

A session on psycho-education may have been provided, but is it enough for the young person? Do they need this explained again in different ways or in greater detail so that they fully understand the rationale for the intervention?

▶ Is the pace appropriate?

Trauma-focused exposure can be distressing for both the young person and the clinician. The young person may have had several explanations about the intervention, but has a direct trauma discussion occurred, or is this being avoided?

▶ Have all the techniques been fully implemented?

Exposure is an important part of many interventions but can be difficult. Whilst imaginal exposure has been undertaken during clinical sessions, have real-life exposure tasks been undertaken?

▶ Have the techniques been implemented well?

The process of thought challenging may have been undertaken, but the emphasis may have been on disproving the young person's unhelpful thoughts rather than on the development of 'balanced thoughts'. Should the clinician consider how they might introduce this idea in a more balanced way?

It is essential to constantly reflect on clinical practice in order to ensure that safe and effective interventions are provided, and that professional skills and competencies continue to develop. The CORE philosophy, PRECISE process, and ABC of specific techniques provide a framework for reflection. This is best undertaken during clinical supervision as an ongoing, curious, supportive, reflective conversation. This should focus on both cases where there have been difficulties as well as those which have been successful. This encourages strengths and success to be acknowledged whilst addressing specific competencies which need to be developed.

Clinical supervision is essential for continuing development and good practice. However, if this is not possible, an open, honest, self-reflective approach should be adopted. This involves reflecting on clinical practice (see Figure 11.3) as well as exploring personal thoughts, feelings, and behaviours that might impact on the intervention (Sburlati & Bennett-Levy 2014). For example, a trauma-focused discussion maybe delayed because the clinician

Young person:
GK   Age: 14   Gender: Male

Primary problem:
OCD

Routine outcome monitoring:
No change over past four sessions.

Session rating:
All high (4) but slightly lower (3) on understanding.

Session focus:
Dropping safety behaviours (touch door handles without washing hands).

What did I do well?
Worked through the chain of events and highlighted how unlikely it was that GK would contract a serious health condition.

What could I do better?
Although he saw that the risk was exceptionally low, I didn't manage to address his concerns and move to a stage of GK touching the door handle without washing his hands.

What will I do differently next time?
Review the OCD hierarchy and identify a less anxiety-provoking ritual to target.

Figure 11.3   Example of a personal reflection log.

feels anxious about hearing the specific content of the young person's trauma. Similarly, the clinician may worry that they will be unable to cope with the young person's distress during a real-life exposure task and so avoid undertaking this.

Personal refection can be significantly enhanced by reviewing video or audio recordings of clinical sessions. If this is not possible, then at the very least, 5–10 minutes after each session should be allocated to a brief review which celebrates positive practice and identifies areas for improvements and an action plan to address any shortfalls (Sburlati & Bennett-Levy 2014). This reflection should also involve information from routine outcome measures and the session rating scale and a brief summary of the session focus. Reflection involves asking:

- ▶ 'What did I do well in that session?'

- ▶ 'What could I have done better?'

- ▶ 'What will I do differently next time?'

This information should be kept together in a reflective log, which can help identify themes both within and across different clients.

Personal reflection requires the adoption of an open mindset and acknowledgement that this is an ongoing process of self-development. Like many new skills, the practice of CBT will continue to develop over time. Personal reflection facilitates this dynamic process of honing skills and ongoing competency development. It is a positive process, central to the development of good practice, and not a sign of failure or inadequacy. It celebrates what has gone well but also encourages continued development and experimentation with different ideas to improve clinical practice.

CHAPTER TWELVE

Resources

A variety of resources are included which are *available free, in colour, to purchasers* of the print version. To find out how to access and download these, visit the website:

www.wiley.com/go/cliniciansguide2e

The online facility provides an opportunity to download and print relevant sections of the guide that can be used in clinical sessions with young people or by the clinician to develop and reflect on their practice.

The online materials can be used flexibly and can be accessed and used as often as required.

A Clinician's Guide to CBT for Children to Young Adults: A Companion to Think Good, Feel Good and Thinking Good, Feeling Better, Second Edition. Paul Stallard.
© 2021 John Wiley & Sons Ltd. Published 2021 by John Wiley & Sons Ltd.
Companion website: www.wiley.com/go/cliniciansguide2e

The Chain of Events

Sometimes we worry that if we don't do something, bad things will happen. Because we think it, we believe that it is true without checking out whether it is possible.

Start at the top and write down the bad thing that you think will happen. Now go to the bottom of the chain and fill in all the links that would have to be there before this could happen.

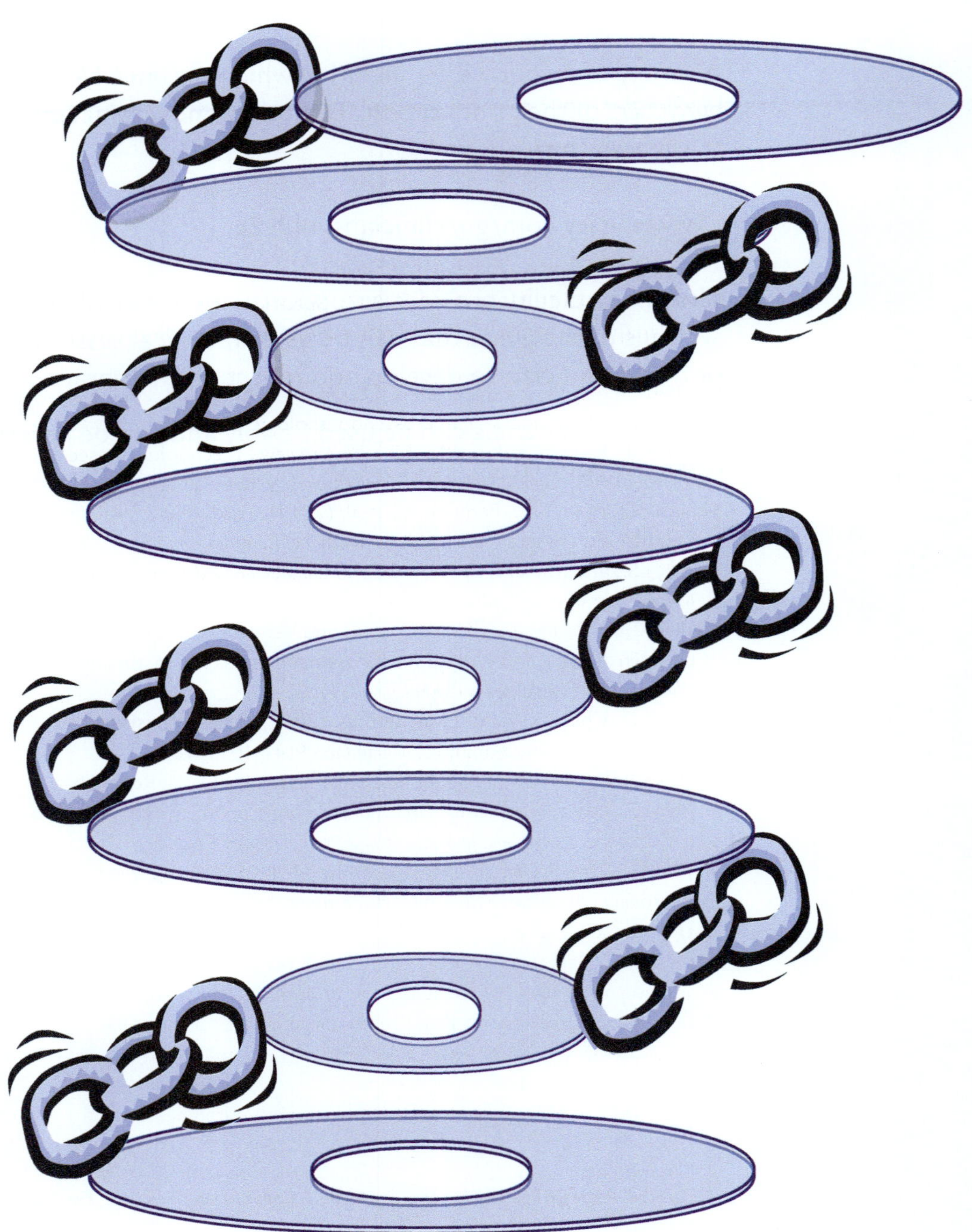

The Negative Trap

Think about one of your difficult situations and write or draw in the boxes below.

- ▶ What was the **TRIGGER?** – Where did this happen, who was there, what occurred?

- ▶ What were you **THINKING?** – What were the thoughts tumbling through your head?

- ▶ How did you **FEEL?** – Describe your feelings and body signals.

- ▶ What did you **DO?** – What happened?

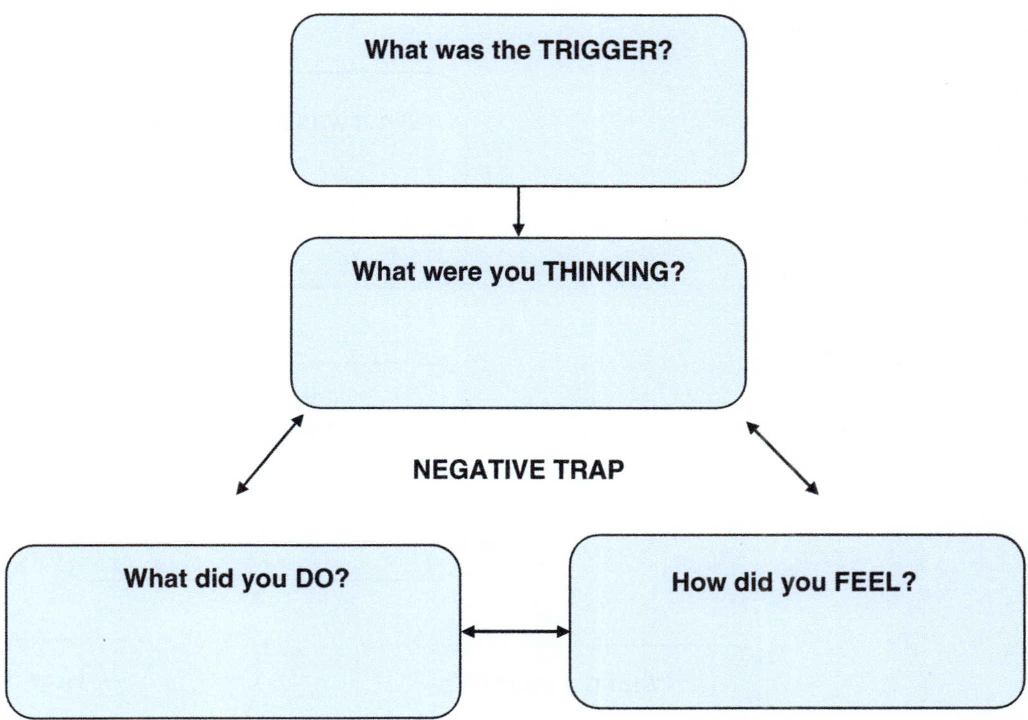

Which of your skills or strengths can help you to break out of this Negative Trap?

Four systems

Think of a recent situation or event that was difficult and draw or write it in the 'What was the **TRIGGER?**' box.

When this happened:

▶ What were you **THINKING?** – What were the thoughts tumbling through your head?

▶ How did you **FEEL?** – Describe your feelings.

▶ What were your **BODY** signals? – What changes did you notice in your body?

▶ What did you **DO?** – What happened?

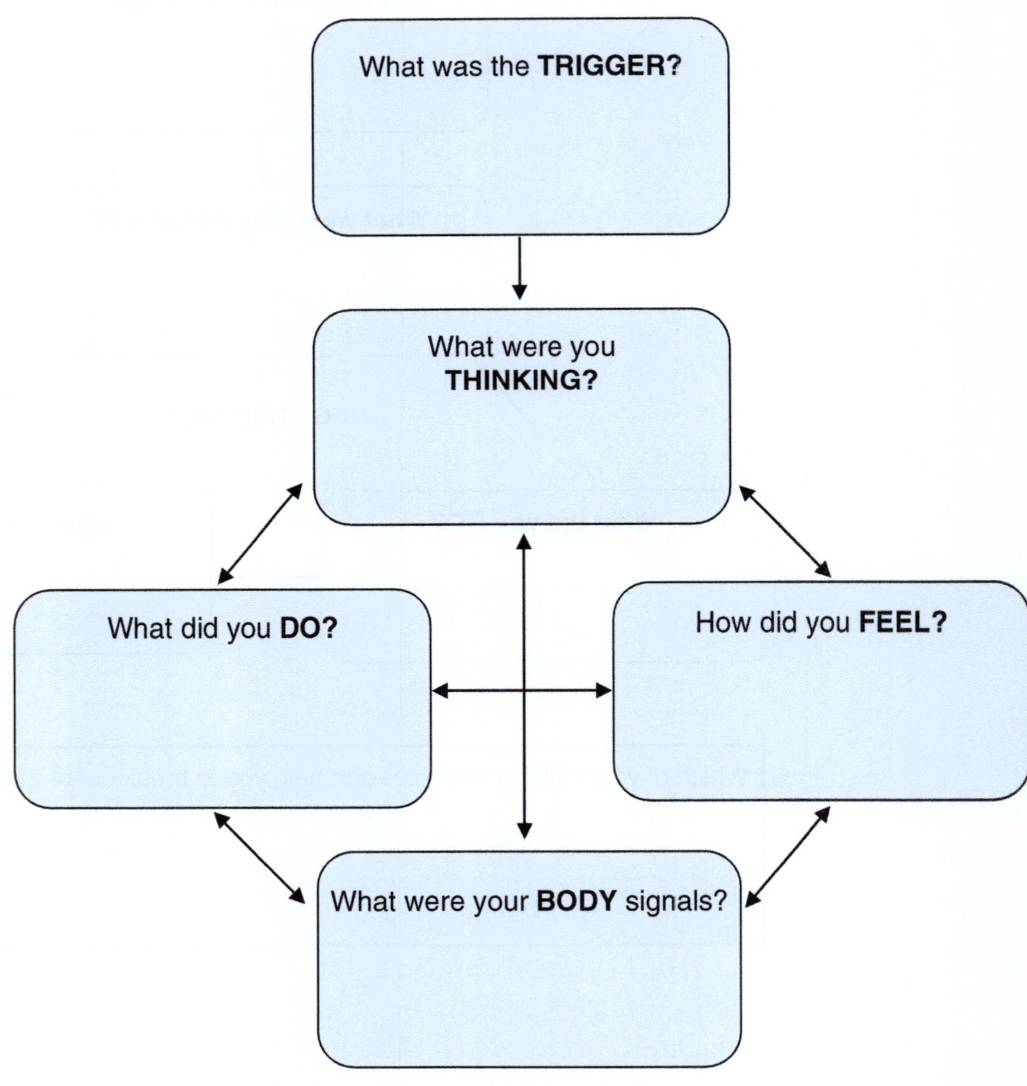

How did this happen?

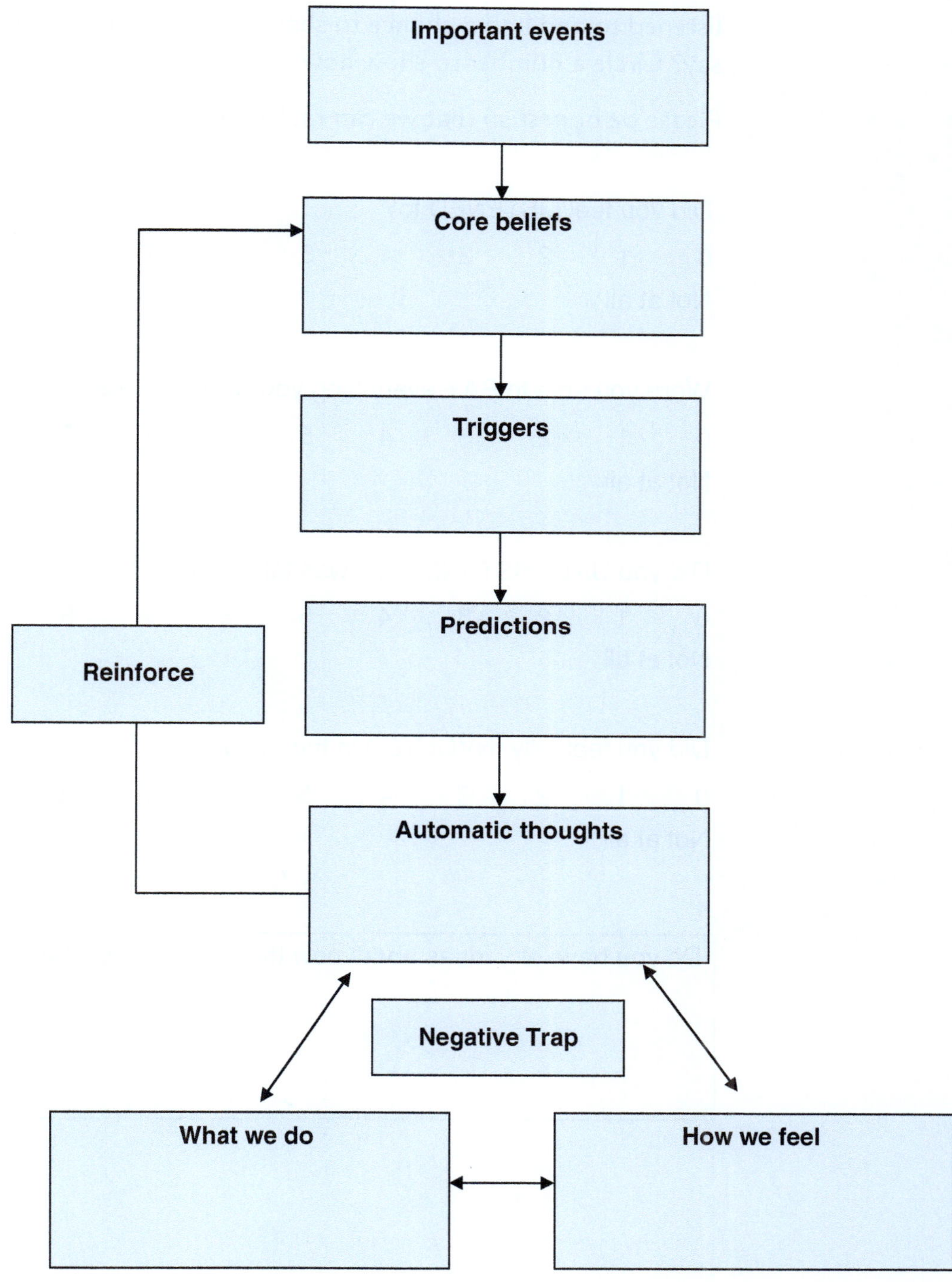

Session rating scale

How have you have found your meeting today? Have you felt involved and listened to and had a chance to share your ideas and say what you wanted to say? Circle a number to show how it has been for you.

Please be honest so that we can make these meetings as helpful as we can.

Did you feel LISTENED to?

0   1   2   3   4   5   6   7   8   9   10

Not at all   Totally

Were you able to SAY everything you wanted to say?

0   1   2   3   4   5   6   7   8   9   10

Not at all   Totally

Did you UNDERSTAND what was talked about?

0   1   2   3   4   5   6   7   8   9   10

Not at all   Totally

Did you feel fully INVOLVED in the meeting?

0   1   2   3   4   5   6   7   8   9   10

Not at all   Totally

Do you have any ideas about how the meetings can be made better for you?

Scales of change

Sometimes it can be helpful to weigh up the benefits and disadvantages of trying to do something. At the top of the scale, write what you are thinking about doing. On one side, write all the reasons to do it and the benefits you will gain, and on the other, all the reasons not to do it.

What I am thinking of doing

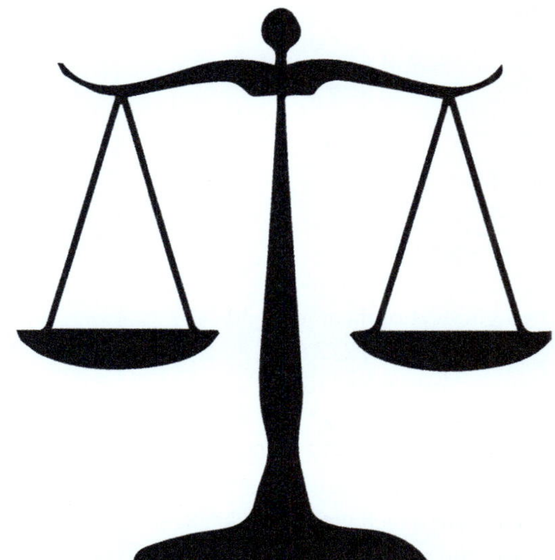

Reasons to do it

Reasons not to do it

Now that you have weighed this up, what will you do?

Anxiety intervention plan

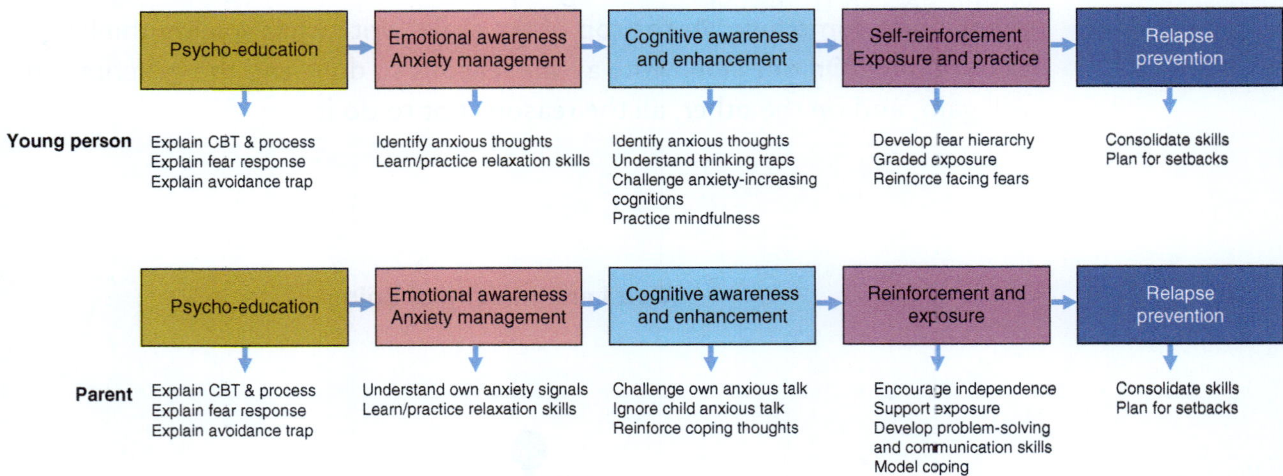

Depression intervention plan

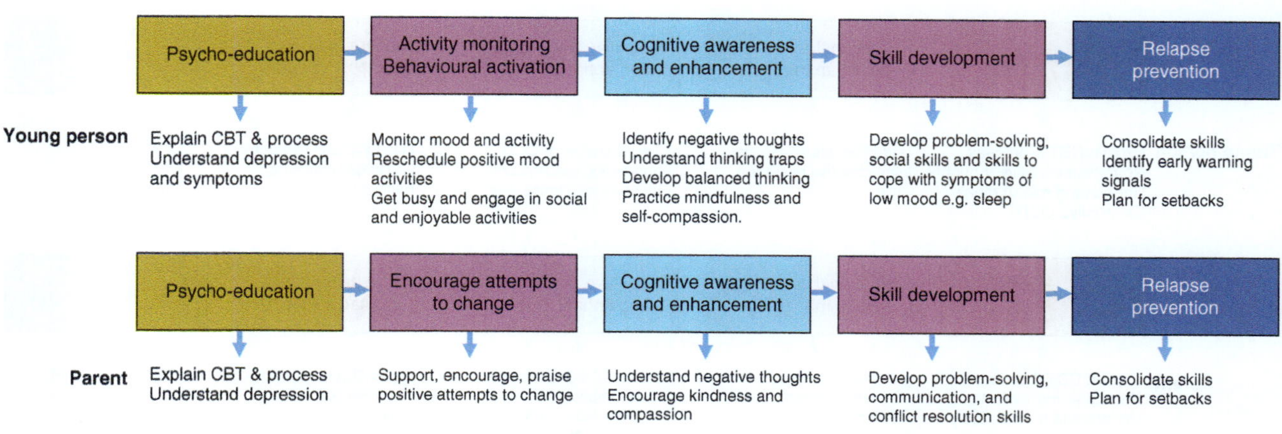

OCD intervention plan

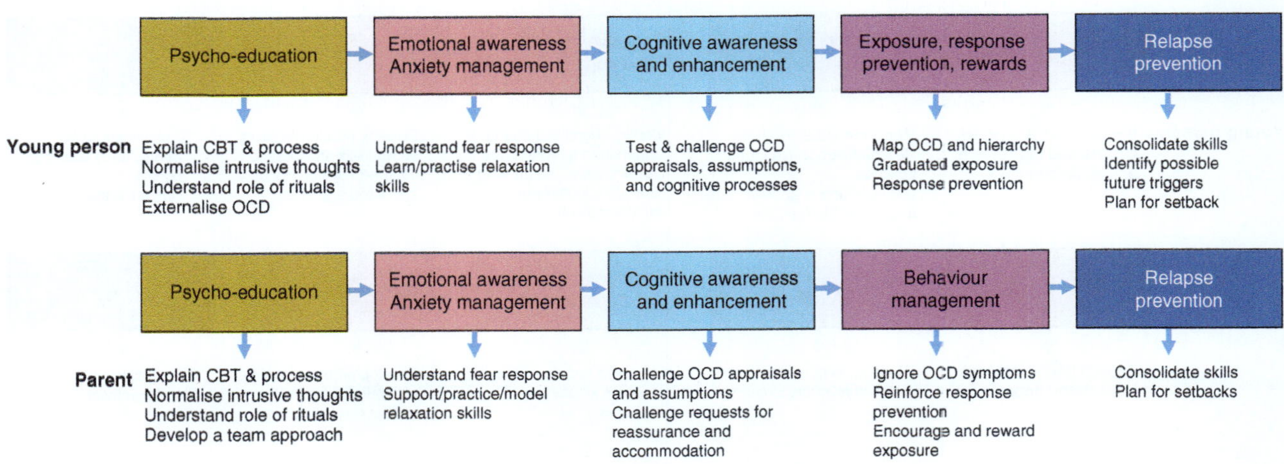

PTSD intervention plan

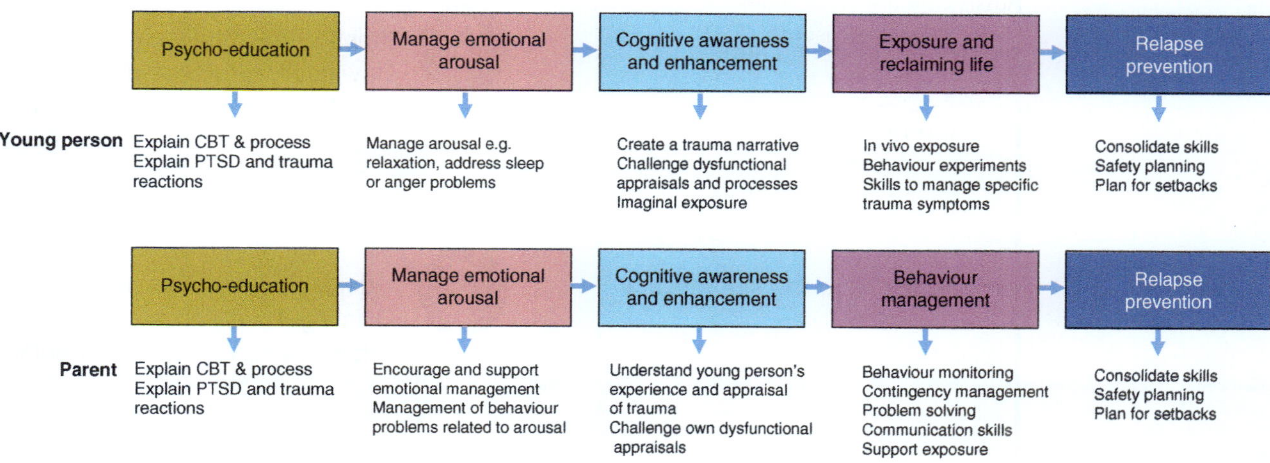

Motivation

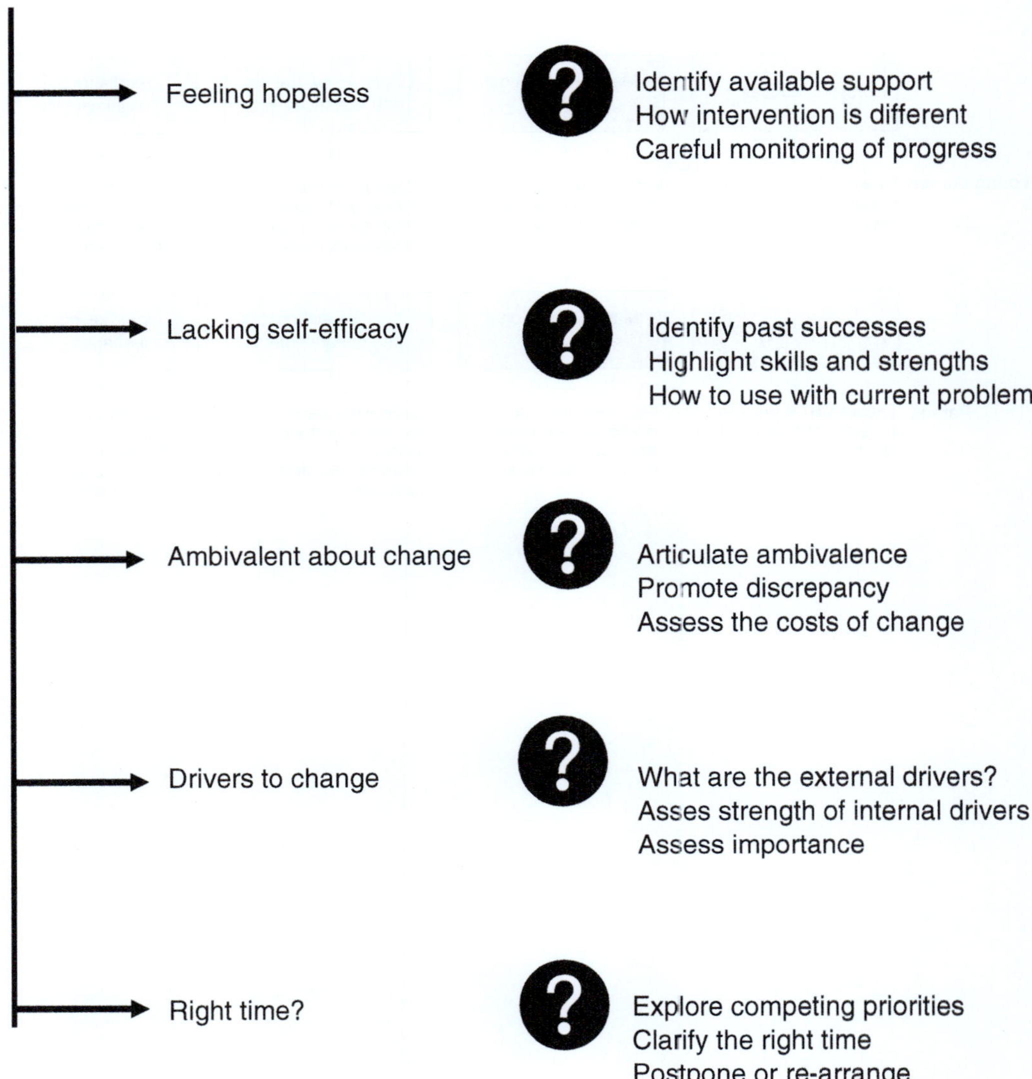

The aim is to explore barriers and beliefs that affect motivation and commitment to change. The approach aims to enable those who feel hopeless, empower those who doubt their self-efficacy, and help those who are ambivalent to identify the benefits of change.

Engagement

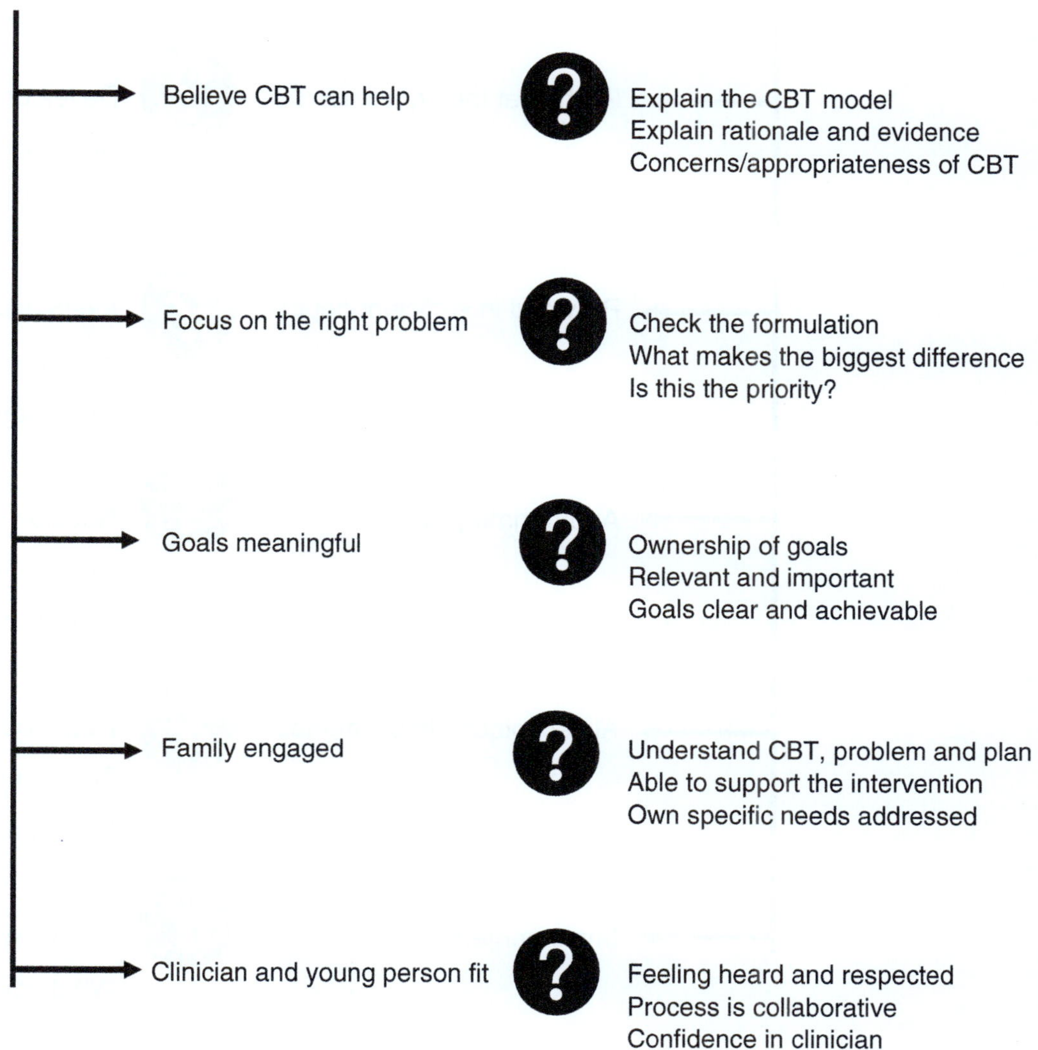

The aim is to explore issues of engagement that might interfere with progress. The primary problem needs to be clarified, the young person's goals confirmed, belief in CBT as helpful strengthened, parental support engaged, and the therapeutic relationship explored in an open and honest way.

Intervention delivery

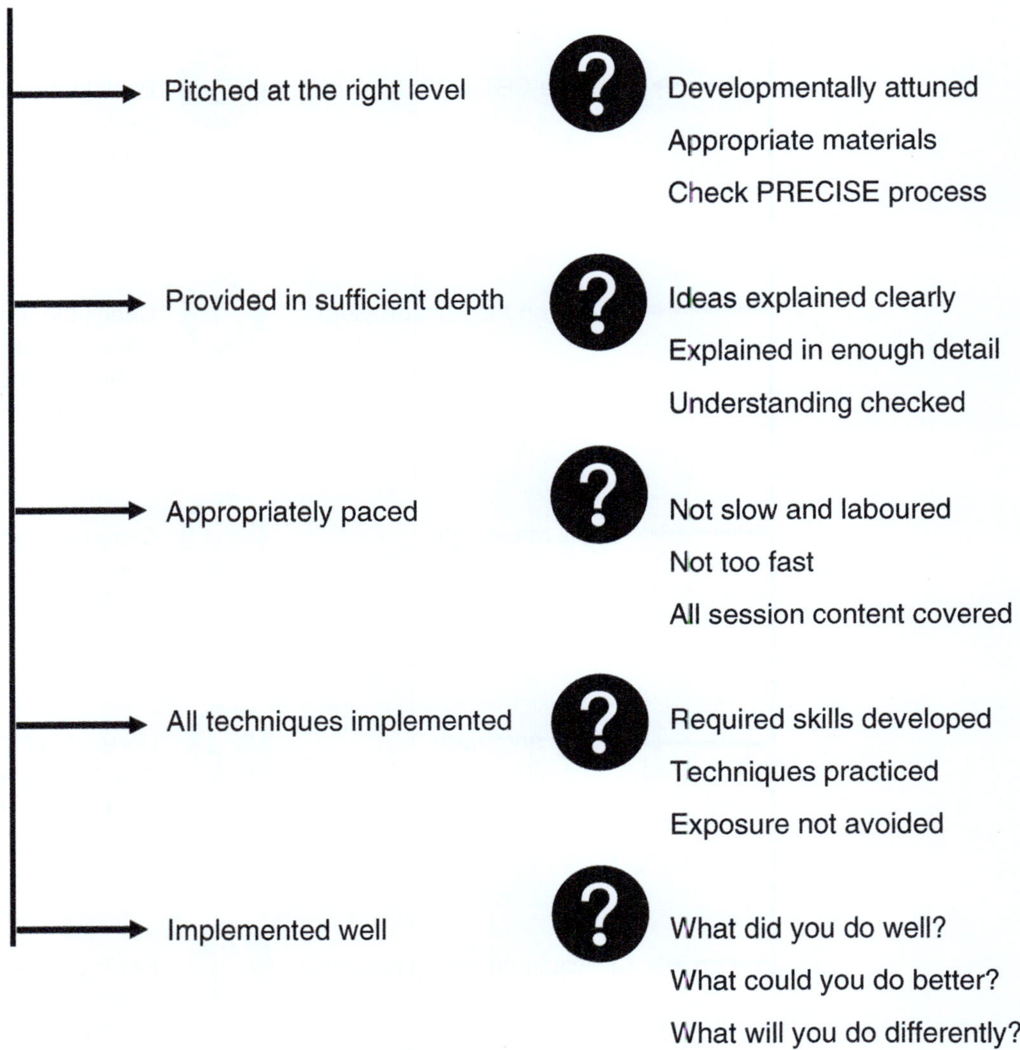

The aim is to develop a curious, open, and honest self-reflective approach to clinical practice. The way that the intervention is pitched, the depth of information provided, the pace of delivery, the coverage of planned content, and the way it is implemented should all be considered.

Reflective practice

Young person initials: Age: Gender:

Primary problem:

Routine outcome monitoring change:

Session rating:

Primary focus of session:

What did I do well in this session?

What could I do better?

What will I do differently next time?

The Cognitive Behaviour Therapy Scale for Children and Young People (CBTS-CYP)

PROCESS - PRECISE

1   Partnership working – collaboration and learning together

Establishes a collaborative and respectful partnership with the child/young person (and, as appropriate, their parents/carers) in which they are actively engaged in working towards a set of joint goals and targets.

This may be evidenced by:

▶ eliciting the child/young person's and parents/carers' understanding and views;

▶ encouraging and inviting the child/young person to participate in discussions, option appraisal, and decision making;

▶ involving the child/young person and parent/carer in goal and target setting, intervention planning, home assignments, and experiments;

▶ encouraging the child/young person to provide open and honest feedback about sessions.

Competence level		Examples (score according to features, not examples)
Incompetent	0	Didactic therapist style, collaboration not encouraged, child views not sought or ignored
Incompetent	1	Therapist too controlling, domineering, or passive and a partnership is not established
Novice	2	Occasional attempts at collaboration but domineering or passive style of therapist limits the establishment of a collaborative partnership
Advanced beginner	3	Collaborative partnership evident but **major** problems, e.g. not enough opportunities for child or carer participation
Competent	4	Collaborative partnership established but **not consistent** or some **minor** problems fully involving child or carers
Proficient	5	Good collaborative partnership established with all involved throughout most of the session; minimal problems
Expert	6	Highly effective and respectful partnership, even in the face of difficulties

2   **Right developmental level – pitch, methods, family involvement**

Engages with the child/young person and family at a level and in a manner that is consistent with their developmental level and understanding.

This may be evidenced by:

► ensuring an optimal balance between cognitive and behavioural techniques;

► using simple, clear, jargon-free language that is respectful and not patronising;

► appropriately using a variety of verbal (direct and indirect approaches) and non-verbal techniques;

► appropriately involving parents/carers/others in sessions.

Competence level		Examples (score according to features, not examples)
Incompetent	0	Therapist shows no recognition/awareness of the developmental stage of the child/family
Incompetent	1	Therapist adopts a 'standardised approach' that is not pitched at the right level
Novice	2	Occasional recognition of developmental issues, but the majority of the intervention is not modified or consistent with the child/parents' level of understanding
Advanced beginner	3	Demonstrates some awareness of developmental issues, but **major** problems, e.g. in ensuring that communication is pitched at the child/parents' level of understanding
Competent	4	Developmental issues recognised and intervention suitably tailored, but **not consistent** or some **minor** problems evident
Proficient	5	Intervention appropriately pitched and tailored to the developmental stage /understanding of all involved throughout most of the session; minimal problems
Expert	6	Highly effective, even in the face of significant developmental difficulties or limited understanding

3   Empathy – genuine, warm, understanding

Empathises with the child/young person and their carers/family through the development of a genuine, warm, and respectful relationship.

This may be evidenced by:

▶ conveying interest and concern through use of specific skills such as active listening, reflection, and summaries;

▶ acknowledging and appropriately responding to the child/young person's and carers/parents' verbal and non-verbal expressions and emotional responses such as distress, excitement, or anxiety;

▶ demonstrating an open, respectful, non-judgemental, caring approach;

▶ appropriately empathising with carers/parents about their own difficulties and the impact of these on their ability to help their child.

Competence level		Examples (score according to features, not examples)
Incompetent	0	Therapist appears preoccupied with techniques and does not show any empathy
Incompetent	1	Therapist appears cold and detached and has difficulty showing warmth and empathy
Novice	2	Occasional attempts at empathy, but overly focused upon techniques/intellectualisation
Advanced beginner	3	Limited attempts at empathy, but **major** problems, e.g. overlooking non-verbal emotional responses or often appearing disinterested/unconcerned.
Competent	4	The therapist is warm, respectful, and shows empathy, but **not consistent** or some **minor** problems evident
Proficient	5	The therapist demonstrates appropriate empathy with all involved throughout most of the session; minimal problems
Expert	6	Highly effective and remains empathic, warm, and respectful in the face of difficulties

4   Creative – verbal and non-verbal techniques

Adapts the ideas and concepts of CBT to facilitate the understanding of and engagement in therapy of the child/young person and their parents/carers.

This may be evidenced by:

▶ tailoring and adapting concepts and methods of CBT around the interests of the child/young person;

▶ using an appropriate range of verbal and non-verbal methods to facilitate understanding and engagement;

▶ creatively using a range of methods, e.g. talking, drawing, questionnaires, metaphor, role play, puppets, etc., to convey ideas and concepts;

▶ utilising the preferred media of the child/young person, e.g. verbal, visual, computer.

Competence level		Examples (score according to features, not examples)
Incompetent	0	Therapist makes no attempts to adapt or explain CBT in a way that facilitates engagement or understanding
Incompetent	1	Therapist inappropriately communicates and conveys concepts in a formulaic way that does not facilitate understanding or engagement
Novice	2	Occasional attempts to tailor the intervention to the child's interests and preferences, but overall delivery is formulaic and is not adapted to the child or their family
Advanced beginner	3	Limited attempts at creativity with **major** problems, e.g. inappropriately relying on verbal techniques or not using different media or creative methods
Competent	4	The therapist appropriately uses materials and media, but **not consistent** or some **minor** problems
Proficient	5	The therapist appropriately uses materials and media as required to facilitate understanding and engagement; minimal problems
Expert	6	Highly flexible and creative use of media and methods to facilitate understanding and engagement, even in the face of difficulties

5   Investigation – reflection and insight

Adopts an open and curious stance that facilitates guided discovery and reflection.

This may be evidenced by:

▶ creating a process of collaborative inquiry in which the child/young person's and/or parents/carers' cognitions, beliefs, and assumptions are subject to objective evaluation;

▶ involving the child/young person in the design of experiments;

▶ helping the child/young person and/or parents/carers to consider alternative explanations about events;

▶ encouraging the child/young person and/or parent/carer to reflect on the outcomes of experiments.

Competence level		Examples (score according to features, not examples)
Incompetent	0	Therapist adopts an 'expert stance' that does not facilitate self-discovery or reflection
Incompetent	1	Therapist is directive and provides no opportunities for self-discovery and reflection
Novice	2	Occasional attempts to be curious, but a predominantly directive style, with the therapist leading the session and providing their interpretations and ideas
Advanced beginner	3	Some opportunities for discovery and the use of a reflective questioning style, but **major** problems, e.g. child not involved in design of experiments or reflecting on outcomes
Competent	4	Curious approach is evident, with questioning and experimentation aiding the discovery of new information, but **not consistent** or some **minor** problems
Proficient	5	Therapist demonstrates skilful use of questioning and experimentation to facilitate reflection, discovery, and synthesis; minimal problems
Expert	6	Highly effective reflective approach that facilitates deep understanding, even in the face of difficulties

6 Self-efficacy – build on strengths and ideas

Adopts an empowering and enabling approach in which self-efficacy and positive attempts at change are promoted.

This may be evidenced by:

- ▶ identifying and highlighting the child/young person's and/or parents/carers' strengths and personal resources;

- ▶ helping the child/young person and/or parents/carers to identify skills and strategies that have shown some past success;

- ▶ developing and shaping the child/young person's and/or parents/carers' ideas and coping strategies;

- ▶ praising and reinforcing the child/young person's and/or parents/carers' use of new skills.

Competence level		Examples (score according to features, not examples)
Incompetent	0	Therapist is disempowering, rejects, ignores, or criticises suggestions from children/carers
Incompetent	1	Therapist is overly deficit-focused, and does not invite or reinforce positive contributions
Novice	2	Occasional acknowledgement and praise of contributions, but overall approach is not empowering
Advanced beginner	3	Some attempts to promote self-efficacy, but **major** problems, e.g. child's ideas are not systematically explored and developed
Competent	4	Overall approach is positive and empowering with contributions being appropriately developed, but **not consistent** or some **minor** problems
Proficient	5	Therapist demonstrates a positive and empowering approach in which contributions are acknowledged, explored, and developed; minimal problems
Expert	6	Highly effective and empowering approach that promotes self-efficacy, even in the face of difficulties

7 **Enjoyable – fun and engaging**

Makes therapy sessions appropriately interesting and engaging.

This may be evidenced by:

▶ using an appropriate mix of materials, activities, humour;

▶ maintaining an appropriate balance between task and non-task (relationship strengthening) activities;

▶ attending to the child/young person's interests and appropriately incorporating these into the intervention;

▶ presenting as positive and hopeful.

Competence level		Examples (score according to features, not examples)
Incompetent	0	Therapist appears bored, distracted, or overly serious
Incompetent	1	Therapist is too formal, and session is not interesting, enjoyable, or engaging
Novice	2	Occasional attempts to make the session interesting, but overall approach does not facilitate interest
Advanced beginner	3	Some attempts to make the session enjoyable and interesting, but **major** problems, e.g. not sufficiently focusing upon child's interests or engaging in non-task activities
Competent	4	Overall, the session is fun and engaging, but **not consistent** or some **minor** problems
Proficient	5	Therapist appropriately attends to the child's interest, uses their preferred medium, and maintains their engagement; minimal problems
Expert	6	Highly effective and able to make the session interesting and engaging, even in the face of difficulties

SKILLS... the ABCs...

A   Assessments and goals – ratings, diaries, questionnaires

Establishes clear goals for the intervention and appropriately uses diaries, questionnaires, and rating scales for assessment.

This may be evidence by:

- undertaking a full assessment of the presenting problem, involving, as appropriate, reports from others;

- complimenting assessment with routine outcome measures (ROMs);

- negotiating goals and the dates when progress will be reviewed;

- using diaries, tick charts, thought bubbles, and rating scales to identify and assess symptoms, emotions, thoughts, and behaviour;

- assessing motivation and readiness to change.

Competence level		Examples (score according to features, not examples)
Incompetent	0	No goals set; questionnaires, assessments, ratings not used
Incompetent	1	Inappropriate goals (unrealistic/inappropriate) and ratings/assessments not used or referred to
Novice	2	Occasional reference to goals/ratings, but overall approach is not embedded in use of assessments or routine outcome monitoring
Advanced beginner	3	Some reference to goals/ratings, but **major** problems, e.g. not using this information or building upon it to inform and shape the session/intervention
Competent	4	Overall demonstrates awareness of goals and ratings, but **not consistent** or some **minor** problems (e.g. explaining to younger children)
Proficient	5	Therapist has clear goals and appropriately incorporates diaries, questionnaires, scales, and ratings within the session; minimal problems
Expert	6	Highly effective use of goals and targets and measures/scales, even in the face of difficulties

B   Behavioural techniques – awareness, triggers, techniques of change

Demonstrates appropriate use of a variety of behavioural techniques to facilitate therapeutic change.

This may be evidenced by:

▶ using behavioural techniques such as developing hierarchies, graded exposure, and response prevention;

▶ using behavioural techniques such as activity rescheduling and behavioural activation;

▶ providing a clear rationale for using behavioural strategies;

▶ identifying and implementing reward and contingency plans;

▶ modelling, use of role play, structured problem-solving approaches, or skills training.

Competence level		Examples (score according to features, not examples)
Incompetent	0	Therapist fails to use or misuses behavioural techniques, fails to elicit relevant behaviours
Incompetent	1	Inappropriate behaviours focused upon or behavioural techniques inappropriately used
Novice	2	Occasional attempts to use behavioural techniques, but with limited skills/flexibility
Advanced beginner	3	Some attempts to appropriately use behavioural techniques, but **major** problems, e.g. rationale and relationship to problems, goals, and targets is not clear
Competent	4	Behavioural techniques used as required (e.g. during session praising child/carer or modelling), but **not consistent** or some **minor** problems
Proficient	5	Therapist demonstrates good awareness and use of behavioural techniques; minimal problems
Expert	6	Highly effective and appropriate use of behavioural techniques, even in the face of difficulties

C Cognitive – awareness, identification, challenge, cognitive reframe

Demonstrates appropriate use of a variety of cognitive techniques to facilitate therapeutic change.

This may be evidenced by:

▶ facilitating cognitive awareness and the use of appropriate techniques such as thought records and bubbles;

▶ identification of cognitions that are functional/dysfunctional and helpful/unhelpful;

▶ identifying important dysfunctional cognitions and common cognitive biases, 'thinking traps';

▶ facilitating the generation of alternative balanced cognitions by thought challenging and alternative perspective taking;

▶ facilitating continuum work and use of rating scales;

▶ promoting mindfulness, acceptance, and compassion.

Competence level		Examples (score according to features, not examples)
Incompetent	0	Therapist fails to use or misuses cognitive techniques, fails to elicit relevant cognitions
Incompetent	1	Inappropriate cognitions focused upon or cognitive techniques inappropriately used
Novice	2	Occasional attempts to promote cognitive awareness or use cognitive techniques, but with limited skills/flexibility
Advanced beginner	3	Some attempts to appropriately use cognitive techniques, but **major** problems, e.g. unclear about purpose, not fully understood, difficulty generating alternative cognitions
Competent	4	Cognitive awareness promoted, and techniques used as required, but **not consistent** or some **minor** problems, e.g. generating alternative cognitions, identifying thinking traps
Proficient	5	Therapist demonstrates good awareness and use of cognitive techniques; minimal problems
Expert	6	Highly effective and appropriate use of cognitive techniques, even in the face of difficulties

D   Discovery – strengths, new information and meanings

Appropriately uses a variety of methods to facilitate self-discovery and understanding.

This may be evidenced by:

- facilitating self-discovery and reflection through use of the Socratic dialogue;

- facilitating self-discovery through alternative perspective taking and attending to new information;

- evaluating beliefs, assumptions, and cognitions through behavioural experiments or prediction testing.

Competence level		Examples (score according to features, not examples)
Incompetent	0	No attempt at facilitating self-discovery, with overall approach being very directive
Incompetent	1	No evidence of Socratic questioning or behavioural experiments
Novice	2	Minimal opportunity for discovery; some use of Socratic questioning and experiments, but unhelpful in facilitating understanding or making connections between themes
Advanced beginner	3	Some attempts at promoting the discovery of new information through experiments, but **major** problems, e.g. experiments poorly planned or disorganised
Competent	4	Therapists uses Socratic questioning and discovery experiments to promote self-discovery, but **not consistent** or some **minor** problems
Proficient	5	Therapist uses skilful questioning and experimentation to facilitate understanding and to challenge cognitions; minimal problems
Expert	6	Highly effective and appropriate use of questioning and experiments to promote a new understanding, even in the face of difficulties

E **Emotional – awareness, identification, management**

Appropriately uses a variety of emotional techniques to facilitate therapeutic change.

This may be evidenced by:

- developing emotional literacy by facilitating the identification of a range of emotions;

- helping to distinguish between different emotions and identifying key bodily signals;

- developing emotional management skills such as relaxation, guided imagery, controlled breathing, and calming activities;

- developing emotional management skills such as physical activity, letting the feelings go, emotional metaphors, emotive imagery, and change the feeling;

- developing emotional management skills such as self-soothing, mind games, and mindfulness.

Competence level		Examples (score according to features, not examples)
Incompetent	0	Therapist fails to use or misuses emotional techniques, fails to elicit relevant emotions
Incompetent	1	Inappropriate emotions focused upon or emotional techniques inappropriately used
Novice	2	Minimal opportunity for emotional recognition and awareness and many relevant opportunities missed
Advanced beginner	3	Some attempts at promoting emotional awareness and management, but some **major** problems, e.g. management techniques poorly demonstrated, inadequate differentiation of emotions
Competent	4	Therapists shows good emotional awareness and promotes recognition and management, but **not consistent** or some **minor** problems
Proficient	5	Therapist skilful at facilitating emotional recognition and management; minimal problems
Expert	6	Highly effective facilitation of emotional awareness and management, even in the face of difficulties

F   Formulation – integration of CBT model

Facilitates the development of a coherent understanding which highlights the relationships between events, cognitions, emotions, physiological responses, and behaviours.

This may be evidenced by:

- providing a coherent and understandable rationale for the use of CBT;

- providing a collaborative understanding of events in which the links between specific events, thoughts, emotions, and behaviour are highlighted (maintenance formulations);

- providing an understanding of important past events and relationships in the development of the current problems (onset formulations);

- including, as appropriate, the role of parents/carers in the onset or maintenance of the child/young person's problems;

- clearly linking activities and goals/targets to the formulation.

Competence level		Examples (score according to features, not examples)
Incompetent	0	No attempt to integrate thoughts, feelings, physiological reactions, and behaviour
Incompetent	1	No reference to the cognitive model
Novice	2	Limited reference to the cognitive model, poorly explained, and not integrated with the problems and goals of therapy
Advanced beginner	3	Some references to the cognitive model and attempts at formulation, but **major** problems, e.g. not distinguishing between thoughts and feelings or identifying key cognitions
Competent	4	Cognitive model referred to and problem formulation developed, but **not consistent** or some **minor** problems, e.g. too complex or not understandable by child
Proficient	5	Therapist demonstrates an ability to develop cognitive formulations which aid understanding and inform the intervention; minimal problems
Expert	6	Highly effective integration of the cognitive model and use of formulations, even in the face of difficulties

G   **General skills – session planning and organisation**

Sessions are well prepared and conducted in a calm and organised way.

This may be evidenced by:

- preparing and bringing the necessary materials and equipment to the meeting;

- managing the child/young person's behaviour during sessions;

- ensuring that sessions have an agenda and clear goals and are appropriately structured;

- ensuring good timekeeping so that all tasks are completed;

- ensuring that sessions are appropriately paced, flexible, and responsive to the needs of the child/young person;

- preparing for endings and relapse prevention.

Competence level		Examples (score according to features, not examples)
Incompetent	0	Session is disorganised, no agenda, poor time keeping
Incompetent	1	Management of child's or carers' behaviour in session is ineffective
Novice	2	Few attempts to organise and structure the session, which overall appears chaotic
Advanced beginner	3	Some attempts at session planning and management, but **major** problems, e.g. not covering all topics, key materials forgotten
Competent	4	Session has many good features, but **not consistent** or some **minor** problems
Proficient	5	Therapist is well prepared and skilfully manages the session and the behaviour of child and parents; minimal problems
Expert	6	Highly effective session preparation and management with good pacing, even in the face of difficulties

H   Home assignments – transfer knowledge and skills to everyday life

Uses home assignments to gather data and transfer skills between clinical sessions and everyday life.

This may be evidenced by:

- negotiating and agreeing assignment tasks;

- ensuring assignments are meaningful and clearly related to the formulation and clinical session;

- ensuring assignments are consistent with the young person's developmental level, interests, and ability;

- agreeing realistic, achievable, and safe assignments;

- referring to goals when planning home assignments and to rating scales when reviewing progress;

- encouraging review and reflection of learning.

Competence level		Examples (score according to features, not examples)
Incompetent	0	Home assignments are not used, or previous assignments are ignored
Incompetent	1	Assignments are occasionally used but are not collaboratively agreed
Novice	2	Occasional use of assignments, but they are random and not clearly linked to the formulation
Advanced beginner	3	Attempts at collaborative assignment setting, but **major** problems, e.g. purpose and instructions poorly described and not clearly linked to the formulation
Competent	4	Collaboratively agreed assignments, but **not consistent** or some **minor** problems, e.g. explaining purpose or defining the task
Proficient	5	Good, clear, collaboratively agreed assignments; minimal problems
Expert	6	Highly effective at negotiating and agreeing creative and clear experiments and encouraging self-reflection, even in the face of difficulties

Beating anxiety

There are times when we all feel worried, anxious, uptight, or stressed. Often there is a reason. It might be:

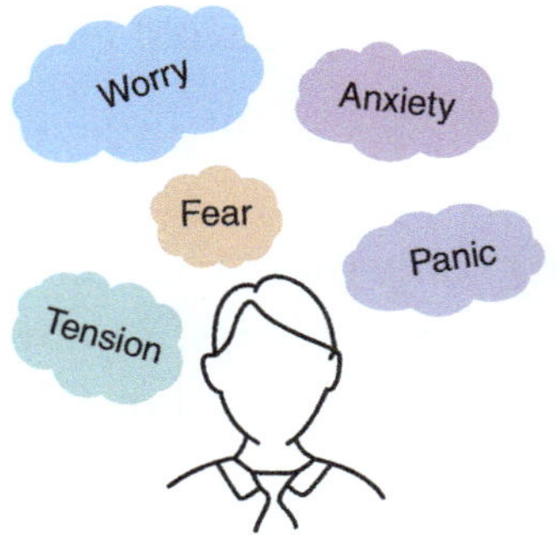

▶ doing something new or difficult, such as having a trial for a sports team

▶ telling someone something they won't like, such as 'I don't want go out with you tonight'

▶ preparing for something important, such as an exam or audition

Usually, you feel better once you have faced the worry. At other times, these uncomfortable feelings seem very strong, come often, or seem to last a long time. You may not be able to find a clear reason, so it may seem hard to know what is making you feel anxious. You may find that these unpleasant feelings stop you from doing the things you would like to do. At these times, it may be useful to learn how you can **beat your anxiety**.

Understand your anxious feelings

When people become anxious or scared, they often notice several changes in their body. This is called the **FLIGHT or FIGHT** reaction. Your body prepares itself to run away or to face and fight the thing that is scaring you. Some common signals are listed below. Understanding which of these are strongest will help you to become better at noticing when you become anxious.

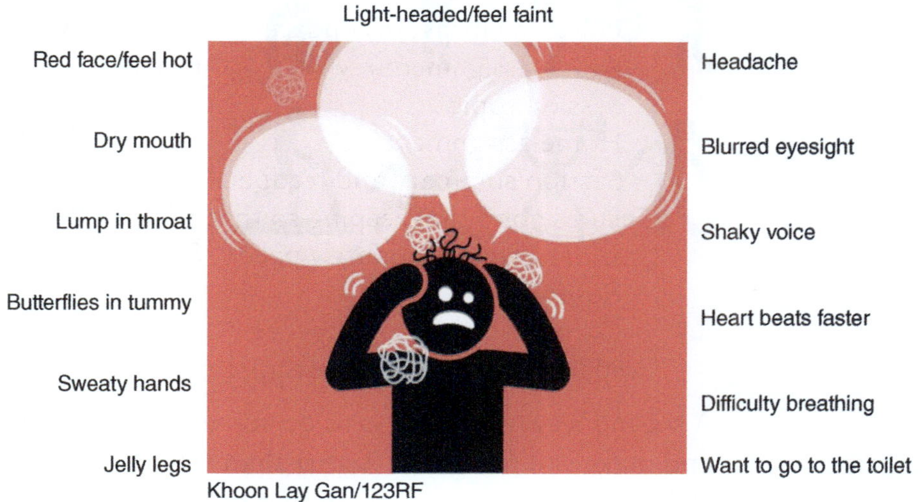

Khoon Lay Gan/123RF

The avoidance trap

Anxiety is an unpleasant feeling, and so we try to avoid situations that create it.

▶ If you are anxious talking with people, you might avoid social situations.

▶ If you are anxious about change, you might avoid going somewhere new.

▶ If you are anxious about dogs, you might avoid places where they might be.

Avoiding these situations may bring some short-term relief, but you never learn that you can cope with your anxious feelings. You become stuck in an avoidance trap and need to learn to break out and **reclaim your life**.

Learn to relax

You can control your anxious feelings by learning to relax. You can do this in different ways, but remember:

▶ There is **no one way** of controlling your anxious feelings.

▶ **Different methods** may be useful at different times.

▶ It is important to **find what works for you**.

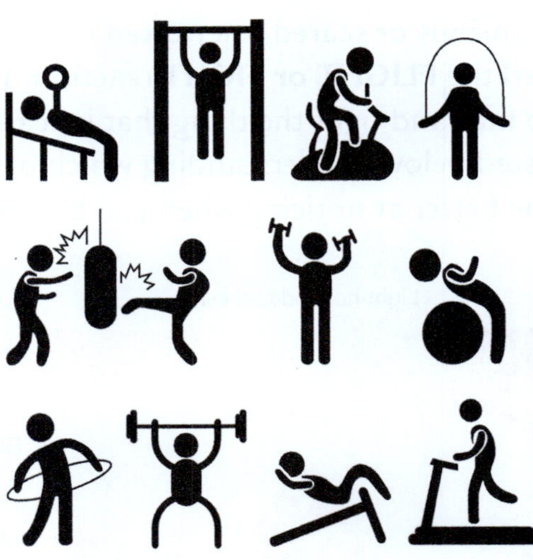

Physical exercise

Sometimes you may notice that you have felt anxious for most of the day. You may have had lots of feelings of anxiety, and when this happens, physical exercise can be a good way of relaxing.

A workout, walk, cycle, run, or swim can help you get rid of any anxious feelings and can make you feel better.

Relaxing activities

A second way of relaxing is to do some activities that change how you feel and make you feel good. Rather than listening to your negative thoughts and feeling anxious, do something that helps you to relax.

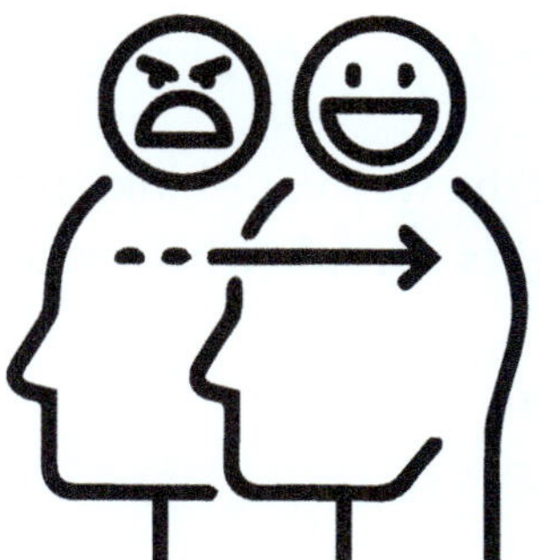

Different activities can help you to unwind and could include computer games, reading, watching the TV or a DVD, playing an instrument, listening to music, a long bath, drawing, or painting your nails.

When you notice that you are feeling anxious or listening to your worrying thoughts, do something to change the feeling.

▶ Instead of lying in bed listening to your negative thoughts, put on your personal stereo and listen to some music.

▶ Instead of worrying whether your friend will call, read a magazine.

The more you practise, the easier you will find it to help yourself feel better.

Controlled breathing

There are times when you may suddenly notice that you have become anxious and need a quick way to relax and regain control.

Controlled breathing is a quick method you can use anywhere, and often people don't even notice what you are doing!

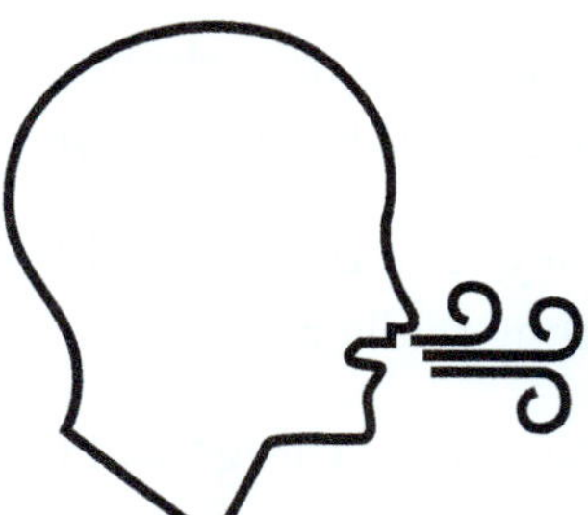

Slowly draw in a deep breath through your nose to the count of 4. Hold it for 5 seconds and then slowly breathe out through your mouth to the count of 6. As you breathe out, say to yourself 'relax'. Doing this a few times will help you regain control of your body and help you feel calmer.

Quick relaxation

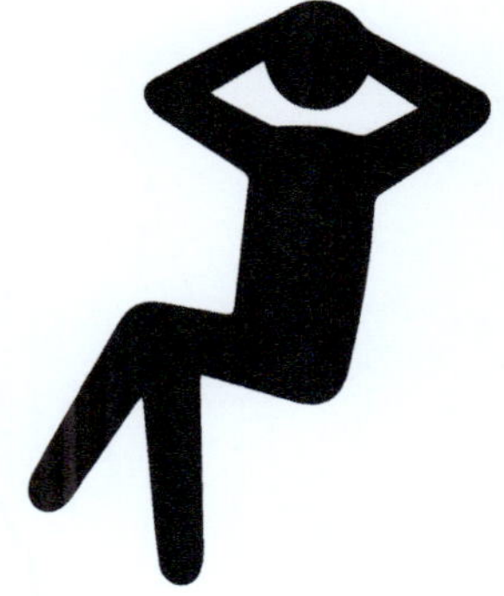

Many famous celebrities, athletes, and musicians use relaxation exercises to help them manage their anxiety and prepare for challenges. This involves tensing each of the major muscle groups for a few seconds and then letting the tension go and relaxing.

Try tensing your arms and hands, legs and feet, stomach, shoulders, and neck, and then your face.

Quick relaxation can help if you get very anxious before doing something. It can help you prepare yourself so that you feel more relaxed before you face your challenge. Remember, the more you practise, the more it will help.

Identify your anxious thoughts

It is important to learn more about the way you think and to identify your negative, critical, or worrying thoughts. People who feel anxious often:

▶ expect negative things to happen

▶ are very critical of what they do

▶ are always looking for signs of threat and danger

▶ are less likely to think that they can successfully cope

▶ tend to avoid challenging situations

For some, this way of thinking takes over. Their thoughts become mainly negative and critical, and they often feel anxious.

Are you stuck in a thinking trap?

You may notice that you are thinking in negative ways. These are thinking traps, and there are five very common traps to look out for:

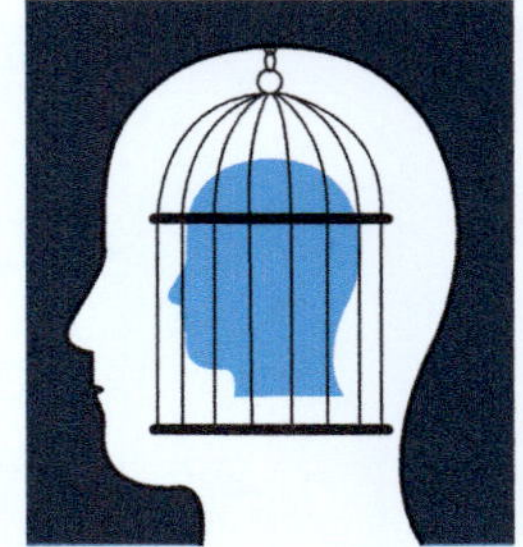

▶ NEGATIVE FILTER – you only see the negative things that happen and ignore or overlook anything positive

▶ BLOWING THINGS UP – small negative things are blown up to become bigger or more important than they really are

▶ PREDICTING FAILURE – you expect that things will go wrong

▶ BEING DOWN ON YOURSELF – you are very critical of what you do and blame yourself for things that go wrong

▶ SETTING YOURSELF UP TO FAIL – you set yourself very high standards and unrealistic expectations that you can seldom achieve

Check your thoughts

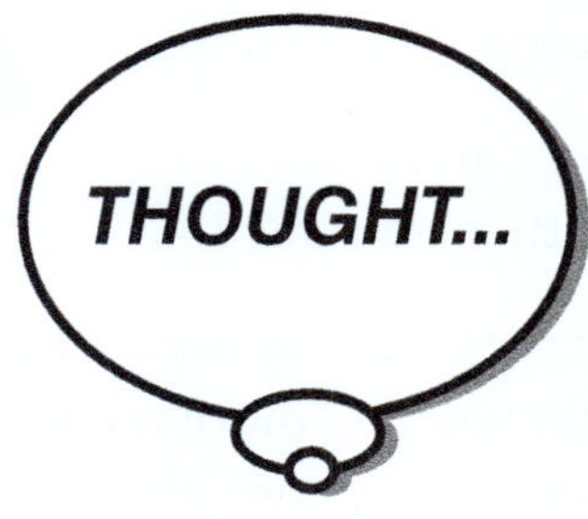

You can make sure that you haven't become stuck in a negative thinking trap by testing your thoughts. This can help you to find some of the things that you may have ignored or overlooked and to realise that there might be another, more helpful way of thinking about things.

- Firstly, CATCH and write down the worrying thoughts that are tumbling around your head.

- Now CHECK them and see if you have fallen into a thinking trap.

- CHALLENGE these thoughts and see if there is something that you have overlooked.

- Now CHANGE them and see if there is a more balanced and helpful way of thinking.

Step back from your worrying thoughts

We spend too much time in our heads. We rehearse what has happened and worry about what will happen but don't really notice what is happening here and now. Mindfulness is a way of getting out of your head. You can learn to connect with the here and now by learning to focus your attention and observe what is happening in an open and curious way. Paying more attention to the present moment can help you to feel less anxious.

You can practise mindfulness in different ways, such as mindful eating, breathing, walking, or observing.

Face your fears

When we feel anxious, we avoid the things that worry us and never learn that we can cope. Learning to **face your fears** can help you to overcome your anxiety and to reclaim your life. You can do this by:

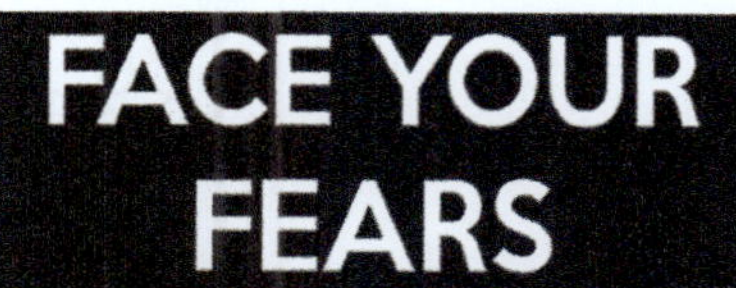

- making a list of the situations or events that you avoid

- arrange them in order of difficulty, with the most anxiety-provoking at the top and the least at the bottom

- start with the least anxiety-provoking, decide when you will face your fear, and think about the support you might need and the skills that will help you to be successful

- use your skills to face your fears, and learn that you can be successful

Once you have been successful, move on to the next step and continue until you have overcome your fears.

Remember to praise yourself

We are not always very good at praising ourselves and saying, 'well done'. So, when you try to beat your anxiety and face your fears, remember to praise yourself. After all, you deserve it for having a try!

Fighting back depression

Everyone feels down, fed up, or unhappy at some time. These feelings usually come and go, but sometimes they last and take over, and you can't seem to shift them. You might notice that you:

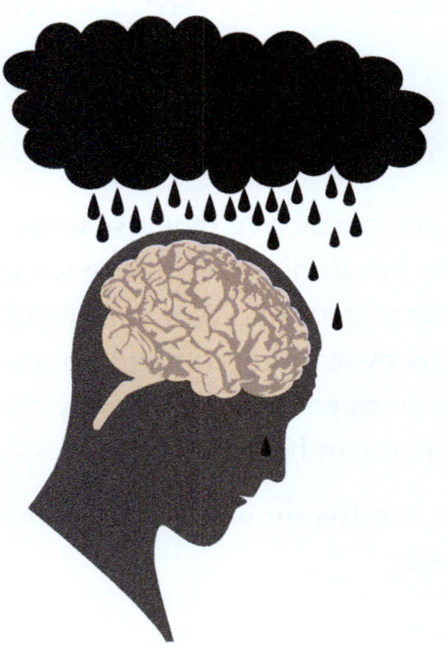

- are often tearful
- cry for no clear reason or over small things
- wake up early in the morning
- have difficulty falling asleep at night
- feel constantly tired and lacking in energy
- comfort eat or have lost your appetite
- have problems concentrating
- stopped doing the things you used to enjoy
- go out less often and just want to be on your own

These are some of the many signals that depression has taken over and that it is **time to fight back!**

Getting started is hard work

When you feel down, it can be very hard to get yourself going again. Everything seems impossible or feels really hard work, and you may feel tired and that you can't be bothered to even try.

This is part of depression, and one of the hardest jobs is to take the first step. Two things might help you to get going.

- Tell other people that you are going to start fighting your depression. They can **help**, **support**, and **encourage** you.

- Remind yourself that **you** can make a difference to how you feel. It is hard work, but there are things you can do to make yourself feel better.

Check what you do and how you feel

When people feel down in their mood, they stop doing things. They don't go out so much and may sit around or stay in bed all day. A useful first step is to check what you are doing and to see if there are any times during the day when you feel worse than other times.

Keep a diary throughout the day, and for each hour, write down what you were doing and how you were feeling and chose a number from 1 (very weak) to 10 (very strong) to rate the feeling. Do you notice any patterns or times when you feel better or worse?

Lisa's diary looked like this:

- 10.00 – In bed. Mood 7

- 11.00 – In bed. Mood 8

- 12.00 – Sitting in my room, thinking. Mood 10

- 1.00 – Downstairs, had lunch with mum. Mood 4

- 2.00 - In my bedroom listening to music. Mood 4

- 3.00 - In my bedroom. Sitting around. Mood 9.

This helped Lisa to see that the times she felt worse were when she was sitting in her room not doing anything.

Change what you do

Once you understand the times you feel particularly bad and the activities that make you feel better or worse, you can plan to do things differently.

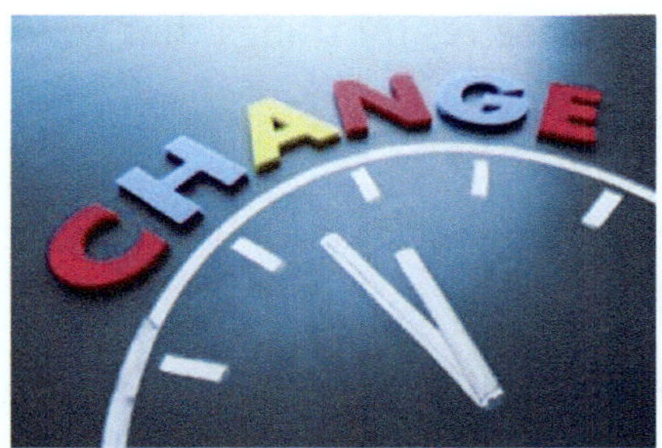

lawren/123RF

Lisa's diary showed that she felt better when she was downstairs with others or listening to music. She decided to change what she did. When she woke, instead of lying in bed, she would go downstairs and be with her family. If she became aware that she was feeling particularly low, she would try to listen to some music to see if it helped.

Get busy

When you feel down you often feel tired and stop doing things, even those things that you used to like doing! Hobbies, interests, activities, or visiting places you used to like (e.g. cinema) happen less often.

One of the first steps in helping yourself is to get busy and to start doing things again. Make a list of the things that you used to enjoy but have now stopped, don't do very often, or haven't done but would like to do. Some of the best activities are those that involve people, give you a sense of achievement, or are important and meaningful to you.

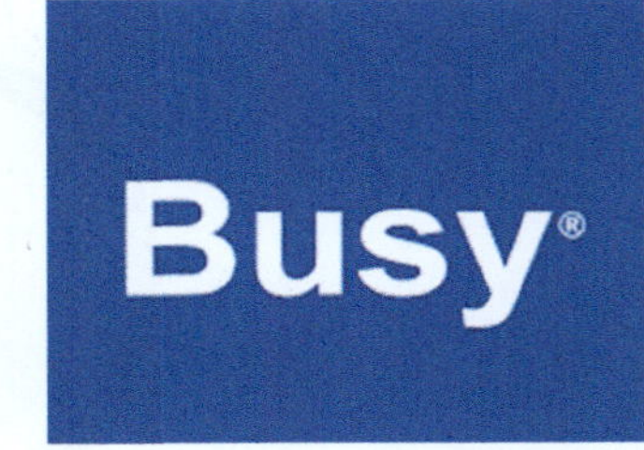

To be successful, make sure that your first step is small. If you haven't been for a run for several months, it is better to get dressed in your running kit and do a short warm-up rather than setting yourself a goal of running 5 kilometres. Once you have achieved your first step, stretch yourself a little as you work towards your goal.

As you start to become busier, you may find that things don't seem as much fun as they used to be. Don't worry, the fun may take a little longer to return. Keep reminding yourself that you are doing well, and remember that being busy gives you less time to listen to your negative thoughts.

Identify your unhelpful thoughts

It is important to learn more about the way you think and to identify your negative, critical, or worrying thoughts. People who are depressed often:

▶ look for, and find, the negative or bad things that happen

▶ are very critical of themselves, what they do, and their future

▶ apply things that go wrong in one area (e.g. not winning a race) to other parts of their life (e.g. 'I am a loser')

▶ personalise and blame themselves for things that go wrong

▶ ignore the good things that happen

Are you stuck in a thinking trap?

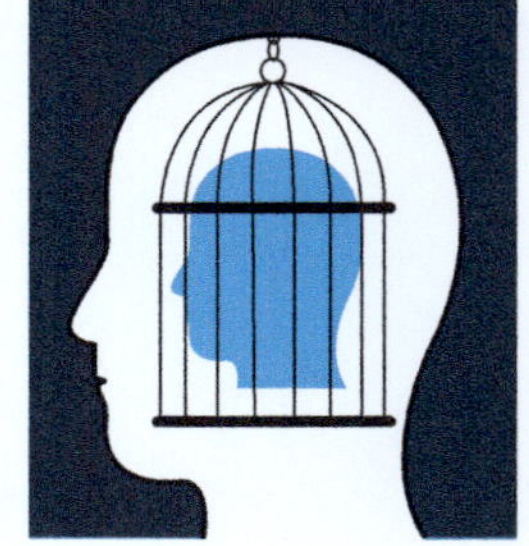

You may notice that you are thinking in negative ways. These are thinking traps, and there are five very common traps to look out for:

▶ NEGATIVE FILTER – you only see the negative things that happen and ignore or overlook anything positive

- BLOWING THINGS UP – small negative things are blown up to become bigger or more important than they really are

- PREDICTING FAILURE – you expect that things will go wrong

- BEING DOWN ON YOURSELF – you are very critical of what you do and blame yourself for things that go wrong

- SETTING YOURSELF UP TO FAIL – you set yourself very high standards and unrealistic expectations that you can seldom achieve

Challenge the way you think

Once you find your negative thoughts and thinking traps, you can learn to challenge yourself.

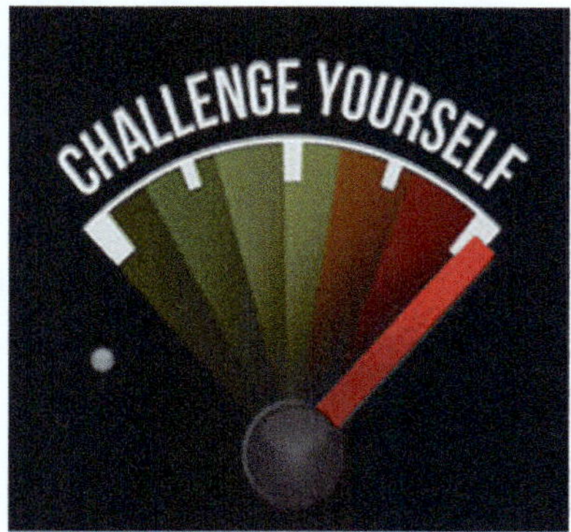

alexmillos/123RF

- If you are looking through a negative filter, learn to stop, look again, and find any positives that you have overlooked.

- If you blow things up, keep things in proportion and stop them growing too big.

- If you predict bad things will happen, do an experiment to check out what really happens.

- If you are down on yourself, develop a more caring and compassionate inner voice.

- If you set yourself up to fail, focus on and celebrate what you achieve rather than what you haven't done.

If you find this hard, it can be helpful to think what you would say to your best friend if you heard them thinking this way?

Step back from your thoughts

We spend too much time in our heads. We go over what has happened and worry that things will go wrong or that we will be unsuccessful. Mindfulness is a way of clearing this clutter out of your head by learning to connect with the here and now in an open and curious way. Paying more attention to the present moment can help you to stop beating yourself up.

You can practise mindfulness in different ways, such as mindful eating, breathing, walking, or observing. In fact, you can do anything mindfully. Try to practise mindfully focusing your attention for a couple of minutes a few times each day.

Be kind to yourself

When we are depressed, we are often very critical and unkind to ourselves. We beat ourselves up, criticise what we do, blame ourselves for the things that go wrong, and are seldom satisfied with what we do. The more critical we are, the worse we feel.

Try a different approach and be kinder to yourself and others.

▶ Practise talking kindly to yourself.

▶ Look after yourself if you have had a bad day.

▶ Forgive mistakes.

▶ Celebrate what you achieve.

▶ Be kind to others.

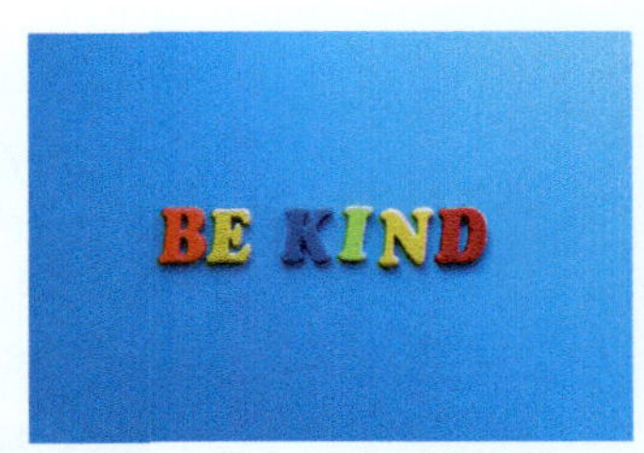

Alexander Zhenzhirov/123 RF

Learn to problem solve

It can often feel a hassle to make decisions or sort out problems, and so we might put them off. Unfortunately, they don't go away. The longer we leave them, the bigger they become and the more overwhelming they feel.

Try a five-step problem-solving approach.

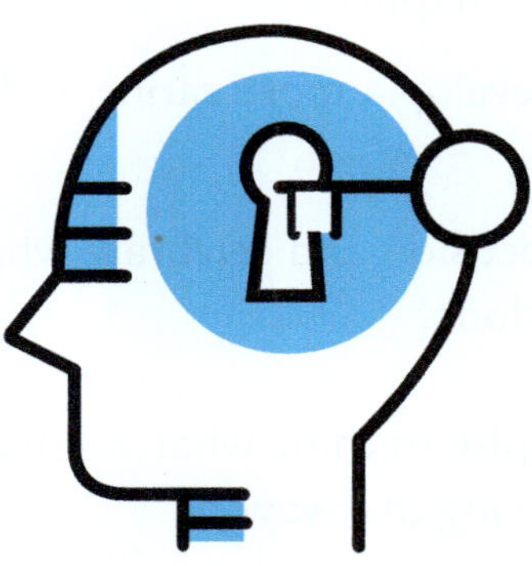

▶ What is the decision you need to make or the problem you must solve?

▶ What are your options or choices? Try to think of as many as you can.

▶ Now look at each choice and think about the consequences. These could be for you or others involved, and could be the immediate or short-term consequences.

▶ The fourth step is to decide. Based on what you now know, what decision will you chose?

▶ After you have tried it, the final step is to consider whether it worked. If you were confronted with a similar problem again, would you make the same decision?

Find the positives

When you feel down, it seems that only negative things happen. This is because you have become trained to be negative and critical and to ignore many of the positive things that occur.

Try to break out of this cycle and to actively search for the positive things that happen. It can help to write down at least one positive thing each day. These could be things that you enjoyed, coped with, achieved, or that made you feel good. Watching the list grow will help you to develop a more balanced view and to recognise that positive things do happen.

Controlling worries and habits

Some people have thoughts that get stuck and keep going around and around in their heads. Sometimes these are about worrying things like germs, danger, or other bad things, for example:

▶ that people will be hurt or involved in accidents

▶ that you will catch or give germs or diseases to others

▶ that you will be rude or behave inappropriately

These are **obsessional thoughts**, and because they are so worrying, people often feel very anxious. To feel better, people try to stop or cancel these thoughts by undertaking 'safety behaviours', habits, or **compulsive behaviours**. These could be things like:

▶ washing hands or clothes

▶ checking things like doors, light switches, windows

▶ doing things (like getting washed or dressed) in a special way

▶ repeating words, phrases, or numbers a set number of times

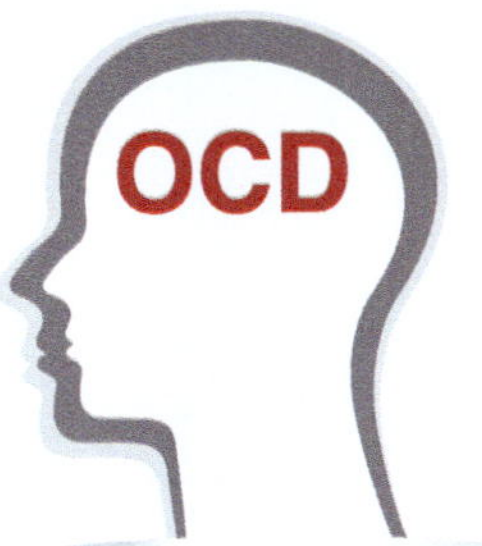

Compulsive behaviours like these can take over. Each day becomes a struggle as more and more time is spent undertaking them. This is called obsessive-compulsive disorder, or OCD for short. When this happens, you need to learn how to **regain control of your life**.

We all have worries

We don't usually tell anyone about our worrying or spooky thoughts. We may worry that other people won't understand, will become cross, or will think that we are silly or mad, and so we keep them locked up in our heads.

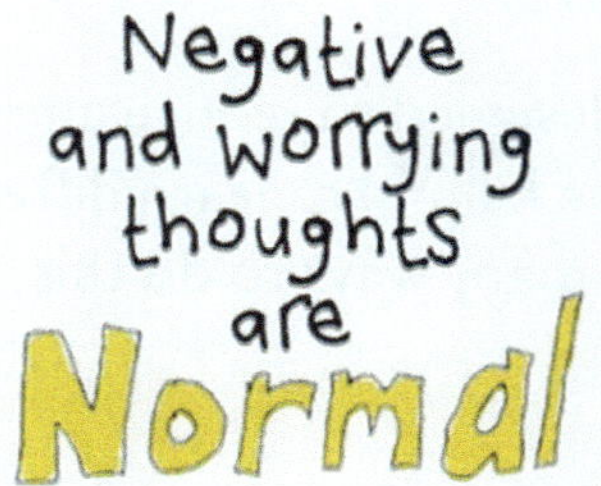

The first thing you need to know is that you are not silly or mad. We all have worrying thoughts at some time or another.

- You may spill or touch something and wonder if you might catch any germs.

- You may forget to unplug the TV and worry that it will catch fire.

- You may have an argument with somebody and wish that something horrible would happen to them.

Because you think it, doesn't mean it will happen

Worrying thoughts are very common, but the difference for people with OCD is that they believe their thoughts will come true. So, someone with OCD might:

- think that their mum will have a car crash and believe that this will happen

- think that they have a serious illness and believe that they will give it to other people if they touch them

It is only the bad things that we believe we can make happen. Thinking that you will win the National Lottery or that you will get an 'A' grade in maths doesn't make it happen.

The second thing we need to know is that just because we think something, doesn't mean it will happen!

Trying to stop your thoughts makes them worse

Some people try very hard not to think about their obsessional thoughts. It may seem to make sense, but we know that this doesn't work. The harder you try not to think about them, the more they will happen.

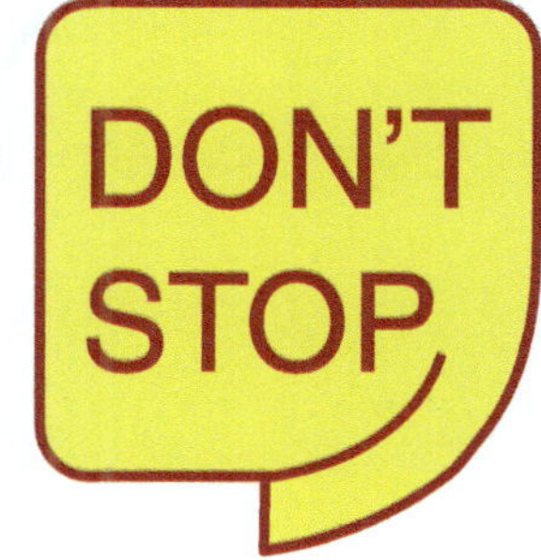

Don't try to stop them. Let them happen and **learn to live with them**.

Learn to manage your anxiety

Safety behaviours or habits are designed to reduce anxiety. Instead of engaging in these habits, it can be helpful to learn different ways to manage these anxious feelings. There are many ways to do this, and it is important to discover what works for you.

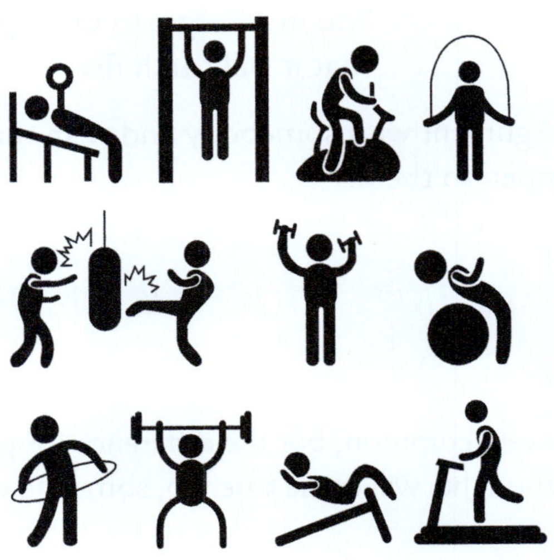

Physical exercise

There may be times when you have become stuck in your habits, having to repeat them several times to make yourself feel better. Physical exercise can be a good way of breaking out of this and managing your anxious feelings.

Relaxing activities

When you become trapped in your habits, see if you can switch to an activity that helps you to unwind. We all have activities we find relaxing; it could be playing computer games, reading, watching the TV or a DVD, playing an instrument, listening to music, a long bath, drawing, or painting your nails.

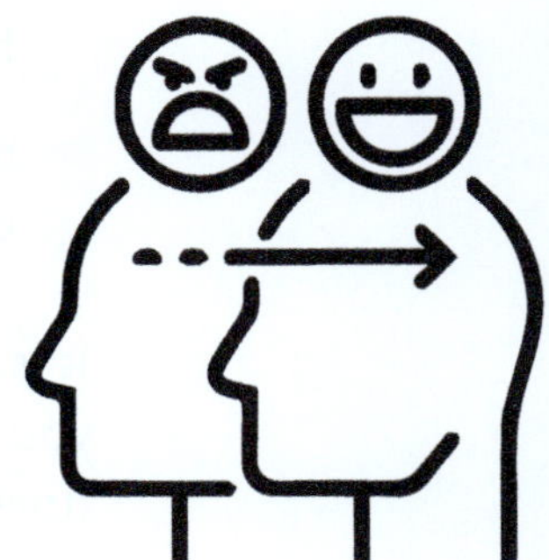

Controlled breathing

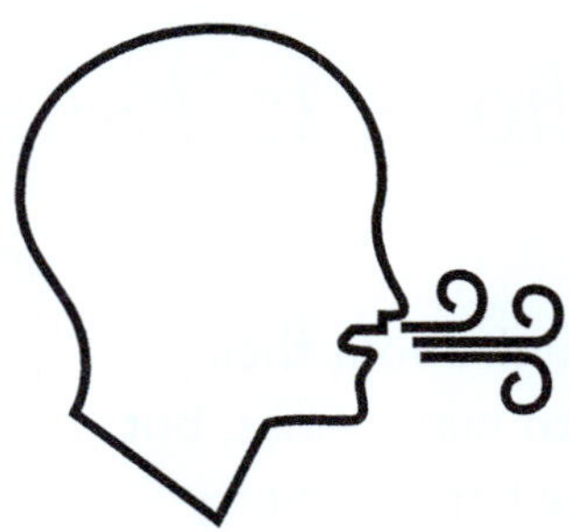

Controlled breathing is a quick way of regaining control. Slowly draw in a deep breath through your nose to the count of 4. Hold it for 5 seconds and then slowly breathe out through your nose to the count of 6. As you breathe out, say to yourself 'relax'. Doing this a few times will help you regain control of your body and help you feel calmer.

Relaxation exercises

Relaxation exercises where each of the muscle groups in the body are tensed for a few seconds and then relaxed can be helpful. Try tensing your arms and hands, legs and feet, stomach, shoulders and neck, and then your face.

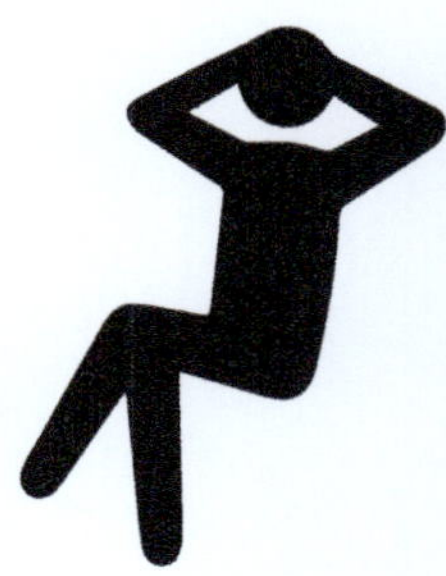

Identify your unhelpful thoughts

People with OCD often:

▶ believe that they are responsible for preventing harm coming to themselves or others

▶ overestimate threat and believe that things are riskier than they are

▶ believe that thinking bad or distressing thoughts is as terrible as actually doing these things

▶ think that having a distressing thought will make them act on it

For people with OCD, it is not the thoughts themselves that are the problem. We all have spooky thoughts. The problem is the way these thoughts are interpreted and responded to, and it is this that creates the difficulties.

Check them out

Experiments are powerful ways of testing thoughts. Check whether your spooky thoughts are playing tricks on you and find out what really happens.

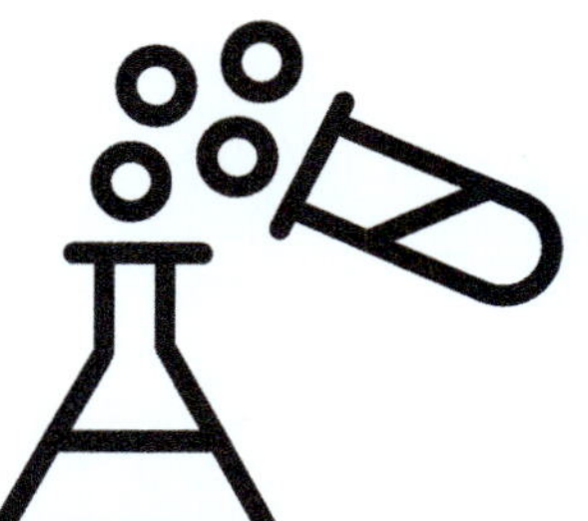

If you keep checking your work before handing it in, check out what happens if you hand it in straight away without checking.

If you feel responsible for causing bad things to happen, check out if you can make someone ill or have an accident.

If you believe that you can make someone have a heart attack and die, create a responsibility pie to identify what other factors can cause heart attacks.

Dump your habits

To beat OCD, you need to learn that you don't have to do your habits or safety behaviours when you have a worrying thought.

▶ Make a list of all your habits and routines and rate how anxious you would be if you couldn't do each one.

▶ Arrange them in order from the lowest (least anxious) to the highest (most anxious).

▶ Starting with the habit that makes you feel least anxious, plan how you will be successful and dump this habit. Try to boss back your worries and repeat positive messages to yourself: 'I am going to beat my habits' or 'I have managed not to do this for 5 minutes, so I can do another 5'.

▶ Now face your fear and let the worrying thought happen. This time, dump the habit and try not to use it to make your fear go away.

You will feel anxious, but it will get easier

When you try to dump your habits, you will worry that your obsessive thoughts will become true and you will feel anxious or uncomfortable. Don't give in! What you will find is that these anxious feelings will reduce over time without doing your habits.

Coping with trauma

Being involved in a trauma can be very frightening, and it is not surprising that most people will be upset for a few days afterwards. You may notice some changes in what you are thinking, how you are feeling, and how you are behaving.

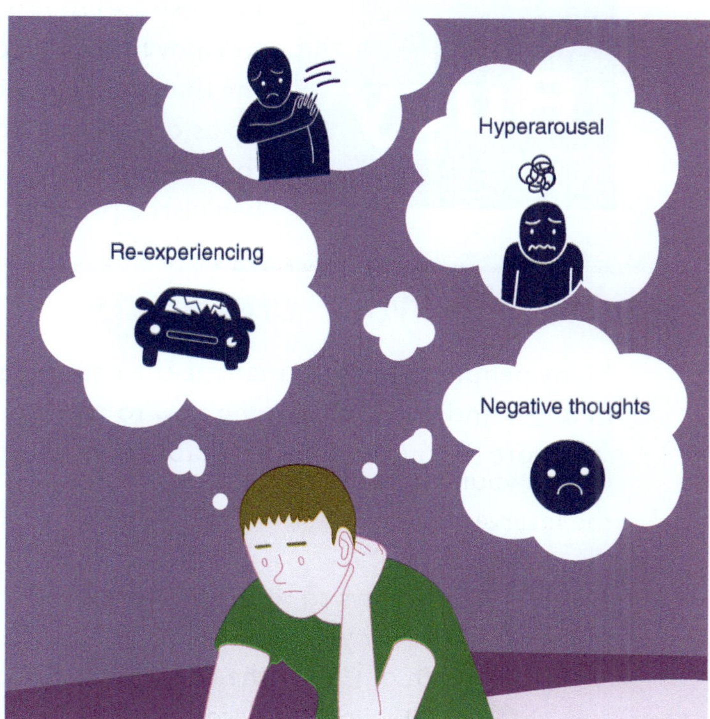

> ▶ You may find that you can't stop thinking about the trauma. You keep going over it in your mind as you try to make sense of what has happened.

> ▶ You may feel anxious, alert, angry, irritable, and very aware of any possible danger. You may have problems sleeping, feel jumpy, and have bad dreams or nightmares

> ▶ You may try to keep yourself safe by avoiding things or places associated with the trauma.

These are normal reactions. For most people, these changes last only a couple of weeks, although for a few, the effects of the trauma will last longer. If your symptoms last longer than four weeks and are interfering with your daily life, you may want to try some new ways to **cope with your trauma**.

Reclaim your life

People often stop doing things after a trauma. They may feel scared to go out or reluctant to do things on their own as life becomes frozen around the time of the trauma.

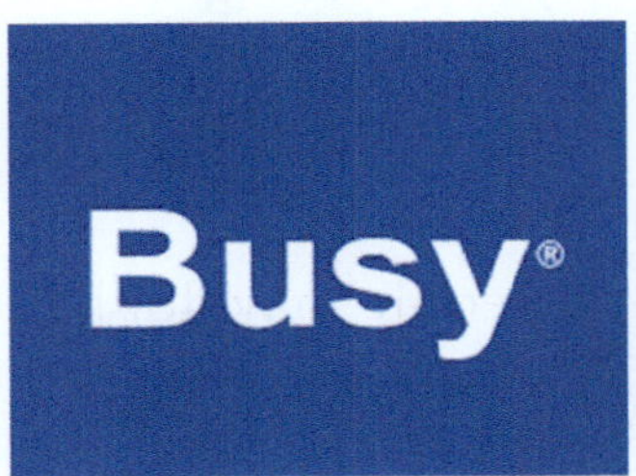

One of the first steps to reclaiming your life is to get busy and to restart the activities that you used to enjoy but have now stopped. Make a list of all the things that you have stopped, put off, or don't do as often. Select one or two that are important for you and plan them back into your life. This begins the process of moving on.

Manage your emotions

Many people struggle to manage their strong emotions, particularly feelings of anger and anxiety. Learning how to manage these feelings can make you feel more in control and better able to deal with your trauma.

Relaxation

There are many ways to relax and manage strong emotions. You need to find out what works for you, but this could include:

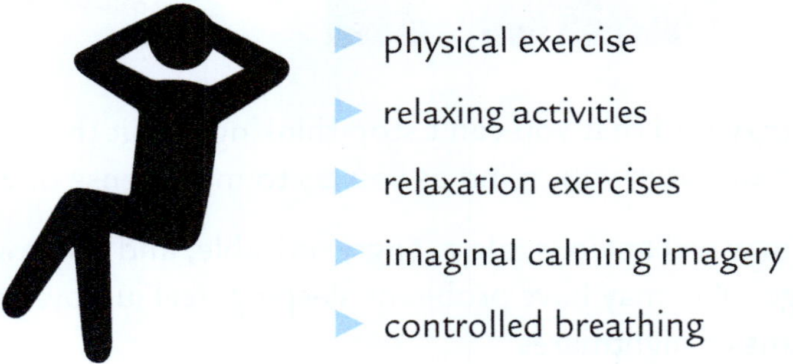

- ▶ physical exercise
- ▶ relaxing activities
- ▶ relaxation exercises
- ▶ imaginal calming imagery
- ▶ controlled breathing

Like all skills, these will become more helpful the more you practise.

Sleep

People who have experienced traumas may find that their sleep is disrupted. They may find it difficult to fall asleep or experience trauma images or nightmares or early morning waking. Poor sleep can then result in tiredness, poor concentration, and irritability.

If you are having problems with your sleep, you may want to try some of these ideas.

▶ Develop a calming night-time routine with a quiet wind-down time before bed.

▶ Avoid sugary and caffeine-heavy drinks.

▶ Don't use bluescreen devices in the hour before bed.

▶ Practise some relaxation techniques before bed.

▶ Listen to audio books or podcasts as you fall asleep.

▶ Try not to worry about trauma nightmares. They will pass.

Anger

People may feel angry after a trauma. They may be angry about what happened, why they were involved, or how they reacted. Sometimes these angry feelings bubble up and you may explode.

Find ways to manage your anger build-up so that you can prevent verbal or physical outbursts.

▶ Taking a few deep breaths and slowly letting them go might help you to ground yourself and stay in control.

▶ Being aware of your anger build-up may help you to walk away before you blow your top.

▶ Find alternative ways of getting rid of the angry feelings, such as hitting a cushion or popping bubble wrap.

Tell your story

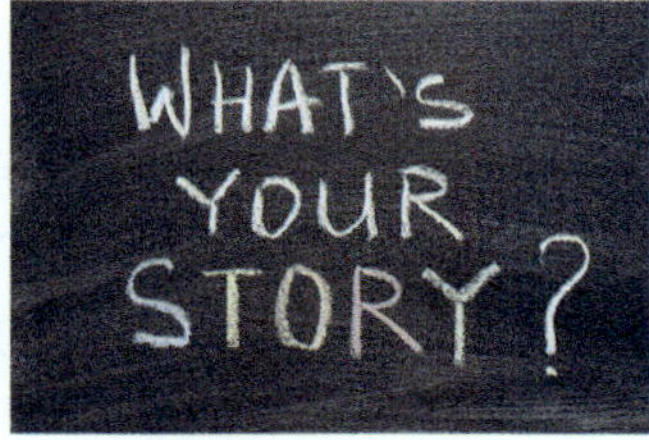

yuriz/123RF

People often experience random thoughts or images about their trauma and understandably find these upsetting. Because of this, people often avoid or stop thinking about the trauma. The trauma is never processed, and you never make sense of what happened.

To help you process the trauma, you will be asked to tell your story about what happened. This will help to identify those parts of the trauma that are unclear or associated with particularly strong emotions. It will also help to understand the way you are thinking about the trauma and the sense you have made of what took place.

Check out what you think

People involved in traumas often have unhelpful thoughts about their role in the trauma, their symptoms, and the effect of the trauma on their life.

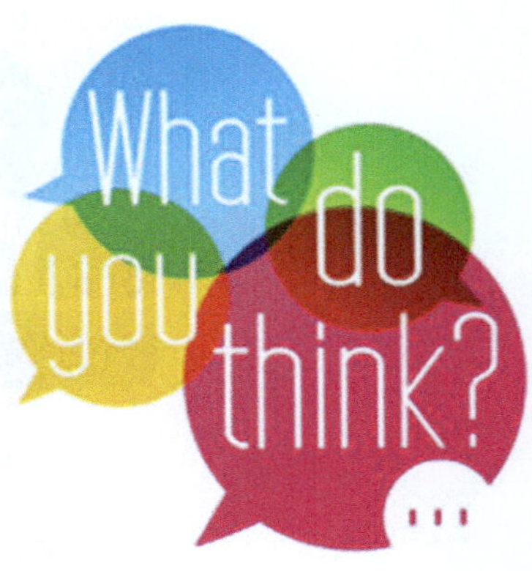

- ► They may feel guilty and blame themselves for what happened: 'If I had stayed with my friends, this wouldn't have happened.'

- ► They may feel ashamed of how they behaved: 'I should have tried to stop this happening.'

- ► They may misunderstand their symptoms: 'There is something seriously wrong with me. I am going crazy.'

- ► They may expect their trauma to happen again: 'If I go back there, it will happen again.'

- ► They may assume their trauma to be life changing: 'I will never get over this. My life is ruined.'

You will be helped to explore these thoughts and to discover new information that will help you to question them. This will help you to update your story, and this may help to reduce your emotional distress.

Face your fears

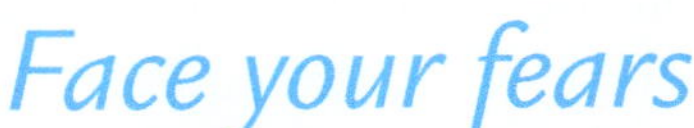
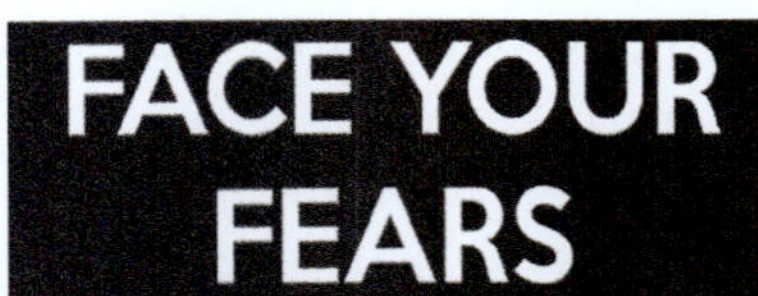

People involved in traumas often avoid the place where the trauma happened, reminders of it, or things that trigger trauma memories. You may feel that this will keep you safe or will stop you experiencing your trauma again and becoming upset.

To move on and reclaim your life, it is helpful to confront and to face these reminders. This will help you discover that whilst they were associated with your trauma, that was in the past. Facing your fears helps you to break this link and to understand that **here and now** these triggers are harmless.

References

Attwood, T., and Scarpa, A. (2013). Modifications of cognitive-behavioral therapy for children and adolescents with high-functioning ASD and their common difficulties. In *CBT for Children and Adolescents with High-functioning Autism Spectrum Disorders*(eds. A. Scarpa, S. Williams White, and T. Attwood.), 27–44. New York: Guilford Press.

Barrett, P. (2010). Friends for Life. www.friendsresilience.org.

Barrett P., and Healy, L.J. (2003). An examination of the cognitive processes involved in childhood obsessive-compulsive disorder. *Behaviour Research and Therapy* 41(3): 285–299.

Barrett P., and Pahl, K.M. (2006). School-based intervention: examining a universal approach to anxiety management. *Journal of Psychologists and Counsellors in Schools* 16(1): 55–75.

Barrett, P., Dadds, M., and Rapee, R. (1996). Family treatment of childhood anxiety: a controlled trial. *Journal of Consulting and Clinical Psychology* 64(2): 333–342.

Barrett, P., Healy-Farrell, L., and March, J.S. (2004). Cognitive behavioral family treatment of childhood obsessive-compulsive disorder: a controlled trial. *Journal of the American Academy of Child & Adolescent Psychiatry* 43(1): 46–62.

Barrett, P., Rapee, R.M., Dadds, M.M., and Ryan S.M. (1996). Family enhancement of cognitive style in anxious and aggressive children. *Journal of Abnormal Child Psychology* 24(2): 187–203.

Beck, A.T. (1976). *Cognitive Therapy and the Emotional Disorders*. New York: International Universities Press.

Beck, A.T., and Dozois, D.J. (2011). Cognitive therapy: current status and future directions. *Annual Review of Medicine* 62: 397–409.

Beck, J.S., Broder, F., and Hindman, R. (2016). Frontiers in cognitive behaviour therapy for personality disorders. *Behaviour Change* 33(2): 80–93.

Bennett, K., Manassis, K., Duda, S., et al. (2016). Treating child and adolescent anxiety effectively: overview of systematic reviews. *Clinical Psychology Review* 50: 80–94.

Bennett-Levy, J., Westbrook, D., Fennell, M., et al. (2004). Behavioural experiments: historical and conceptual underpinnings. In: *Oxford Guide to Behavioural Experiments in Cognitive Therapy* (eds. J. Bennett-Levy, G. Butler, M. Fennell, et al.), 1–20. New York: Oxford University Press.

Bickman, L., Kelley, S.D., Breda, C., et al. (2011). Effects of routine feedback to clinicians on mental health outcomes of youths: results of a randomized trial. *Psychiatric Services* 62(12): 1423–1429.

Birmaher, B., Brent, D., and AACAP Work Group on Quality Issues. (2007). Practice parameter for the assessment and treatment of children and adolescents with depressive disorders. *Journal of the American Academy of Child & Adolescent Psychiatry* 46(11): 1503–1526.

Bishop, S.R., Lau, M., Shapiro, S., et al. (2004). Mindfulness: a proposed operational definition. *Clinical psychology: Science and practice* 11(3): 230–241.

Bjaastad, J.F., Haugland, B.S., Fjermestad, K.W., et al. (2016). Competence and Adherence Scale for Cognitive Behavioral Therapy (CAS-CBT) for anxiety disorders in youth: psychometric properties. *Psychological Assessment* 28(8): 908–916.

Blackburn, I.M., James, I.A., Milne, D.L., et al. (2001). The revised cognitive therapy scale (CTS-R): psychometric properties. *Behavioural and Cognitive Psychotherapy* 29(4): 431–446.

Bögels, S.M., and Zigterman, D. (2000). Dysfunctional cognitions in children with social phobia, separation anxiety disorder, and generalized anxiety disorder. *Journal of Abnormal Child Psychology* 28(2): 205–211.

Bolton, D. (2004). Cognitive behaviour therapy for children and adolescents: some theoretical and developmental issues. In: *Cognitive Behaviour Therapy for Children and Families* (ed. P.J. Graham), 9–24. Cambridge: Cambridge University Press.

Borquist-Conlon, D.S., Maynard, B.R., Brendel, K.E., and Farina, A.S. (2019). Mindfulness-based interventions for youth with anxiety: a systematic review and meta-analysis. *Research on Social Work Practice* 29(2): 195–205.

Bradley, J., Murphy, S., Fugard, A.J., et al. (2013). What kind of goals do children and young people set for themselves in therapy? Developing a goals framework using CORC data. *Child and Family Clinical Psychology Review* 1(1): 8–18.

Breinholst, S., Esbjørn, B.H., Reinholdt-Dunne, M.L., and Stallard, P. (2012). CBT for the treatment of child anxiety disorders: a review of why parental involvement has not enhanced outcomes. *Journal of Anxiety Disorders* 26(3): 416–424.

Bromley, C., and Westwood, S. (2013). Young people's participation: views from young people on using goals. *Clinical and Family Psychology Review* 1: 41–60.

Burns, D.D. (1981). *Feeling Good*. New York: Signet Books.

Butler, G. (1998). Clinical formulation. In: *Comprehensive Clinical Psychology* (eds. A.S. Bellack and M. Hersen), 1–23. New York: Pergamon Press.

Calear, A.L., and Christensen, H. (2010). Review of internet-based prevention and treatment programs for anxiety and depression in children and adolescents. *Medical Journal of Australia* 192(S11): S12–S14.

Carlier, I.V., Meuldijk, D., Van Vliet, I.M., et al. (2012). Routine outcome monitoring and feedback on physical or mental health status: evidence and theory. *Journal of Evaluation in Clinical Practice* 18(1): 104–110.

Carnes, A., Matthewson, M., and Boer, O. (2019). The contribution of parents in childhood anxiety treatment: A meta-analytic review. *Clinical Psychologist* 23(3): 183–195.

Cartwright-Hatton, S., Laskey, B., Rust, S., and McNally, D. (2010). *From Timid to Tiger*. Chichester, UK: Wiley-Blackwell.

Cartwright-Hatton, S., McNally, D., Field, A.P., et al. (2011). A new parenting-based group intervention for young anxious children: results of a randomized controlled trial. *Journal of the American Academy of Child & Adolescent Psychiatry* 50(3): 242–251.

Chalder, T., and Hussain, K. (2002). *Self-Help for Chronic Fatigue Syndrome: A Guide for Young People*. Oxford: Blue Stallion Publications.

Charlesworth, G.M., and Reichelt, F,K. (2004). Keeping conceptualisation simple: examples with family carers of people with dementia. *Behavioural and Cognitive Psychotherapy* 32(4): 401–409.

Cheang, R., Gillions, A., and Sparkes, E. (2019). Do mindfulness-based interventions increase empathy and compassion in children and adolescents: a systematic review. *Journal of Child and Family Studies* 28: 1765–1779.

Chiu, A.W., McLeod, B.D., Har, K., and Wood, J.J. (2009). Child–therapist alliance and clinical outcomes in cognitive behavioral therapy for child anxiety disorders. *Journal of Child Psychology and Psychiatry* 50(6): 751–758.

Chorpita, B.F. (2007). *Modular Cognitive-Behavioral Therapy for Childhood Anxiety Disorders*. New York: Guilford Press.

Chorpita, B.F., Moffitt, C.E., and Gray, J. (2005). Psychometric properties of the Revised Child Anxiety and Depression Scale in a clinical sample. *Behaviour Research and Therapy* 43(3): 309–322.

Chu, B.C., and Kendall, P.C. (2004). Positive association of child involvement and treatment outcome within a manual-based cognitive-behavioral treatment for children with anxiety. *Journal of Consulting and Clinical Psychology* 72(5): 821–829.

Chu, B.C., and Kendall, P.C. (2009). Therapist responsiveness to child engagement: flexibility within manual-based CBT for anxious youth. *Journal of Clinical Psychology* 65(7): 736–754.

Chu, B.C., Skriner, L.C., and Zandberg, L.J. (2014). Trajectory and predictors of alliance in cognitive behavioral therapy for youth anxiety. *Journal of Clinical Child & Adolescent Psychology* 43(5): 721–734.

Clark, D.M., Canvin, L., Green, J., et al. (2018). Transparency about the outcomes of mental health services (IAPT approach): an analysis of public data. *The Lancet* 391(10121): 679–686.

Clarke, A.M., Kuosmanen, T., and Barry, M.M. (2015). A systematic review of online youth mental health promotion and prevention interventions. *Journal of Youth and Adolescence* 44(1): 90–113.

Clarke, G., Lewinsohn, P., and Hops, H. (1990). Adolescent Coping with Depression Course. Available from https://research.kpchr.org/Research/Research-Areas/Mental-Health/Youth-Depression-Programs.

Cohen, J.A., Issues, T.W., and AACAP Work Group on Quality Issues. (2010). Practice parameter for the assessment and treatment of children and adolescents with posttraumatic stress disorder. *Journal of the American Academy of Child & Adolescent Psychiatry* 49(4): 414–430.

Cohen, J.A., Deblinger, E., Mannarino, A.P., and Steer, R.A. (2004). A multisite, randomized controlled trial for children with sexual abuse–related PTSD symptoms. *Journal of the American Academy of Child & Adolescent Psychiatry* 43(4): 393–402.

Cohen, J.A., Mannarino, A.P., and Deblinger, E. (2006). *Treating Trauma and Traumatic Grief in Children and Adolescents*. New York: Guilford Press.

Compton, S.N., March, J.S., Brent, D., et al. (2004). Cognitive-behavioral psychotherapy for anxiety and depressive disorders in children and adolescents: an evidence-based medicine review. *Journal of the American Academy of Child & Adolescent Psychiatry* 43(8): 930–959.

Creed, T.A., and Kendall, P.C. (2005). Therapist alliance-building behavior within a cognitive-behavioral treatment for anxiety in youth. *Journal of Consulting and Clinical Psychology* 73(3): 498–505.

Creed, T.A., Reisweber, J., Beck, A.T., et al. (2011). *Cognitive Therapy for Adolescents in School Settings*. New York: Guilford Press.

Creswell, C. and Willetts, L. (2018). *Helping Your Child with Fears and Worries*. Oxford: Blackwell.

Creswell, C., Violato, M., Fairbanks, H., et al. (2017). Clinical outcomes and cost-effectiveness of brief guided parent-delivered cognitive behavioural therapy and solution-focused brief therapy for treatment of childhood anxiety disorders: a randomised controlled trial. *The Lancet Psychiatry* 4(7): 529–539.

Curry, J.F., and Craighead, W.E. (1990). Attributional style in clinically depressed and conduct disordered adolescents. *Journal of Clinical and Consulting Psychology* 58(1): 109–116.

Dalgleish, T., Goodall, B., Chadwick, I., et al. (2015). Trauma-focused cognitive behaviour therapy versus treatment as usual for post-traumatic stress disorder (PTSD) in young children aged 3 to 8 years: study protocol for a randomised controlled trial. *Trials* 16(1): 116.

Dardas, L.A., van de Water, B., and Simmons, L.A. (2018). Parental involvement in adolescent depression interventions: a systematic review of randomized clinical trials. *International Journal of Mental Health Nursing* 27(2): 555–570.

Davis III, T.E., Ollendick, T.H., and Öst, L.G. (2019). One-session treatment of specific phobias in children: recent developments and a systematic review. *Annual Review of Clinical Psychology* 15: 233–256.

Donoghue, K., Stallard, P., and Kucia, J. (2011). The clinical practice of cognitive behavioural therapy for children and young people with a diagnosis of Asperger's syndrome. *Clinical Child Psychology and Psychiatry* 16(1): 89–102.

Dray, J., Bowman, J., Campbell, E., et al. (2017). Systematic review of universal resilience-focused interventions targeting child and adolescent mental health in the school setting. *Journal of the American Academy of Child & Adolescent Psychiatry* 56(10): 813–824.

Dreyfus, H.L. (1986). The Dreyfus model of skill acquisition. In *Competency Based Education and Training* (ed. J. Burke). London: Falmer Press.

Duncan, B.L., Miller, S.D., Sparks, J.A., et al. (2003). The Session Rating Scale: preliminary psychometric properties of a 'working' alliance measure. *Journal of Brief Therapy* 3(1): 3–12.

Dunning, D.L., Griffiths, K., Kuyken, W., et al. (2019). Research review: the effects of mindfulness-based interventions on cognition and mental health in children and adolescents – a meta-analysis of randomized controlled trials. *Journal of Child Psychology and Psychiatry* 60(3): 244–258.

Durlak, J.A., Fuhrman, T., and Lampman, C. (1991). Effectiveness of cognitive-behavior therapy for maladapting children: a meta-analysis. *Psychological Bulletin* 110(2): 204–214.

Edbrooke-Childs, J., Jacob, J., Law, D., et al. (2015). Interpreting standardized and idiographic outcome measures in CAMHS: what does change mean and how does it relate to functioning and experience? *Child and Adolescent Mental Health* 20(3): 142–148.

Ellis, A. (1977). The basic clinical theory of rational-emotive therapy. In *Handbook of Rational-Emotive Therapy* (eds. A. Ellis & R. Grieger), 3–34. New York: Springer.

Elvins, R., and Green, J. (2008). The conceptualization and measurement of therapeutic alliance: an empirical review. *Clinical Psychology Review* 28(7): 1167–1187.

Ewing, D.L., Monsen, J.J., Thompson, E.J., et al. (2015). A meta-analysis of transdiagnostic cognitive behavioural therapy in the treatment of child and young person anxiety disorders. *Behavioural and Cognitive Psychotherapy* 43(5): 562–577.

Fairburn, C.G., and Cooper, Z. (2011). Therapist competence, therapist quality, and therapist training. *Behaviour Research and Therapy* 49(6–7): 373–378.

Fjermestad, K.W., Lerner, M.D., McLeod, B.D., et al. (2016). Therapist-youth agreement on alliance change predicts long-term outcome in CBT for anxiety disorders. *Journal of Child Psychology and Psychiatry* 57(5): 625–632.

Fjermestad, K.W., Mowatt Haugland, B.S., Heiervang, E., and Öst, L.G. (2009). Relationship factors and outcome in child anxiety treatment studies. *Clinical Child Psychology and Psychiatry* 14(2): 195–214.

Flavell, J.H., Flavell, E.R., and Green, F.L. (2001). Development of children's understanding of connections between thinking and feeling. *Psychological Science* 12(5): 430–432.

Forti-Buratti, M.A., Saikia, R., Wilkinson, E.L., and Ramchandani, P.G. (2016). Psychological treatments for depression in pre-adolescent children (12 years and younger): systematic review and meta-analysis of randomised controlled trials. *European Child & Adolescent Psychiatry* 25(10): 1045–1054.

Franklin, M.E., Kratz, H.E., Freeman, J.B., et al. (2015). Cognitive-behavioral therapy for pediatric obsessive-compulsive disorder: empirical review and clinical recommendations. *Psychiatry Research* 227(1): 78–92.

Freeman, J., Benito, K., Herren, J., et al. (2018). Evidence base update of psychosocial treatments for pediatric obsessive-compulsive disorder: evaluating, improving, and transporting what works. *Journal of Clinical Child and Adolescent Psychology* 47(5): 669–698.

Freeman, J.B., Garcia, A.M., Coyne, L., et al. (2008). Early childhood OCD: preliminary findings from a family-based cognitive-behavioral approach. *Journal of the American Academy of Child & Adolescent Psychiatry* 47(5): 593–602.

Freeman, J., Sapyta, J., Garcia, A., et al. (2014). Family-based treatment of early childhood obsessive-compulsive disorder: the Pediatric Obsessive-Compulsive Disorder Treatment Study for Young Children (POTS Jr) – a randomized clinical trial. *JAMA Psychiatry* 71(6): 689–698.

Friedberg, R.D., and McLure, J.M. (2002). *Clinical Practice of Cognitive Therapy with Children and Adolescents: The Nuts and Bolts*. New York: Guilford Press.

Friedberg, R.D., and McClure, J.M. (2015). *Clinical Practice of Cognitive Therapy with Children and Adolescents: The Nuts and Bolts*, 2nd edn. New York: Guilford Press.

Fuggle, P., Dunsmuir, S., and Curry, V. (2012). *CBT with Children, Young People and Families*. London: Sage.

Garcia, J.A., and Weisz, J.R. (2002). When youth mental health care stops: therapeutic relationship problems and other reasons for ending youth outpatient treatment. *Journal of Consulting and Clinical Psychology* 70(2): 439–443.

Geller, D.A., March, J., and AACAP Committee on Quality Issues (CQI). (2012). Practice parameter for the assessment and treatment of children and adolescents with obsessive-compulsive disorder. *Focus* 10(3): 360–373.

Gilbert, P. (2013). *The Compassionate Mind*. London: Constable Robinson.

Goodman, R. (1997). The Strengths and Difficulties Questionnaire: a research note. *Journal of Child Psychology and Psychiatry* 38(5): 581–586.

Goodyer, I., Dubicka, B., Wilkinson, P., et al. (2007). Selective serotonin reuptake inhibitors (SSRIs) and routine specialist care with and without cognitive behaviour therapy in adolescents with major depression: randomised controlled trial. *BMJ* 335(7611): 142.

Graham, P. (2005) Jack Tizard lecture: cognitive behaviour therapies for children: passing fashion or here to stay? *Child and Adolescent Mental Health* 10(2): 57–62.

Greenberger, D., and Padesky, C.A. (1995). *Mind over Mood: A Cognitive Therapy Treatment Manual for Clients*. New York: Guilford Press.

Grist, R., Porter, J., and Stallard, P. (2017). Mental health mobile apps for preadolescents and adolescents: a systematic review. *Journal of Medical Internet Research* 19(5): e176.

Grist, R., Croker, A., Denne, M., and Stallard P. (2019). Technology delivered interventions for depression and anxiety in children and adolescents: a systematic review and meta-analysis. *Clinical Child and Family Psychology Review* 22(2): 147–171.

Gutermann, J., Schreiber, F., Matulis, S., et al. (2015). Therapeutic adherence and competence scales for developmentally adapted cognitive processing therapy for adolescents with PTSD. *European Journal of Psychotraumatology* 6(1): 26632.

Gutermann, J., Schreiber, F., Matulis, S., et al. (2016). Psychological treatments for symptoms of posttraumatic stress disorder in children, adolescents, and young adults: a meta-analysis. *Clinical Child and Family Psychology Review* 19(2): 77–93.

Hall, C.L., Moldavsky, M., Baldwin, L., et al. (2013). The use of routine outcome measures in two child and adolescent mental health services: a completed audit cycle. *BMC Psychiatry* 13(1): 270.

Hancock, K.M., Swain, J., Hainsworth, C.J., et al. (2018). Acceptance and commitment therapy versus cognitive behavior therapy for children with anxiety: outcomes of a randomized controlled trial. *Journal of Clinical Child & Adolescent Psychology* 47(2): 296–311.

Harrington, R., Whittaker, J., Shoebridge, P., and Campbell, F. (1998). Systematic review of efficacy of cognitive behaviour therapies in childhood and adolescent depressive disorder. *BMJ* 316(7144): 1559–1563.

Hetrick, S.E., Cox, G.R., and Merry, S.N. (2015). Where to go from here? An exploratory meta-analysis of the most promising approaches to depression prevention programs for children and adolescents. *International Journal of Environmental Research and Public Health* 12(5): 4758–4795.

Higa-McMillan, C.K., Francis, S.E., Rith-Najarian, L., and Chorpita, B.F. (2016). Evidence base update: 50 years of research on treatment for child and adolescent anxiety. *Journal of Clinical Child & Adolescent Psychology* 45(2): 91–113.

Hirshfeld-Becker, D.R., Masek, B., Henin, A., et al. (2008). Cognitive-behavioral intervention with young anxious children. *Harvard Review of Psychiatry* 16(2): 113–125.

Hirshfeld-Becker, D.R., Masek, B., Henin, A., et al. (2010). Cognitive behavioral therapy for 4-to 7-year-old children with anxiety disorders: a randomized clinical trial. *Journal of Consulting and Clinical Psychology* 78(4): 498–510.

Hollis, C., Falconer, C.J., Martin, J.L., et al. (2017). Annual research review: digital health interventions for children and young people with mental health problems – a systematic and meta-review. *Journal of Child Psychology and Psychiatry* 58(4): 474–503.

Hudson, J.L., Rapee, R.M., Lyneham, H.J., et al. (2015). Comparing outcomes for children with different anxiety disorders following cognitive behavioural therapy. *Behaviour Research and Therapy* 72: 30–37.

James, A.C., James, G., Cowdrey, F.A., et al. (2015). Cognitive behavioural therapy for anxiety disorders in children and adolescents. *Cochrane Database of Systematic Reviews*. doi: 10.1002/14651858.CD004690.pub3.

Jaycox, L.H., Reivich, K.J., Gillham, J., and Seligman, M.E. (1994). Prevention of depressive symptoms in school children. *Behaviour Research and Therapy* 32(8): 801–816.

Johnson, K.R., Fuchs, E., Horvath, K.J., and Scal, P. (2015). Distressed and looking for help: internet intervention support for arthritis self-management. *Journal of Adolescent Health* 56(6): 666–671.

Kabat-Zinn, J. (2005). *Full Catastrophe Living: Using the Wisdom of Your Body and Mind to Face Stress, Pain, and Illness*, 15th (anniversary) edn. New York: Delta Trade Paperback/Bantam Dell.

Karver, M.S., De Nadai, A.S., Monahan, M., and Shirk, S.R. (2018). Meta-analysis of the prospective relation between alliance and outcome in child and adolescent psychotherapy. *Psychotherapy* 55(4): 341–355.

Karver, M.S., Handelsman, J.B., Fields, S., and Bickman, L. (2006). Meta-analysis of therapeutic relationship variables in youth and family therapy: the evidence for different relationship variables in the child and adolescent treatment outcome literature. *Clinical Psychology Review* 26(1): 50–65.

Kaslow, N.J., Rehm, I.P., Pollack, S.L., and Siegel, A.W. (1988). Attributional style and self-control behaviour in depressed and non-depressed children and their parents. *Journal of Abnormal Child Psychology* 16(2): 163–175.

Kazantzis, N. (2003). Therapist competence in cognitive-behavioural therapies: review of the contemporary empirical evidence. *Behaviour Change* 20(1): 1–12.

Keen, A.J.A., and Freeston, M.H. (2008). Assessing competence in cognitive behaviour therapy. *British Journal of Psychiatry* 193(1): 60–64.

Kendall, P.C. (1990). Coping Cat Manual. Ardmore, PA: Workbook Publishing.

Kendall, P.C. (1994). Treating anxiety disorders in children: results of a randomized clinical trial. *Journal of Consulting and Clinical Psychology* 62(1): 100–110.

Kendall, P.C., and Ollendick, T.H. (2004). Setting the research and practice agenda for anxiety in children and adolescence: a topic comes of age. *Cognitive and Behavioral Practice* 11(1): 65–74.

Kendall, P.C., Stark, K.D., and Adam, T. (1990). Cognitive deficit or cognitive distortion in childhood depression. *Journal of Abnormal Child Psychology* 18(3): 255–270.

Kendall, P.C., Flannery-Schroeder, E., Panichelli-Mindel, S.M., et al. (1997). Therapy for youths with anxiety disorders: a second randomized clinical trial. *Journal of Consulting and Clinical Psychology* 65(3): 366–380.

Kennard, B.D., Clarke, G.N., Weersing, V.R., et al. (2009). Effective components of TORDIA cognitive-behavioral therapy for adolescent depression: preliminary findings. *Journal of Consulting and Clinical Psychology* 77(6): 1033–1041.

Kennedy, S.J., Rapee, R.M., and Edwards, S.L. (2009). A selective intervention program for inhibited preschool-aged children of parents with an anxiety disorder: effects on current anxiety disorders and temperament. *Journal of the American Academy of Child & Adolescent Psychiatry* 48(6): 602–609.

Khanna, M.S., and Kendall, P.C. (2010). Computer-assisted cognitive behavioral therapy for child anxiety: results of a randomized clinical trial. *Journal of Consulting and Clinical Psychology* 78(5): 737–745.

King, N.J., Heyne, D., and Ollendick, T.H. (2005). Cognitive-behavioral treatments for anxiety and phobic disorders in children and adolescents: a review. *Behavioral Disorders* 30(3): 241–257.

Klingbeil, D.A., Renshaw, T.L., Willenbrink, J.B., et al. (2017). Mindfulness-based interventions with youth: a comprehensive meta-analysis of group-design studies. *Journal of School Psychology* 63: 77–103.

Knaup, C., Koesters, M., Schoefer, D., et al. (2009). Effect of feedback of treatment outcome in specialist mental healthcare: meta-analysis. *The British Journal of Psychiatry* 195(1): 15–22.

Kroenke, K., Spitzer, R.L., and Williams, J.B. (2001). The PHQ-9: validity of a brief depression severity measure. *Journal of General Internal Medicine* 16(9): 606–613.

Kuyken, W., and Beck, A.T. (2007). Cognitive therapy. In: *Handbook of Evidence-Based Psychotherapy: A Guide for Research and Practice* (eds. V. Freeman & M.J. Power), 15–40. Chichester, UK: Wiley.

Kuyken, W., Padesky, C.A, and Dudley. R. (2008). The science and practice of case conceptualization. *Behavioural and Cognitive Psychotherapy* 36(6): 757–768.

Lambert, M.J., and Archer, A. (2006). Research findings on the effects of psychotherapy and their implications for practice. In *Evidence-Based Psychotherapy: Where Practice and Research Meet* (eds. C.D. Goodheart, A.E. Kazdin, and R.J. Sternberg), 111–130. Washington, DC: American Psychological Association.

Lambert, M.J., and Shimokawa, K. (2011). Collecting client feedback. *Psychotherapy* 48(1): 72–79.

Lansford, J.E., Malone, P.S., Dodge, K.A., et al. (2006). A 12-year prospective study of patterns of social information processing problems and externalizing behaviors. *Journal of Abnormal Child Psychology* 34(5): 715–724.

Law, D., and Jacob, J. (2013). *Goals and Goal-Based Outcomes (GBOs)*. London: CAMHS Press.

Law, D., and Wolpert, M. (2014). *Guide to Using Outcomes and Feedback Tools*. London: Child Outcomes Research Consortium (CORC).

Lazarus, A.A., and Abramovitz, A. (1962). The use of 'emotive imagery' in the treatment of children's phobias. *Journal of Mental Science* 108(453): 191–195.

Leigh, E., and Clark, D.M. (2018). Understanding social anxiety disorder in adolescents and improving treatment outcomes: applying the cognitive model of Clark and Wells (1995). *Clinical Child and Family Psychology Review* 21(3): 388–414.

Lewinsohn, P.M., Clarke, G.N., Hops, H., and Andrews, J. (1990). Cognitive-behavioral group treatment of depression in adolescents. *Behaviour Therapy* 21(4): 385–401.

Libby, S., Reynolds, S., Derisley, J., and Clark, S. (2004). Cognitive appraisals in young people with obsessive-compulsive disorder. *Journal of Child Psychology and Psychiatry* 45(6): 1076–1084.

Liber, J.M., McLeod, B.D., Van Widenfelt, B.M., et al. (2010). Examining the relation between the therapeutic alliance, treatment adherence, and outcome of cognitive behavioral therapy for children with anxiety disorders. *Behavior Therapy* 41(2): 172–186.

Lumley, M.N., and Harkness, K.L. (2007). Specificity in the relations among childhood adversity, early maladaptive schemas, and symptom profiles in adolescent depression. *Cognitive Therapy and Research* 31(5): 639–657.

MacBeth, A., and Gumley, A. (2012). Exploring compassion: a meta-analysis of the association between self-compassion and psychopathology. *Clinical Psychology Review* 32(6): 545–552.

MacDonell, K.W., and Prinz, R.J. (2017). A review of technology-based youth and family-focused interventions. *Clinical Child and Family Psychology Review* 20(2): 185–200.

Manassis, K., Lee, T.C., Bennett, K., et al. (2014). Types of parental involvement in CBT with anxious youth: a preliminary meta-analysis. *Journal of Consulting and Clinical Psychology* 82(6): 1163–1172.

March, J.S., and Mulle, K. (1998). *OCD in Children and Adolescents: A Cognitive-Behavioral Treatment Manual*. New York: Guilford Press.

Marker, C.D., Comer, J.S., Abramova, V., and Kendall, P.C. (2013). The reciprocal relationship between alliance and symptom improvement across the treatment of childhood anxiety. *Journal of Clinical Child & Adolescent Psychology* 42(1): 22–33.

Marsh, I.C., Chan, S.W., and MacBeth, A. (2018). Self-compassion and psychological distress in adolescents – a meta-analysis. *Mindfulness* 9(4): 1011–1027.

Mavranezouli, I., Megnin-Viggars, O., Daly, C., et al. (2020). Research review: psychological and psychosocial treatments for children and young people with post-traumatic stress disorder: a network meta-analysis. *Journal of Child Psychology and Psychiatry* 61(1): 18–29.

Maynard, B.R., Solis, M., Miller, V., and Brendel, K.E. (2017). Mindfulness-based interventions for improving cognition, academic achievement, behavior and socio-emotional functioning of primary and secondary students. *Campbell Systematic Reviews* 13: 1–147.

McCauley, E., Berk, M.S., Asarnow, J.R., et al. (2018). Efficacy of dialectical behavior therapy for adolescents at high risk for suicide: a randomized clinical trial. *JAMA Psychiatry* 75(8): 777–785.

McGrath, C.A., and Abbott, M.J. (2019). Family-based psychological treatment for obsessive compulsive disorder in children and adolescents: a meta-analysis and systematic review. *Clinical Child and Family Psychology Review* 22(4): 478–501.

McLeod, B.D. (2011). Relation of the alliance with outcomes in youth psychotherapy: a meta-analysis. *Clinical Psychology Review* 31(4): 603–616.

McLeod, B.D., and Weisz, J.R. (2005). The therapy process observational coding system-alliance scale: measure characteristics and prediction of outcome in usual clinical practice. *Journal of Consulting and Clinical Psychology* 73(2): 323–333.

McLeod, B.D., Southam-Gerow, M.A., Rodríguez, A., et al. (2018). Development and initial psychometrics for a therapist competence instrument for CBT for youth anxiety. *Journal of Clinical Child & Adolescent Psychology* 47(1): 47–60.

McLeod, B.D., Southam-Gerow, M.A., Jensen-Doss, A., et al. (2019). Benchmarking treatment adherence and therapist competence in individual cognitive-behavioral treatment for youth anxiety disorders. *Journal of Clinical Child & Adolescent Psychology* 48(sup1): S234–S246.

Merry, S.N., Hetrick, S.E., Cox, G.R., et al. (2012). Cochrane Review: psychological and educational interventions for preventing depression in children and adolescents. *Evidence-Based Child Health: A Cochrane Review Journal* 7(5): 1409–1685.

Merry, S.N., Stasiak, K., Shepherd, M., et al. (2012). The effectiveness of SPARX, a computerised self-help intervention for adolescents seeking help for depression: randomised controlled non-inferiority trial. *BMJ* 344: e2598.

Monga, S., Rosenbloom, B.N., Tanha, A., et al. (2015). Comparison of child–parent and parent-only cognitive-behavioral therapy programs for anxious children aged 5 to 7 years: short-and long-term outcomes. *Journal of the American Academy of Child & Adolescent Psychiatry* 54(2): 138–146.

Morina, N., Koerssen, R., and Pollet, T. (2016). Interventions for children and adolescents with posttraumatic stress disorder: a meta-analysis of comparative outcome studies. *Clinical Psychology Review* 47: 41–54.

Neil, A.L., and Christensen, H. (2009). Efficacy and effectiveness of school-based prevention and early intervention programs for anxiety. *Clinical Psychology Review* 29(3): 208–215.

NICE. (2005). Obsessive-compulsive disorder: core interventions in the treatment of obsessive-compulsive disorder and body dysmorphic disorder. CG31. https://www.nice.org.uk/guidance/cg31. London: NICE.

NICE. (2018). *Post-traumatic stress disorder (update): NG116*. https://www.nice.org.uk/guidance/ng116. London: NICE.

NICE. (2019). *Depression in children and young people: identification and management.* NG134. https://www.nice.org.uk/guidance/indevelopment/gid-ng10106/documents. London: NICE.

O'Kearney, R. (1998). Responsibility appraisals and obsessive-compulsive disorder: a critique of Salkovskis's cognitive theory. *Australian Journal of Psychology* 50(1): 43–47.

Öst, L.G., and Ollendick, T.H. (2017). Brief, intensive and concentrated cognitive behavioral treatments for anxiety disorders in children: a systematic review and meta-analysis. *Behaviour Research and Therapy* 97: 134–145.

Öst, L.G., Riise, E.N., Wergeland, G.J., et al. (2016). Cognitive behavioral and pharmacological treatments of OCD in children: a systematic review and meta-analysis. *Journal of Anxiety Disorders* 43: 58–69.

Oud, M., de Winter, L., Vermeulen-Smit, E., et al. (2019). Effectiveness of CBT for children and adolescents with depression: a systematic review and meta-regression analysis. *European Psychiatry* 57: 33–45.

Overholser, J.C. (1993a). Elements of the Socratic method: I. systematic questioning. *Psychotherapy: Theory, Research, Practice, Training* 30(1): 67–74.

Overholser, J.C. (1993b). Elements of the Socratic method: II. inductive reasoning. *Psychotherapy: Theory, Research, Practice, Training* 30(1): 75–85.

Padesky, C.A., and Mooney, K.A. (2012). Strengths-based cognitive-behavioural therapy: a four-step model to build resilience. *Clinical Psychology & Psychotherapy* 19(4): 282–290.

Pahl, K.M., and Barrett, P.M. (2010). Preventing anxiety and promoting social and emotional strength in preschool children: a universal evaluation of the Fun FRIENDS program. *Advances in School Mental Health Promotion* 3(3): 14–25.

Pediatric OCD Treatment Study (POTS) Team. (2004). Cognitive-behavior therapy, sertraline, and their combination for children and adolescents with obsessive-compulsive disorder: the Pediatric OCD Treatment Study (POTS) randomized controlled trial. *JAMA* 292(16): 1969.

Pennant, M.E., Loucas, C.E., Whittington, C., et al. (2015). Computerised therapies for anxiety and depression in children and young people: a systematic review and meta-analysis. *Behaviour Research and Therapy* 67: 1–8.

Perihan, C., Burke, M., Bowman-Perrott, L., et al. (2019). Effects of cognitive behavioral therapy for reducing anxiety in children with high functioning ASD: a systematic review and meta-analysis. *Journal of Autism and Developmental Disorders.* doi: 10.1007/s10803-019-03949-7.

Peris, T.S., Rozenman, M.S., Sugar, C.A., et al. (2017). Targeted family intervention for complex cases of pediatric obsessive-compulsive disorder: a randomized controlled trial. *Journal of the American Academy of Child & Adolescent Psychiatry* 56(12): 1034–1042.

Peris, T.S., Compton, S.N., Kendall, P.C., et al. (2015). Trajectories of change in youth anxiety during cognitive-behavior therapy. *Journal of Consulting and Clinical Psychology* 83(2): 239–252.

Perrin, S., Meiser-Stedman, R., and Smith, P. (2005). The Children's Revised Impact of Event Scale (CRIES): validity as a screening instrument for PTSD. *Behavioural and Cognitive Psychotherapy* 33(4): 487–498.

Perry, Y., Werner-Seidler, A., Calear, A., et al. (2017). Preventing depression in final year secondary students: school-based randomized controlled trial. *Journal of Medical Internet Research* 19(11): e369.

Piacentini, J., and Bergman, R.L. (2001). Developmental issues in cognitive therapy for childhood anxiety disorders. *Journal of Cognitive Psychotherapy* 15(3): 165–182.

Piacentini, J., Bergman, R.L., Chang, S., et al. (2011). Controlled comparison of family cognitive behavioral therapy and psychoeducation/relaxation training for child obsessive-compulsive disorder. *Journal of the American Academy of Child & Adolescent Psychiatry* 50(11): 1149–1161.

Piaget, J. (1952). *The Origins of Intelligence in the Child.* London. Routledge & Kegan Paul.

Platt, B., Waters, A.M., Schulte-Koerne, G., et al. (2017). A review of cognitive biases in youth depression: attention, interpretation and memory. *Cognition and Emotion* 31(3): 462–483.

Prochaska, J.O., DiClemente, C.C., and Norcross, J.C. (1992). In search of how people change. *American Psychologist* 47(9): 1102–1104.

Quakley, S., Reynolds, S., and Coker, S. (2004). The effects of cues on young children's abilities to discriminate among thoughts, feelings and behaviours. *Behaviour Research and Therapy* 42(3): 343–356.

Reynolds, S., and Parkinson, M. (2015). *Teenage Depression – A CBT Guide for Parents: Help Your Child Beat Their Low Mood.* London: Robinson.

Reynolds, S., Wilson, C., Austin, J., and Hooper, L. (2012). Effects of psychotherapy for anxiety in children and adolescents: a meta-analytic review. *Clinical Psychology Review* 32(4): 251–262.

Richardson, T., Stallard, P., and Velleman, S. (2010). Computerised cognitive behavioural therapy for the prevention and treatment of depression and anxiety in children and adolescents: a systematic review. *Clinical Child and Family Psychology Review* 13(3): 275–290.

Rijkeboer, M.M., and de Boo, G.M. (2010). Early maladaptive schemas in children: development and validation of the schema inventory for children. *Journal of Behavior Therapy and Experimental Psychiatry* 41(2): 102–109.

Roberts, C.M. (2006). Embedding mental health promotion programs in school contexts: the Aussie Optimism Program. *International Society for the Study of Behavior Newsletter* 2(50): 1–4.

Russell, R., Shirk, S., and Jungbluth, N. (2008). First-session pathways to the working alliance in cognitive-behavioral therapy for adolescent depression. *Psychotherapy Research* 18(1): 15–27.

Salkovskis, P.M. (1985). Obsessional compulsive problems: a cognitive-behavioural analysis. *Behaviour Research and Therapy* 23(5): 571–583.

Salkovskis, P.M. (1989). Cognitive behavioural factors and the persistence of intrusive thoughts in obsessional problems. *Behaviour Research and Therapy* 27(6): 677–682.

Salloum, A., Wang, W., Robst, J., et al. (2016). Stepped care versus standard trauma-focused cognitive behavioral therapy for young children. *Journal of Child Psychology and Psychiatry* 57(5): 614–622.

Sburlati, E.S., and Bennett-Levy, J. (2014). Self-assessment of our competence as therapists. In: *Evidence-Based CBT for Anxiety and Depression in Children and Adolescents: A Competencies-Based Approach* (eds. E.S. Sburlati, H.J. Lyneham, C.A. Schniering, and R.M. Rapee), 25–35. Chichester, UK: John Wiley.

Sburlati, E.S., Schniering, C.A., Lyneham, H.J., and Rapee, R.M. (2011). A model of therapist competencies for the empirically supported cognitive behavioral treatment of child and adolescent anxiety and depressive disorders. *Clinical Child and Family Psychology Review* 14(1): 89–109.

Scarpa, A., Hassenfeldt, T.A., and Attwood, T. (2017). Cognitive-behavioral treatment for children with autism spectrum disorder. In: *Clinical Handbook of Psychological Disorders in Children and Adolescents: A Step-by-Step Treatment Manual* (eds. C.A. Flessner and J.C. Piacentini), chapter 16. New York: Guilford Press.

Scheeringa, M.S., Weems, C.F., Cohen, J.A., et al. (2011). Trauma-focused cognitive-behavioral therapy for posttraumatic stress disorder in three through six year-old children: a randomized clinical trial. *Journal of Child Psychology and Psychiatry* 52(8):853–860.

Seligman, L.D., Goza, A.B., and Ollendick, T.H. (2004). Treatment of depression in children and adolescents. In: *Handbook of Interventions that Work with Children and Adolescents: Prevention and Treatment* (eds. P.M. Barrett and T.H. Ollendick), 301–328. Chichester, UK: Wiley.

Seligman, M.E., Abramson, L.Y., Semmel, A., and Von Baeyer, C. (1979). Depressive attributional style. *Journal of Abnormal Psychology* 88(3): 242–247.

Shafran, R., Fonagy, P., Pugh, K.A., and Myles, P. (2014). Transformation of mental health services for children and young people in England. In: *Dissemination and Implementation of Evidence-Based Practices in Child and Adolescent Mental Health*, vol. 158 (eds. R.S. Beidas and P.C. Kendall), 158–178. New York: Oxford University Press.

Shirk, S.R., and Karver, M. (2003). Prediction of treatment outcome from relationship variables in child and adolescent therapy: a meta-analytic review. *Journal of Consulting and Clinical Psychology* 71(3): 452–464.

Shirk, S., Burwell, R., and Harter, S. (2003). Strategies to modify low self-esteem in adolescents. *Cognitive Therapy with Children and Adolescents* 32(2): 189–213.

Shochet, I.M., Whitefield, K., and Holland, D. (1997). *Resourceful Adolescent Program: Participant Workbook*. Brisbane: Queensland University of Technology.

Smith, P., Dalgleish, T., and Meiser-Stedman, R. (2019). Practitioner review: posttraumatic stress disorder and its treatment in children and adolescents. *Journal of Child Psychology and Psychiatry* 60(5): 500–515.

Smith, P., Yule, W., Perrin, S., et al. (2007). Cognitive behavior therapy for PTSD in children and adolescents: a randomized controlled trial. *Journal of the American Academy of Child & Adolescent Psychiatry* 46(8): 1051–1061.

Smith, P., Scott, R., Eshkevari, E., et al. (2015). Computerised CBT for depressed adolescents: randomised controlled trial. *Behaviour Research and Therapy* 73: 104–110.

Šouláková, B., Kasal, A., Butzer, B., and Winkler, P. (2019). Meta-review on the effectiveness of classroom-based psychological interventions aimed at improving student mental health and well-being, and preventing mental illness. *The Journal of Primary Prevention* 40(3): 255–278.

Spence, S.H. (1995). *Social Skills Training: Enhancing Social Competence in Children and Adolescents*. Windsor, UK: NFER-Nelson.

Spence, S.H., Donovan, C.L., March, S., et al. (2011). A randomized controlled trial of online versus clinic-based CBT for adolescent anxiety. *Journal of Consulting and Clinical Psychology* 79(5): 629–642.

Spitzer, R.L., Kroenke, K., Williams, J.B., and Löwe, B. (2006). A brief measure for assessing generalized anxiety disorder: the GAD-7. *Archives of Internal Medicine* 166(10): 1092–1097.

Stallard, P. (2002a). *Think Good, Feel Good. A Cognitive Behaviour Therapy Workbook for Children and Young People*. Chichester, UK: Wiley.

Stallard, P. (2002b). Cognitive behaviour therapy with children and young people: a selective review of key issues. *Behavioural and Cognitive Psychotherapy* 30(3): 297–309.

Stallard, P. (2005). *A Clinician's Guide to Think Good-Feel Good: Using CBT with Children and Young People*. Chichester, UK: Wiley.

Stallard, P. (2007). Early maladaptive schemas in children: stability and differences between a community and a clinic referred sample. *Clinical Psychology & Psychotherapy* 14(1): 10–18.

Stallard, P. (2009). Cognitive behaviour therapy with children and young people. In: *Clinical Psychology in Practice* (eds. H. Beinart, P. Kennedy, and S. Llewelyn), 117–126. Oxford: BPS Blackwell.

Stallard, P. (2019a). *Think Good, Feel Good: A Cognitive Behavioural Therapy Workbook for Children and Young People*. Chichester, UK: Wiley.

Stallard, P. (2019b). *Thinking Good, Feeling Better: A Cognitive Behavioural Therapy Workbook for Adolescents and Young Adults*. Chichester, UK: Wiley.

Stallard, P., and Rayner, H. (2005). The development and preliminary evaluation of a schema questionnaire for children (SQC). *Behavioural and Cognitive Psychotherapy* 33(2): 217–224.

Stallard, P., Myles, P., and Branson, A. (2014). The cognitive behaviour therapy scale for children and young people (CBTS-CYP): development and psychometric properties. *Behavioural and Cognitive Psychotherapy* 42(3): 269–282.

Stallard, P., Skryabina, E., Taylor, G., et al. (2014). Classroom-based cognitive behaviour therapy (FRIENDS): a cluster randomised controlled trial to Prevent Anxiety in Children through Education in Schools (PACES). *The Lancet Psychiatry* 1(3): 185–192.

Stockings, E.A., Degenhardt, L., Dobbins, T., et al. (2016). Preventing depression and anxiety in young people: a review of the joint efficacy of universal, selective and indicated prevention. *Psychological Medicine* 46(1): 11–26.

Storch, E.A., Arnold, E.B., Lewin, A.B., et al. (2013). The effect of cognitive-behavioral therapy versus treatment as usual for anxiety in children with autism spectrum disorders: a randomized, controlled trial. *Journal of the American Academy of Child & Adolescent Psychiatry* 52(2): 132–142.

Tarrier, N., and Calam, R. (2002). New developments in cognitive-behavioural case formulation. Epidemiological, systemic and social context: an integrative approach. *Behavioural and Cognitive Psychotherapy* 30(3): 311–328.

Thornton, S. (2002). *Growing Minds: An Introduction to Cognitive Development*. London: Palgrave Macmillan.

Twohig, M.P., and Levin, M.E. (2017). Acceptance and commitment therapy as a treatment for anxiety and depression: a review. *Psychiatric Clinics* 40(4): 751–770.

Van Steensel, F.J., and Bögels, S.M. (2015). CBT for anxiety disorders in children with and without autism spectrum disorders. *Journal of Consulting and Clinical Psychology* 83(3): 512–523.

Van Vlierberghe, L., and Braet, C. (2007). Dysfunctional schemas and psychopathology in referred obese adolescents. *Clinical Psychology & Psychotherapy* 14(5): 342–351.

Van Vlierberghe, L., Braet, C., Bosmans, G., et al. (2010). Maladaptive schemas and psychopathology in adolescence: on the utility of Young's schema theory in youth. *Cognitive Therapy and Research* 34(4): 316–332.

Vause, T., Jaksic, H., Neil, N., et al. (2018). Functional behavior-based cognitive-behavioral therapy for obsessive compulsive behavior in children with autism spectrum disorder: a randomized controlled trial. *Journal of Autism and Developmental Disorders*. doi: 10.1007/s10803-018-3772-x.

Vigerland, S., Lenhard, F., Bonnert, M., et al. (2016). Internet-delivered cognitive behavior therapy for children and adolescents: a systematic review and meta-analysis. *Clinical Psychology Review* 50: 1–10.

Visagie, L., Loxton, H., Stallard, P., and Silverman, W.K. (2017). Insights into the feelings, thoughts, and behaviors of children with visual impairments: a focus group study prior to adapting a cognitive behavior therapy–based anxiety intervention. *Journal of Visual Impairment & Blindness* 111(3): 231–246.

Waite, P., Codd, J., and Creswell, C. (2015). Interpretation of ambiguity: differences between children and adolescents with and without an anxiety disorder. *Journal of Affective Disorders* 188: 194–201.

Wang, Z., Whiteside, S.P., Sim, L., et al. (2017). Comparative effectiveness and safety of cognitive behavioral therapy and pharmacotherapy for childhood anxiety disorders: a systematic review and meta-analysis. *JAMA Pediatrics* 171(11): 1049–1056.

Watson, H.J., and Rees, C.S. (2008). Meta-analysis of randomized, controlled treatment trials for pediatric obsessive-compulsive disorder. *Journal of Child Psychology and Psychiatry* 49(5): 489–498.

Weisz, J.R., Hawley, K.M., and Doss, A.J. (2004). Empirically tested psychotherapies for youth internalizing and externalizing problems and disorders. *Child and Adolescent Psychiatric Clinics* 13(4): 729–815.

Weisz, J.R., Chorpita, B.F., Frye, A. et al. (2011). Youth top problems: using idiographic, consumer-guided assessment to identify treatment needs and to track change during psychotherapy. *Journal of Consulting and Clinical Psychology* 79(3): 369–380.

Wellman, H.M., Hollander, M., and Schult, C.A. (1996). Young children's understanding of thought bubbles and thoughts. *Child Development* 67(3): 768–788.

Werner-Seidler, A., Perry, Y., Calear, A.L., et al. (2017). School-based depression and anxiety prevention programs for young people: a systematic review and meta-analysis. *Clinical Psychology Review* 51: 30–47.

Wood, A., Kroll, L., Moore, A., and Harrington, R. (1995). Properties of the Mood and Feelings Questionnaire in adolescent psychiatric outpatients: a research note. *Journal of Child Psychology and Psychiatry* 36(2):327–334.

Wood, J.J., Drahota, A., Sze, K., et al. (2009). Cognitive behavioral therapy for anxiety in children with autism spectrum disorders: a randomized, controlled trial. *Journal of Child Psychology and Psychiatry* 50(3): 224–234.

Wozney, L., McGrath, P.J., Gehring, N.D., et al. (2018). eMental healthcare technologies for anxiety and depression in childhood and adolescence: systematic review of studies reporting implementation outcomes. *JMIR Mental Health* 5(2): e48.

Wright, B., Tindall, L., Littlewood, E., et al. (2017). Computerised cognitive–behavioural therapy for depression in adolescents: feasibility results and 4-month outcomes of a UK randomised controlled trial. *BMJ Open* 7(1): e012834.

Wuthrich, V.M., Rapee, R.M., Cunningham, M.J., et al. (2012). A randomized controlled trial of the Cool Teens CD-ROM computerized program for adolescent anxiety. *Journal of the American Academy of Child & Adolescent Psychiatry* 51(3): 261–270.

Yang, L., Zhou, X., Zhou, C., et al. (2017). Efficacy and acceptability of cognitive behavioral therapy for depression in children: a systematic review and meta-analysis. *Academic Pediatrics* 17(1): 9–16.

Yaros, A., Lochman, J.E., Rosenbaum, J., and Jimenez-Camargo, L.A. (2014). Real-time hostile attribution measurement and aggression in children. *Aggressive Behavior* 40(5): 409–420.

Young, J. (1990). *Cognitive Therapy for Personality Disorder: A Schema-Focused Approach*. Sarasota, FL: Professional Resource Press.

Young, J.E., and Beck, A.T. (1988). Cognitive therapy scale: rating manual. Unpublished manuscript, University of Pennsylvania, Philadelphia, PA.

Zenner, C., Herrnleben-Kurz, S., and Walach, H. (2014). Mindfulness-based interventions in schools – a systematic review and meta-analysis. *Frontiers in Psychology* 5: 603.

Zhou, X., Hetrick, S.E., Cuijpers, P., et al. (2015). Comparative efficacy and acceptability of psychotherapies for depression in children and adolescents: a systematic review and network meta-analysis. *World Psychiatry* 14(2): 207–222.

Zhou, X., Zhang, Y., Furukawa, T.A., et al. (2019). Different types and acceptability of psychotherapies for acute anxiety disorders in children and adolescents: a network meta-analysis. *JAMA Psychiatry* 76(1): 41–50.

Zoogman, S., Goldberg, S.B., Hoyt, W.T., and Miller, L. (2015). Mindfulness interventions with youth: a meta-analysis. *Mindfulness* 6(2): 290–302.

Index

Page numbers in *italics* refer to Figures and **bold** refer to Tables

Wiley The manufacturer's authorized representative according to the EU
General Product Safety Regulation is Wiley-VCH GmbH, Boschstr. 12,
69469 Weinheim, Germany, e-mail: Product_Safety@wiley.com.

Printed and bound by CPI Group (UK) Ltd, Croydon, CR0 4YY

20/03/2025

01835006-0002